Psychodynamic Psychotherapy

Psychodynamic Psychotherapy

A Clinical Manual

Second Edition

By

Deborah L. Cabaniss

and

Sabrina Cherry

Carolyn J. Douglas

Anna Schwartz

Columbia University Department of Psychiatry, New York, USA

WILEY Blackwell

This second edition first published 2017 © 2017 John Wiley & Sons, Ltd.

Edition history: John Wiley & Sons Ltd. (1e, 2011)

Registered Office John Wiley & Sons Ltd, The Atrium, Southern Gate, Chichester, West Sussex, PO19 8SQ, UK

Editorial Offices 350 Main Street, Malden, MA 02148-5020, USA
9600 Garsington Road, Oxford, OX4 2DQ, UK
The Atrium, Southern Gate, Chichester, West Sussex, PO19 8SQ, UK

For details of our global editorial offices, for customer services, and for information about how to apply for permission to reuse the copyright material in this book please see our website at www.wiley.com/wiley-blackwell.

The right of Deborah L. Cabaniss, Sabrina Cherry, Carolyn J. Douglas, and Anna R. Schwartz to be identified as the authors of this work has been asserted in accordance with the UK Copyright, Designs and Patents Act 1988.

Library of Congress Cataloging-in-Publication Data

Names: Cabaniss, Deborah L., author. | Cherry, Sabrina, author. | Douglas,
    Carolyn J., author. | Schwartz, Anna R., author.
Title: Psychodynamic psychotherapy : a clinical manual / Deborah L. Cabaniss
    and Sabrina Cherry, Carolyn J. Douglas, Anna Schwartz.
Description: Second edition. | Chichester, West Sussex ; Malden, MA : John
    Wiley & Sons Inc., [2017] | Preceded by Psychodynamic psychotherapy : a
    clinical manual / by Deborah L. Cabaniss ... [et al.]. 2011. | Includes
    bibliographical references and index.
Identifiers: LCCN 2016018489| ISBN 9781119141983 (cloth) | ISBN 9781119141990 (epub)
Subjects: | MESH: Psychotherapy, Psychodynamic–methods
Classification: LCC RC480 | NLM WM 420.5.P75 | DDC 616.89/14–dc23 LC record available
at https://lccn.loc.gov/2016018489

A catalogue record for this book is available from the British Library.

Set in 10/12pt PalatinoLTStd-Roman by Thomson Digital, Noida, India

SKY10053403_081523

For our families

Thomas, William and Daniel

Marc, Rebecca and Ruth

Jon, William and Ben

Eric, Lena and Maia

Contents

Preface

In the four years since *Psychodynamic Psychotherapy: A Clinical Manual* was published, we have taken to heart the enormous amount we have learned about it from our students and readers. While the core of our "Listen/Reflect/Intervene" method is largely unchanged, we have worked hard in writing this second edition to produce a manual that truly brings this treatment into the 21st century. Here are the highlights of what's new:

Common factors: Outcome studies indicate that common factors, such as rapport with the therapist and expecting positive results, account for at least some of the efficacy of all talk therapies. This is true of psychodynamic psychotherapy as well. In this edition, the role of common factors is featured as a major theory of therapeutic action, and common factors are highlighted throughout.

Modern language: Using terms like "ego function" and "super-ego" suggested that ego psychology was still the dominant way to think about psychodynamics. In this edition, we introduce new language for a new era. The idea of "domains of function" – self, relationships, adapting, cognition, work/play – echoes current constructions such as the NIMH's Research Domain Criteria (RDoCs). Even the ominous word "termination" is gone.

Current research: This manual includes up-to-date research from epigenetics to outcome studies that impacts the way we think about psychodynamic psycho-therapy today.

Formulation: We have brought our ideas about formulation from our 2013 book *Psychodynamic Formulation* (Wiley 2013) into this edition, including the "Describe/Review/Link" method for teaching and constructing formulations.

New concepts: Important current concepts and techniques, from mentalization to transference-focused treatment, are included. We have also updated our approach to resistance, defenses, and dreams.

Use of this manual: Today, it is critical for both students and educators to have a guide for how to use manuals in conducting and teaching psychotherapy. Our new "Use of this Manual" section is designed to do just that.

Educators' guide: We have included an "Educators' Guide" in this edition, much like the one in *Psychodynamic Formulation*, to help educators use this manual to anchor a psychodynamic curriculum. There are also more "Suggested Activities" to use in class, as well as evaluation tools.

Psychoeducational material for patients: Lastly, we have included the Post-Evaluation Psychodynamic Psychotherapy Educational Resource – the "PEPPER" – to help you help your patients learn about this important treatment.

We hope you'll agree that this new *Psychodynamic Psychotherapy: A Clinical Manual* is truly a psychotherapy manual for today and tomorrow.

Acknowledgments

روان درمانی تحلیلی

That's Farsi for "Psychodynamic Psychotherapy." Five years ago, I wouldn't have dreamed that I would know that. But since we published the first edition of this book, it has been translated into Mandarin, Korean, and Farsi, and has been adopted by training programs from Harvard to Stanford. We've been overwhelmed by the response, and delighted that it has helped students realize that psychodynamic psychotherapy can be taught in a clear way that makes sense to even the most junior learners. We've been particularly pleased that even people who are not in the field have said: "I wish I'd had that book when I was in therapy!" Our heartfelt thanks go to all of our readers, who have added "Listen/Reflect/Intervene" to the lexicon.

Once again, the dream team of Sabrina Cherry, Carolyn Douglas, and Anna Schwartz helped produced a book that no one of us could have done alone. Our "groupthink" propelled us out of ego psychology and into a psychodynamic psycho-therapy manual for the 21st century. I'm sure they won't miss my late-night queries, but I will miss the incredible learning experience of working with a group like this day in and day out.

None of this could have happened without the Columbia University Department of Psychiatry Residency Program. Maria Oquendo and Melissa Arbuckle, our fearless leaders, have allowed us to experiment and innovate in order to produce something really new in psychodynamic training. And, as before, our terrific Columbia residents teach us every day what works and what doesn't.

Steven Roose provided wisdom that got us through many a conceptual sticky wicket. Darren Reed at Wiley gave us the opportunity to dive into this project again. Joshua Gordon and Richard Brockman shared their Columbia "Neuroscience of Psycho-dynamic Psychotherapy" curriculum. Yael Holoshitz, Lauren Havel, and Alison Lenet contributed with the "PEPPER." William Cabaniss was there with technical support during crunch time. And a big shout-out to Maya Nair, who gave us a "pre-read" and was intrepid about offering feedback to her teachers.

Of course, our biggest thanks go to our families, who once again put up with us while we went down the drop-box rabbit hole. We're back, at least until we come up with a new three-step process to explore . . .

DEBORAH L. CABANISS, M.D.
January 2016

Use of This Manual

Psychodynamic Psychotherapy: A Clinical Manual is a manual for conducting psychodynamic psychotherapy. It outlines the techniques used for

- assessment
- beginning the treatment
- conducting psychodynamic psychotherapy using uncovering and supporting techniques

Like all psychotherapy manuals, it is designed to operationalize the techniques clearly so that this treatment can be taught, delivered, and studied in the most effective way. Psychotherapy manuals are not scripts or cookbooks. Rather, they are treatment guides. Here are some suggestions for optimal use of this manual:

For students: Psychotherapy manuals are not meant to be read cover to cover like novels. Approach this manual chapter by chapter. Try to learn all of the terms and concepts, and then try to use them immediately, as appropriate, in your work with patients. Although you can initially use the exact language suggested in the examples, try to adapt the skills outlined in the manual to the patients with whom you are working. Return to chapters at various stages of your training in order to approach the skills in new, more advanced ways. Use the suggested activities to practice the skills you have learned individually, in supervision, or in a classroom setting.

For supervisors: Even if you learned psychodynamic psychotherapy from other materials, read along with your supervisees to learn how to supervise from a manual. Use the Listen/Reflect/Intervene rubric to help your supervisees become aware of the specific skills they are using. Consider adapting the suggested activities to a supervisory setting.

For educators: You can use this manual, as well as its companion book, *Psychodynamic Formulation*, as your primary texts for teaching psychodynamic psychotherapy to students of

- Counseling
- Nursing
- Psychiatry

- Psychoanalytic psychotherapy
- Psychology
- Social work

For more detailed suggestions about the use of this manual in didactics and supervision, see Appendix 1, "How to Use *Psychodynamic Psychotherapy: A Clinical Manual* – A Guide for Educators."

About the Companion Website

This book includes a companion website:

www.wiley.com/go/cabaniss/psychotherapy

with the "Listening Exercise" for Chapter 16 (Learning to Listen).

This is a short recording that will help the reader to learn about different ways we listen. It is designed to accompany a listening exercise, which is found near the beginning of Chapter 16.

Introduction

"Why can't I find a good relationship?"

"Why do I keep bombing out at work?"

"Why can't I have more patience with my children?"

"Why can't I feel good about myself?"

Feeling good about ourselves, having loving relationships with others, and doing satisfying work – for most of us, those are our life goals. We all have certain patterns that guide the way we try to achieve these goals. By the time we are adults, our patterns are fairly fixed, and changing them is not so easy. The habitual nature of these patterns is akin to the way water runs down a hill – after a while, a certain groove gets carved out and the water always flows down that channel. If you want the water to flow another way, you're going to have to do some hard work to alter the path. It's the same with us – after a certain age, we're pretty consistent about the way we think and behave. But for many people, their characteristic ways of thinking about themselves and dealing with others are maladaptive and they need a way to change.

The problem is that although they know they *want* to change, they don't know *what* they want to change. That is because habitual patterns, more often than not, are motivated by wishes, thoughts, fears, and conflicts that are out of awareness. For example, take a person who never advocates for herself and doesn't know why – but who deep down feels that she deserves to be punished. Or a person who is lonely but is unaware that his fear of rejection is actually causing him to avoid others. For these people, learning about their deep-seated thoughts and fears can be unbelievably powerful. The insecure woman can understand that her self-sabotage has been a lifelong form of self-punishment, and the lonely man can begin to understand that he produces his own isolation by denying his need for others. They can start to develop new patterns of behavior. They can change their lives.

This is what psychodynamic psychotherapy is all about. It offers people a chance to create new ways of thinking and behaving in order to improve the quality of their lives. Since most of the ways we think about ourselves and deal with our environment evolved as we grew up, we can think of this process as reactivating development. One thing that is incredibly exciting about this view of psychodynamic psychotherapy is that it fits so well with advances in neural science [1–4]. For example, we now hypothesize that all learning comes with changes in our neural substrate – so adult brains change all the time. In the words of Eric Kandel, "Insofar as psychotherapy works, it works by acting on brain functions, not on single synapses, but on synapses nevertheless" [5]. New growth – new connections – new patterns.

In this model, not all environments foster new growth – you need a particular set of circumstances in which people feel safe enough to allow this to happen. If you've ever worked on changing anything that had become habitual, it's likely that the process involved another person, like a coach, teacher, or parent. In psychodynamic psychotherapy, that person is the therapist. Change happens not only because people learn new things about themselves, but also because they feel safe enough to try out new ways of thinking and behaving in the context of this new relationship.

This manual will teach you to conduct psychodynamic psychotherapy. Because it was first developed as a syllabus for teaching psychiatric residents, it has been classroom tested for many years. It will systematically take you from assessment to ending using straightforward language and carefully annotated examples. Psychodynamic psychotherapy is a specific type of therapy that requires the therapist to carefully and deliberately make a thorough assessment, establish a therapeutic framework, interact with patients in particular ways, and make choices about therapeutic strategies. As you journey through this book, you will learn all of these essential skills. Here's the basic roadmap: Part One (What Is Psychodynamic Psychotherapy?) will introduce you to psychodynamic psychotherapy and to some of the ways we hypothesize that it works. Part Two (Assessment) will teach you to assess patients for psychodynamic psychotherapy, including assessment of domains of function and defenses. In Part Three (Beginning the Treatment), you'll learn the essentials for beginning the treatment, including fostering the therapeutic alliance, setting the frame, and setting goals. Part Four (Listen/Reflect/Intervene) will teach you a systematic way of listening to patients, reflecting on what you've heard, and making choices about what to say and how. Part Five (Conducting a Psychodynamic Psychotherapy: Technique) will teach you to apply the Listen/Reflect/Intervene method to the essential elements of psychodynamic technique – affect, resistance, transference, countertransference, unconscious fantasy, conflict, and dreams. By then you'll be ready to use these methods to meet therapeutic goals, and in Part Six (Meeting Therapeutic Goals) you'll see how these techniques are used to address problems with self-esteem, relationships with others, characteristic ways of adapting, and cognitive functions. Finally, Part Seven (Working Through and Ending) will take you to the end of the treatment, addressing ways in which our technique shifts over time.

Learning is best when it's active – and thus we've included suggested activities at the end of most of the chapters. These are designed to allow you to try out the skills and techniques that you will learn in this book. They can be done alone, with a partner, or as part of a classroom activity. "Comments" are included to guide reflection and discussion; they are not meant to be definitive or "correct" answers.

We have made many deliberate choices about the use of jargon. For example, we do not extensively use terms like "transference" and "resistance" until we formally introduce them in Part Five, both because we want to define our terms carefully and because we want you to think as openly as possible as you begin learning this treatment. We all have preconceived ideas about these concepts and, as much as possible, we are trying to reduce the impact of previously held notions. We have also consciously decided to avoid discussion of particular theoretical schools of psychodynamic psychotherapy, such as object relations theory and self-psychology. Again, this decision reflects our intention to teach the technique of psychodynamic psychotherapy in the most ecumenical way possible.

So, let's begin at the beginning – on to Part One and "What Is Psychodynamic Psychotherapy?"

Introduction: References

1. Peterson B.S. (2005) Clinical neuroscience and imaging studies of core psychoanalytic concepts. *Clinical Neuroscience Research*, **4** (5), 349–365.
2. Rothman J.L., and Gerber A.J. (2009) Neural models of psychodynamic concepts and treatments: Implications for psychodynamic psychotherapy, in *Handbook of Evidence-Based Psychodynamic Psychotherapy* (eds R.A. Levy and J. S. Ablon), Humana Press, New York, p. 305–338.
3. Westen, D. (2002) Implications of developments in cognitive neuroscience for psychoanalytic psychotherapy. *Harvard Review of Psychiatry*, **10** (6), 369–373.
4. Westen, D., and Gabbard, G.O. (2002) Developments in cognitive neuroscience: I. Conflict, compromise, and connectionism. *Journal of the American Psychoanalytic Association*, **50** (1), 53–98.
5. Kandel, E.R. (1979) Psychotherapy and the single synapse: the impact of psychiatric thought on neurobiologic research. *New England Journal of Medicine*, **301** (19), 1028–10.

PART ONE: What Is Psychodynamic Psychotherapy?

1 The Treatment for a Mind in Motion

Key concepts

Psychodynamics means *mind in motion*.

A psychodynamic frame of reference postulates that dynamic (moving) elements in the unconscious affect conscious thoughts, feelings, and behavior.

A psychotherapy that is based on the psychodynamic frame of reference is a psychodynamic psychotherapy.

The basic goal of psychodynamic psychotherapy is to help people with problems and patterns that lead to unhappiness and dissatisfaction in life by uncovering unconscious thoughts and feelings and/or directly supporting function in the context of the relationship with the therapist.

Both uncovering and supporting techniques are used in almost every psychodynamic psychotherapy.

What is psychodynamic psychotherapy?

Literally, **psychotherapy** means *treatment for the mind*. Psychotherapy has its origins in psychoanalysis – the "talking cure" that was first developed by Sigmund Freud [1]. Consequently, the word psychotherapy has come to refer to a treatment that involves talking. But it's not just any talking – in order to be psychotherapy, the talking has to be:

- a treatment
- conducted by a trained professional
- within a set framework
- in order to improve the mental and emotional health of a patient

And what about **psychodynamic**? You've probably heard this word many times – but what does it mean? Psycho comes from the Greek word *psyche*, which meant *soul* but has come to mean *mind*, and dynamic comes from the Greek word *dynamis*, which meant power but has come to mean *physical force in motion*. Simply stated, the word psychodynamics refers to the forces of the mind that are in motion. Freud coined this word when he realized that, as opposed to earlier conceptualizations of a static psyche, the mind was an ever-changing system, rolling with perpetually moving energized

Psychodynamic Psychotherapy: A Clinical Manual, Second Edition. Deborah L. Cabaniss, Sabrina Cherry, Carolyn J. Douglas and Anna Schwartz.
© 2017 John Wiley & Sons, Ltd. Published 2017 by John Wiley & Sons, Ltd.

elements. These unconscious elements could explode into consciousness and vice versa, while powerful wishes and prohibitions could barrel into one another, releasing the psychic equivalent of colliding subatomic particles [2].

Freud realized not only that elements of the mind were in motion, but also that most of this frenzied mental activity was going on outside of awareness. He described this mental activity as **unconscious** and hypothesized that it could affect conscious thoughts, feelings, and behavior. Thus, we arrive at the two definitions that provide the foundation for this manual:

1. A psychodynamic frame of reference is one that postulates that unconscious mental activity affects our conscious thoughts, feelings, and behavior.
2. A psychodynamic psychotherapy is any therapy based on a psychodynamic frame of reference.

The unconscious

We often refer to our unconscious mental activity as **the unconscious**. Feelings, memories, conflicts, ways of relating to others, self-perceptions – all of these can be unconscious and can cause problems with thoughts and behavior. Unconscious thoughts and feelings develop in a person from childhood, and are a unique mix of early experiences and temperamental/genetic factors. We keep certain thoughts, feelings, and fantasies out of awareness because they threaten to overwhelm us if they become conscious. They might be too frightening or stimulating; they might fill us with shame or disgust. Because of this, we make them unconscious but they do not disappear – they remain full of energy and constantly push to reach awareness. Their energy affects us from their unconscious hiding places, and they exert their influence on the way we think, feel, and behave. A good analogy comes from Greek mythology:

> Zeus, the young god, was tired of being ruled by the patriarchal Titans, so he buried them in a big pit called Tartarus. Deep beneath the earth, they no longer posed a threat to Zeus's dominance. Or did they? Though out of sight, they had not disappeared, and their rumblings were thought to cause earthquakes and tidal waves.

So too, unconscious thoughts and feelings are hidden from view but continue to rumble in their own way, causing unhappiness and suffering in the form of maladaptive thoughts and behaviors.

Psychodynamic psychotherapy and the unconscious

In many ways, the psychodynamic psychotherapist is like the plumber you call to fix your leaky ceiling. You see the dripping, but you can't see the source; you can catch the drops in a pail, but that doesn't stop the flow. The plumber knows that the rupture lies behind the plaster, somewhere in pipes that as yet can't be seen. Here, though, the plumber has an advantage over the psychodynamic psychotherapist – he can use a sledgehammer to break through the plaster, reveal the underlying pipes, find and fix the offending leak, and patch the ceiling. But the psychodynamic psychotherapist is working with a human psyche, not a plaster ceiling, and thus requires more subtle tools to seek and mend what's beneath the surface.

Uncovering and supporting

Like the plumber, the psychodynamic psychotherapist's first goal is to understand what lies beneath the surface – that is, to understand what's going on in the patient's unconscious. Many of the techniques of psychodynamic psychotherapy are designed to do just that. Once we think that patients are motivated by thoughts and feelings that are out of their awareness, we then have to decide how to use what we have learned in order best to help them. Sometimes we decide that making patients aware of what's going on in their unconscious will help. We call this **uncovering** – Freud called it "making conscious what has so far been unconscious" [3]. We have many techniques for helping patients to uncover – or become aware of – unconscious material. What we're uncovering are inner thoughts and feelings that they keep hidden from themselves but that nevertheless affect their self-perceptions, relationships with others, ways of adapting, and behavior.

Sometimes, however, we decide that making patients aware of unconscious material will *not* be helpful. We generally make this decision when we judge that the unconscious material could be potentially overwhelming. Then we use what we have learned about the unconscious to **support** functioning without uncovering thoughts and feelings. (See Chapter 18 for discussion of uncovering and supporting techniques.)

Here are two examples – one in which we would choose to *uncover* and one in which we would choose to *support*:

*Ms A is a 32-year-old woman who has a trusting relationship with her husband, many close friends, and a satisfying personal career. In the past, she has used journaling, cooking, and athletics to work through short periods of anxiety. She presents to you complaining of insomnia that she believes has been triggered by a fight she is having with her younger sister, B. Ms A says that she's "mystified" by B's hostile behavior, which began about a month ago in the context of B's impending graduation from medical school. Further exploration reveals that although B wanted to become a dermatologist, she was not offered a position in this field and will have to do an interim year of internal medicine and then reapply. Ms A says that she has been very sympathetic about this setback and does not know why B is so hostile toward her. When you ask about their earlier relationship, you discover that Ms A has cruised effortlessly from one Ivy League institution to another, while B has struggled academically. You hypothesize that B's hostility toward Ms A may be fueled by envy, and that Ms A has been unconsciously keeping herself from becoming aware of this out of guilt. You think that Ms A will benefit from learning about her unconscious guilt and decide to help her **uncover** it. Once she grapples with her guilty feelings, she is able to recognize her sister's hostility and envy. This awareness helps her to understand their recent interpersonal difficulties and resolves the insomnia.*

Ms C is a 32-year-old woman who is isolated, moves frequently from job to job, and often reacts to stress by binge eating and purging. She presents to you complaining of insomnia that she believes has been triggered by a fight with her younger sister, D. She says that she is shouldering the entire burden of caring for their chronically ill mother while D "just sits in her suburban home with the other soccer moms and sends checks." Ms C, who is struggling to make ends meet, tells you that she thinks that her sister, who is married to a very wealthy man, is "shallow and materialistic" and that she "wouldn't switch lives with her if you paid me." She says that she is "enraged" at D for not doing more to help their mother and that ruminations about this are causing her to stay awake at night. You hypothesize that Ms C's rage is fueled by envy of D, but you decide that learning about the way in which this might be contributing to the insomnia will not help her at this time. Instead, you decide to **support** *Ms C's functioning by empathizing with the amount of work she is doing to care for her ailing mother, and by suggesting that she use her mother's Medicare benefits to get some help with eldercare. Once she feels validated, Ms C relaxes, her insomnia resolves, and she is better able to understand many aspects of her current situation.*

In both cases, the first thing that the psychodynamic psychotherapist needed to do was to understand the way in which unconscious thoughts and feelings were affecting the patient's conscious behavior. However, in one situation the therapist decided to *uncover* while in the other the therapist decided to *support*. Thus, we can say that the basic techniques of psychodynamic psychotherapy are to:

1. understand the ways in which the patient is affected by thoughts and feelings that are out of awareness
2. decide whether uncovering or supporting will help most at that moment
3. uncover unconscious material and/or support mental functioning in the way that best helps the patient

Making the decision in Step #2 depends on careful assessment of the patient, both at the beginning and throughout the treatment, to determine what will be most helpful at any given point in time (see Part Two). When psychodynamic psychotherapy primarily uses uncovering techniques, it is often called insight-oriented, expressive, interpretive, exploratory, or psychoanalytic psychotherapy, and when it primarily uses support, it is often called supportive therapy [4]. Unfortunately, these techniques are often seen as completely separate from one another. On the contrary, *uncovering and supporting do not constitute separate therapies, but rather are both used in an oscillating manner in* **all** *psychodynamic psychotherapy*. One patient may benefit from therapy in which mostly uncovering techniques are used, while another may benefit from therapy in which supporting techniques predominate, but all treatments use some of each at different points.

The optimal mix of supporting and uncovering techniques will vary from patient to patient, and sometimes from moment to moment, depending on the individual person's strengths, problems, and needs. Some patients only require the implicit support conveyed in the therapist's attitude of empathy, understanding, and interest. Other patients need more explicit support throughout the treatment. Whatever the overarching goals we choose at the start of treatment, we are prepared to shift our approach flexibly depending on the patient's changing needs.

The importance of the therapeutic relationship

Uncovering and supporting do not happen in a vacuum – they happen in the context of the relationship between therapist and patient. This relationship is central to what defines psychodynamic psychotherapy. It not only provides a safe environment in which patients can talk about their problems, it also allows them to learn about themselves and their relationships through their interaction with the therapist. The therapeutic relationship itself is likely to be an agent of change in psychodynamic psychotherapy, both as a "relationship laboratory" from which the patient can learn, and as a direct source of support that can foster growth and change. Talking about and learning from the therapeutic relationship is called discussion of the **transference** (see Chapters 12 and 21) and is often a major focus of psychodynamic psychotherapy.

With this addition, we can round out our definition of psychodynamic psychotherapy in this way:

> *Psychodynamic psychotherapy is a talk therapy based on the idea that people are affected and motivated by thoughts and feelings that are out of their awareness. Its goals are to help people to change habitual ways of thinking and behaving by helping them learn more about how their minds work, and/or directly supporting their functioning, in the context of the relationship with the therapist.*

But how does this happen? Let's move on to Chapter 2 to explore some of the theories behind the technique.

Chapter 1: References

1. Vaughan, S.C. (1998) *The Talking Cure: The Science behind Psychotherapy*, Henry Holt, New York.
2. Moore, B.E., and Fine, B.D. (eds) (1990) *Psychoanalytic Terms and Concepts*, Yale University Press, New Haven, p. 152.
3. Freud, S. (1894) The neuro-psychoses of defense, in The Standard Edition of the Complete Psychological Works of Sigmund Freud (1893–1899): Early Psycho-Analytic Publications, Vol. **III**, Hogarth Press, London, p. 164.
4. Winston, A., Rosenthal, R.N., and Pinsker, H. (2004) *Introduction to Supportive Psychotherapy*, American Psychiatric Publishing, Washington, DC.

2 How Does Psychodynamic Psychotherapy Work?

Key concepts

A theory of therapeutic action is a theory that tries to explain how psychotherapy works. Basic theories of therapeutic action for psychodynamic psychotherapy include:

- the role of common factors
- making the unconscious conscious
- supporting characteristic patterns of function
- reactivating development

Psychodynamic psychotherapy can be thought of as a process in which development can be reactivated and new growth can occur in the context of the relationship with the therapist. Explaining to patients how therapy works makes it more effective.

Theories of therapeutic action

In order to choose what to say to patients, we have to have some idea about why what we're saying will help them. This means that we have to have theories about how we think therapy works. A theory that tries to explain how psychotherapy works is called a **theory of therapeutic action** [1]. In psychodynamic psychotherapy, we have several theories of therapeutic action that help guide our work.

The role of common factors

Research indicates that the most effective forms of psychotherapy – including psycho-dynamic psychotherapy – share similar elements that at least partially account for therapeutic outcome [2–10]. These are generally called **common factors**. They are closely related to the **therapeutic alliance** between patient and therapist – that is, the trust that is engendered when patients feel safe, heard, and understood in a non-judgmental atmosphere (see Chapter 9). Common factors include:

- the rapport between therapist and patient
- fostering positive expectations of the treatment

Psychodynamic Psychotherapy: A Clinical Manual, Second Edition. Deborah L. Cabaniss, Sabrina Cherry, Carolyn J. Douglas and Anna Schwartz.
© 2017 John Wiley & Sons, Ltd. Published 2017 by John Wiley & Sons, Ltd.

- collaborative goal setting
- role preparation for the treatment
- offering a cogent rationale for the treatment

These elements convey to patients that the therapist is reliable and committed to helping them. They indicate that the therapist is listening and responding to the patient's needs and goals. And they offer hope that the treatment will address the patient's problems and lead to improvement.

We will return to a discussion of common factors in Part Three, "Beginning the Treatment."

Making the unconscious conscious

In psychodynamic psychotherapy, one of the things that we think helps our patients is making the unconscious conscious. This idea was the basis for Freud's first theory of therapeutic action [11]. Drawing on his clinical work, Freud hypothesized that some patients developed symptoms because thoughts and feelings that were not accessible to consciousness nevertheless exerted a pathological effect on their conscious functioning. Freud's idea was that many of these thoughts were memories, and thus he famously said that these patients "suffer mainly from reminiscences" [12]. Although Freud first used hypnosis to bring sequestered memories into consciousness, he and his patients soon realized that simply talking freely brought unconscious thoughts and feelings to the surface. Since that time, ideas about therapeutic action have become more complex. However, the basic ideas that

- thoughts and feelings that are out of awareness can affect and motivate people, often leading to habitual but maladaptive ways of thinking and behaving; and
- becoming aware of these thoughts and feelings can be therapeutic

are still central tenets of psychodynamic psychotherapy.

Why should becoming aware of unconscious thoughts and feelings be therapeutic?

There are many ways to think about this:

- **Lancing the abscess:** One idea is that cloistered-off thoughts and feelings can be harmful and releasing them can be cathartic. The analogy in physical medicine is the pus-filled abscess that causes pain even if it is hidden beneath the skin. This theory suggests that just as the abscess needs to be lanced and debrided, sequestered feelings need to be released. This is often called **abreaction** and remains an important idea in psychodynamic psychotherapy [13].
- **Preventing proliferation in the dark:** Freud said that an element from the unconscious "proliferates in the dark" if it is not brought into consciousness

through speaking, meaning that it will grow to enormous, inappropriate dimensions [14]. Again, we have all had the experience of being less afraid of something once we've talked about it. In this model, talking about something is like turning on the light in your bedroom to find that the giant monster in the corner is really a hat on a chair.

- **Knowing ourselves better helps us make better decisions:** If the forces that govern our thoughts, feelings, and behavior are unconscious, we cannot control them. They guide our decision making, provoke anxiety, and produce feelings. It makes sense, then, that increasing awareness of these forces can help people by giving them more conscious control over how they make decisions, think about themselves, and have relationships with others. Explaining this concept to patients can be a very effective and powerful way to help them understand this treatment and its therapeutic potential.

How do we help people to become aware of things that are out of awareness?

If we think that unconscious thoughts and feelings cause conscious suffering, we have to access them – but the question is *how*. It is like getting to uncharted territory without a map. Even with a map, we might not understand what we found there because the unconscious mind and the conscious mind use different types of thought processes. The unconscious mind is governed by what we call **primary process**, which is non-linear and non-verbal (like dreams), while the conscious mind is governed by **secondary process**, which is linear and verbal (like conscious thought) [15]. Thus, in order to understand unconscious thoughts and feelings, we have to translate them into a form that the conscious mind can understand. We do this with *words*. You can think of words as boats that ferry ideas between the unconscious and conscious parts of the mind. We've all had this experience – when we use a word to shape an inchoate thought, we often have an "a-ha" moment. This is enormously helpful, and can reduce anxiety. Once we have words for a thought or feeling, we can talk about it, subject it to conscious scrutiny, and use it to understand ourselves more fully.

You will learn specific techniques for helping patients to uncover unconscious thoughts and feelings in Parts Four and Five of this manual.

Supporting function

A third theory of therapeutic action is that psychodynamic psychotherapy works by helping patients strengthen function in several domains. Formerly called **ego functions** (see Chapter 4), these domains of function include processes such as reality testing, impulse control, and self-esteem regulation that help us to manage our inner mental life and relationship to the world. They can be weakened globally or selectively, acutely or persistently.

As our understanding of the mind and neuroscience evolves, researchers in this area increasingly find that the best way to understand these functions is to cluster them into dimensions or domains [16,17]. As in our companion book, *Psychodynamic Formulation*, we follow this approach, using five domains of function (see Chapter 4 for more detail):

- Self
- Relationships
- Adapting
- Cognition
- Work and Play

Psychodynamic psychotherapy helps patients by improving function in all of these domains. This theory of therapeutic action suggests that patients can not only derive temporary benefit by "borrowing" function from their therapists, but can also more permanently strengthen function by internalizing new ways of thinking and behaving. All of the supporting techniques described in this manual are designed to improve these functions (Chapter 18).

Reactivating development

Another theory of therapeutic action in psychodynamic psychotherapy is that this treatment reactivates mental and emotional development in order to foster new, healthier growth. A good analogy for this model is what happens when a tennis player stops improving because she is hampered by a weak serve. A new coach diagnoses the problem, helps her to "unlearn" her old serve, teaches her new technique, and improves her game. Similarly, people may have difficulty moving forward as adults because of problematic function that resulted from abuse or neglect in combination with the person's unique temperamental and genetic milieu [18]. Like the coach, a therapist can offer people the opportunity to grow and develop healthier function *in the context of the new relationship with the therapist*. Areas in which new growth can occur include the development of

- new ways of thinking about oneself and of regulating self-esteem
- new ways of relating to others
- more flexible, adaptive coping mechanisms
- improved cognitive function

For example, if a person who believes that no one will take care of him realizes that his therapist does, we hypothesize that this reactivates the development of his self-esteem regulation and capacity for relationships with others, allowing for new, healthier growth. For some patients, putting this experience into words can help them become aware not only of the problem and the potential reasons for it, but also of the ways in which the therapeutic relationship is helping them to develop new patterns of thinking and feeling. With other patients, this process may be more experiential and less verbally explicit. Today, we are even beginning to have a sense of the neurobiological mechanisms through which psychotherapy might reactivate development. Advances in neuroscience suggest that early experiences can result in lasting neurobiological changes that may be reversible in certain circumstances [19]. For example, in animal models, variation in maternal care affects methylation of histones, the proteins around which a cell's DNA is wrapped. Methylation changes the structure of the histones, affecting which parts of the DNA are available for transcription. In this way, maternal care affects gene transcription without changing the genome itself. This is called an **epigenetic** change [20,21]. Although these changes can affect gene transcription for life, they have also been shown to be reversible in rodents when pups raised by neglectful mothers are cross-fostered by attentive ones [22].

Epigenetic changes in response to early parental loss or emotional deprivation may even cluster in particular areas of the brain, such as the amygdala [23]. Fortunately, the brain is a flexible organ that is continually built and rebuilt by our experiences throughout life. We have every reason to expect that this includes the experience of being in psychotherapy. Increasingly, the neuroimaging literature shows measurable changes in brain function after psychotherapeutic intervention [24–27]. Scientists have even suggested that psychotherapy may produce epigenetic changes in genes that affect the chemistry of the brain's neurocircuitry, leading to new synaptic connections [28–30]. In a very real sense, then, therapy may be successful to the degree that therapists create and foster the conditions that allow for neuroplasticity or changes in neural circuits to occur [31–34].

Explaining to patients how psychodynamic psychotherapy works

It is very important for therapists to understand how we think psychodynamic psychotherapy works. But our patients need to understand that, too. As we'll discuss further in Part Three, therapy is more effective when we offer our patients plausible rationales or "narratives" for their symptoms, as well as an explanation about how treatment actually works, early in the treatment [8]. In Appendix 3, we offer an example of the kind of basic information and FAQs (frequently asked questions) about psychodynamic psychotherapy that you can give to patients at the start of treatment. This two-page educational resource includes not only what patients can expect ("Will my therapist talk?") and how they might best participate in therapy (e.g., by saying whatever comes to mind), but also how we think psychodynamic psychotherapy works. We recommend sharing this with your patients during the informed consent process (see Chapter 7). Of course, you may talk about how therapy works differently with different patients. Some of this may vary with the person's problem. For example, you might emphasize the importance of reactivating development with a person who has a history of severe childhood trauma, while you might emphasize the benefit of making the unconscious conscious with someone struggling with unconscious fears about expressing anger.

Now that you have an idea of what psychodynamic psychotherapy is, how we think it works, and how to share this with patients, let's move on to thinking about how we assess patients for this treatment and for whom it is most helpful.

Theories of therapeutic action

- The role of common factors
- Making the unconscious conscious
- Supporting function
- Reactivating development

Chapter 2: References

1. Michels, R. (2005) The theory of therapeutic action. *The Psychoanalytic Quarterly*, **76**, 1725–1733.
2. Frank, J.D. (1982) Therapeutic components shared by all psychotherapies, in *Psychotherapy Research and Behavior Change: Master Lecture Series*, Vol. **1** (eds J. H. Harvey and M. M. Parks), American Psychological Association, Washington, DC, p. 9–37.
3. DeFife, J.A., and Hilsenroth, M.J. (2011) Starting off on the right foot: Common factor elements in early psychotherapy process. *Journal of Psychotherapy Integration*, **21** (2), 172–191.
4. Bordin, E.S. (1994) Theory and research on the therapeutic alliance: New directions, in *The Working Alliance: Theory, Research and Practice* (eds A. O. Horvath and L. S. Greenberg), John Wiley & Sons, New York, p. 13–37.
5. Hilsenroth, M.J., and Cromer, T.D. (2007) Clinician interventions related to the alliance during the initial interview and psychological assessment. *Psychotherapy: Theory, Research, Practice, Training*, **44**, 205–218.
6. Safran, J.D., Muran, J.C., and Eubanks-Carter, C. (2011) Repairing alliance ruptures. *Psychotherapy*, **48** (1), 80–87.
7. Safran, J.D., Muran J.C., and Proskurov B. (2009) Alliance, negotiation and rupture resolution, in *Handbook of Evidence-Based Psychodynamic Psychotherapy* (eds R.A. Levy and J. S. Ablon), Humana Press, New York.
8. Summers, R.F., and Barber, J.P. (2010) *Psychodynamic Therapy: A Guide to Evidence-Based Practice*, Guilford, New York.
9. Horvath, A.O., Del Re, A.C., Fluckiger, C., and Symonds, D. (2011) Alliance in individual psychotherapy. *Psychotherapy*, **48** (1), 9–16.
10. Barber, J.P., Muran, J.C., McCarthy, K.S., and Keefe, J.R. (2013) Research on psychodynamic therapies, in *Bergen and Garfield's Handbook of Psychotherapy and Behavior Change*, 6th ed. (ed. M. J. Lambert), John Wiley & Sons, New York, p. 443–494.
11. Lear, J. (2005) *Freud*, Routledge, New York.
12. Breuer, J., and Freud, S. (1894) On the psychical mechanism of hysterical phenomena: Preliminary communication, in *The Standard Edition of the Complete Psychological Works of Sigmund Freud (1893–1895), Studies on Hysteria*, Vol. **II**, Hogarth, London, p. 7.
13. Auchincloss, E.L., and Samberg, E. (1990) *Psychoanalytic Terms and Concepts*, Yale University Press, New Haven, p. 1.
14. Freud, S. (1915) On the history of the psycho-analytic movement, in *The Standard Edition of the Complete Psychological Works of Sigmund Freud (1914–1916), Papers on Metapsychology and Other Works*, Vol. **XIV**, Hogarth, London, p. 149.
15. Auchincloss, E.L., and Samberg, E. (1990) *Psychoanalytic Terms and Concepts*, Yale University Press, New Haven, p. 199–201.
16. Cloninger, C.R. (2000) Biology of personality dimensions. *Current Opinion in Psychiatry*, **13** (6) 611–616.

17. Widiger, T.A. (2005) Five factor model of personality disorder: Integrating science and practice. *Journal of Research in Personality*, **39** (1), 67–83.
18. Cabaniss, D.L., Cherry, S., Graver, R.L., and Schwartz, A. (2013) *Psychodynamic Formulation*, Wiley Blackwell, Oxford.
19. Kandel, E.R. (1998) A new intellectual framework for psychiatry. *American Journal of Psychiatry*, **155** (4), 457–469.
20. Bagot, R.C., and Meaney, M.J. (2010) Epigenetics and the biological basis of gene X environment interactions. *Journal of the American Academy of Child & Adolescent Psychiatry*, **49** (8), 752–771.
21. Duncan, L.E., and Keller, M.C. (2011) A critical review of the first 10 years of candidate gene-by-environment interaction research in psychiatry. *American Journal of Psychiatry*, **168** (10), 1041–1049.
22. Champagne, F. (2008) Epigenetic mechanisms and the transgenerational effects of maternal care. *Frontiers in Neuroendocrinology*, **29** (3), 386–397.
23. Suderman, M., McGowan, P.O., Sasaki, A., *et al.* (2012) Conserved epigenetic sensitivity to early life experience in the rat and human hippocampus. *Proceedings of the National Acadacdemy of Sciences USA*, **109** (Suppl. 2), 17266–17272.
24. Protopopescu, X., and Gerber, A.J. (2013) Bridging the gap between neuroscientific and psychodynamic models in child and adolescent psychiatry. *Child Adolescent Psychiatric Clinics of North America*, **22**, 1–31.
25. Beutel, M.E., Stark, R., Pan, H., Silbersweig, D., and Dietrich, S. (2010) Changes of brain activation pre- post short-term psychodynamic inpatient psychotherapy: An fMRI study of panic disorder patients. *Psychiatry Research*, **184** (2), 96–104.
26. deGreck, M., Scheidt, L., Bolter, A.F., *et al.* Multimodal psychodynamic psychotherapy induces normalization of reward related activity in somatoform disorder. *World Journal of Biological Psychiatry*, **12** (4), 293–308.
27. Buchheim, A., Viviani, R., Kessler, H., *et al.* (2012) Changes in prefrontal-limbic function in major depression after 15 months of long-term psychotherapy. *PLoS ONE*, **7** (3): e33745. doi: 10.1371/journal.pone.0033745
28. Beauregard, M. (2014) Functional neuroimaging studies of the effects of psychotherapy. *Dialogues in Clinical Neuroscience*, **16** (1), 75–81.
29. Stahl, S. (2012) Psychotherapy as an epigenetic 'drug': Psychiatric therapeutics target symptoms linked to malfunctioning brain circuits with psychotherapy as well as drugs. *Journal of Clinical Pharmacy and Therapeutics*, **37**, 249–253.
30. Perroud, N., Salzmann, A., Prada, P., *et al.* (2013) Response to psychotherapy in borderline personality disorder and methylation status of the BDNF gene. *Translational Psychiatry*, **3** (1) e207. doi: 10.1038/tp.2012.140
31. Yehuda, R., Daskalakis, N.P., Desarnaud, F., *et al.* (2013) Epigenetic biomarkers as predictors and correlates of symptom improvement following psychotherapy in combat veterans. *Frontiers in Psychiatry*, **4** (118). doi: 10.3389/fpsyt.2013.00118
32. Cozolino, L. (2010) *The Neuroscience of Psychotherapy: Healing the Social Brain*, Norton, New York.
33. Barsaglini, A. (2014) The effects of psychotherapy on brain function: A systematic and critical review. *Progress in Neurobiology*, **114**, 1–14.
34. Meaney, M.J. (2001) Maternal care, gene expression, and the transmission of individual differences in stress reactivity across generations. *Annual Review of Neuroscience*, **24**, 1161–1192.

PART TWO:
Assessment

Introduction

Key concepts

There are four basic phases of psychodynamic psychotherapy:

- assessment
- beginning
- middle
- ending

The two major goals of the assessment phase of psychodynamic psychotherapy are:

- gathering information about the patient in order to formulate the case and to make treatment recommendations
- making a connection with the patient and setting the tone for the treatment

Psychodynamic Psychotherapy: A Clinical Manual, Second Edition. Deborah L. Cabaniss, Sabrina Cherry, Carolyn J. Douglas and Anna Schwartz.
© 2017 John Wiley & Sons, Ltd. Published 2017 by John Wiley & Sons, Ltd.

Psychodynamic psychotherapy has four basic phases:

Phase	Goals
Assessment	Includes assessing the acute problems and ongoing patterns of function, taking a history, constructing an initial formulation, and making a recommendation for treatment.
Beginning	Beginning the treatment: includes establishing the frame, developing an alliance, setting goals, and helping patients learn to use therapy. Sometimes called the Induction Phase.
Middle	The main work time of the treatment: patient and therapist are working well together on achieving therapeutic goals. Sometimes called the Midphase.
Ending	Ending the treatment: includes consolidating goals, reviewing the treatment, realistic appraisal of change, possibility for future development, planning for future treatment if necessary, and leave taking. Sometimes called the Termination Phase.

This manual covers all phases of treatment. In this section we begin with the **Assessment**.

In order best to help our patients, we need to understand as much as we can about the problems that have brought them for help and the way in which their minds characteristically work. This is the task of the Assessment Phase. Chapter 3 will teach you how to take a full history while creating conditions of comfort and emotional safety, designed to encourage your patients to talk freely and openly. Chapter 4 focuses specifically on assessment of function, including defense mechanisms. In Chapter 5, you will learn to create an initial formulation that will help you and your patient set specific goals for psychodynamic psychotherapy. Finally, Chapter 6 describes the general indications for psychodynamic psychotherapy so that you can have a clear idea of who will benefit most from this treatment.

3 Creating a Safe Place and Conducting an Assessment

Key concepts

Every psychodynamic psychotherapy begins with an assessment. Depending on the type of treatment and setting, this may last from one to four sessions.
  During this phase, the therapist should:

- create a safe environment for the patient to begin to talk
- start by asking open-ended questions in order to discover the patient's chief complaint
- take a thorough history of the present and past psychiatric illness, as well as the developmental history
- assess:
  - chief complaint and current symptoms, including any disorders from the *Diagnostic and Statistical Manual of Mental Disorders* (DSM)
  - domains of function, including strengths and difficulties
  - reflective capacity and psychological mindedness
  - motivation and resources

Dr Z, an interventional cardiologist at a tertiary care medical center, readies himself for his first angiogram of the day. Mr A, his first patient, was sent by a local internist for assessment of "classic angina." "Good morning, Mr A," says Dr Z. "How are you?" "Fine," says Mr A, "except that I continue to have that pain in my stomach all the time." "All the time?" asks Dr Z. "Let's have a listen." This patient has been "sent" for an angiogram, but Dr Z is skeptical about the diagnosis and makes his own assessment before embarking on the "intervention" that he was asked to perform.

As psychodynamic psychotherapists, we have to do the same thing. There's an old saying: "If you're a carpenter, everything looks like a nail." Just because we're psychodynamic psychotherapists doesn't mean that psychodynamic psychotherapy is always the right treatment. The first thing we need to do with every patient we see is to make a full assessment in order to determine the right treatment for that person. Even if you're a trainee who is "sent" a patient for psychodynamic psychotherapy, you still have to conduct an assessment in order to make an informed recommendation.

Psychodynamic Psychotherapy: A Clinical Manual, Second Edition. Deborah L. Cabaniss, Sabrina Cherry, Carolyn J. Douglas and Anna Schwartz.
© 2017 John Wiley & Sons, Ltd. Published 2017 by John Wiley & Sons, Ltd.

Decades of *New Yorker* cartoons portrayed psychotherapists as passive, waiting for their patients to begin. Nothing could be further from the truth. When we start the assessment phase, we have two major jobs. The first is to create a situation in which the patient feels comfortable enough to talk about extremely personal things. The second is to try to discover:

- who this person is, and
- why he/she is coming for help now

Creating a safe place for talking

Helping patients feel safe, heard, and understood in a non-judgmental atmosphere has been referred to as providing a **holding environment** [1,2]. In the therapeutic relationship, providing a holding environment means establishing conditions that help patients feel secure, safe, and trusting. It is the basic groundwork for the **therapeutic alliance** between the patient and therapist (see Chapter 9).

We try to create this environment of safety in the following ways:

Taking an empathic, non-judgmental stance

As we'll discuss more in Part Three, approaching patients with empathy and a non-judgmental stance is key to creating a safe place. Part of this involves starting with open-ended questions, designed to encourage patients to talk about the problems that brought them to treatment. Even though you have myriad things that you want to know about the patient, start the initial session by following the patient's lead for a while (about 5–10 minutes in a 45–50-minute session) in order to really understand the chief complaint. No topic is too personal for this venue. Some patients will talk freely about everything from their sexual relationships to their deepest fears. Other patients may have more difficulty talking because of shame, fear of judgment, or trouble trusting people. Be prepared for this, listen attentively, and ask appropriate questions in your most non-judgmental tone. Some patients will remain tense and uncomfortable despite your best efforts. Try to address and lessen their discomfort, while remembering that their anxiety may offer you important information about who they are:

Therapist	*I heard from Dr Y that you'd be coming into the clinic, but I don't know more about what brings you here today. Can you tell me about that?*
Ms B	*Well, it's about my boyfriend. We were going to get married but the plans are off. I've been crying for days. I think that I've ruined my life. I can barely talk about it.*
Therapist	*I can see that you're very upset – can you tell me more about what happened?*
Ms B	*It's too embarrassing – I'm such a terrible person – I had too much to drink about three weeks ago and slept with someone else and he found out – I've been distraught since then. You must think that I'm a terrible person.*
Therapist	*This is clearly very hard for you to talk about, but the fact that it has made you so upset is why you've come to talk to me today. I just want to hear about what's happened so that I*

can best help you to feel better and to understand the situation. Let's start from the beginning. When was the wedding supposed to be?

Warmth and interest will carry the day. Getting the whole story conveys your interest to patients and makes them feel safe enough to tell you even the most difficult stories.

Attending to the person's physical comfort

It is very important to offer the patient a clean, quiet place in which to talk to you. Comfortable chairs that are close enough to encourage conversation but not so close that therapist and patient touch in any way are essential. Turning your phone off during sessions or offering to adjust the thermostat are small gestures that can go a long way toward helping patients feel safe and comfortable.

Assuring confidentiality

Making sure that patients know that their conversations with you are confidential is key to making them feel safe. You can convey this explicitly, as well as preventing interruptions during sessions.

Demonstrating understanding

Simply conveying your initial impressions to patients in a way that makes them feel heard, validated, and understood can be immensely therapeutic (see Chapter 9):

Mr C	*So these last two months have been terrible – it's hard to put into words exactly what's been happening – but I've just felt awful since my wife died – not eating, not sleeping – and just dragging around. I don't know why I haven't been able to get back to work.*
Therapist	*It sounds like you've been really depressed. It's really hard to work when you feel that bad.*
Mr C	*Yes – I have been depressed – that's right – my sister keeps telling me to just go back to the office but you're right – it isn't that easy.*

Setting the frame and boundaries

It is said that "good fences make good neighbors," and similarly, a good framework makes for a safe evaluation. Opacity and guessing make people anxious; openness and transparency help people feel secure. Letting patients know who you are, for how long you'll be speaking, and that this is an assessment for psychotherapy gives them the context for the interview. We'll discuss this more in Chapter 8.

Being professional and thorough

Conveying a professional tone will also help patients feel safe. This means being warm without being familiar. Remember that this is a one-way relationship – the art is to keep it that way without being wooden.

>   *Mr D*   *Yeah, I grew up right outside of Rochester.*
>
>   *Therapist*   *Oh really, me too! Where did you go to high school?*

This response is too familiar – the patient doesn't need to know where you're from.

>   *Mr D*   *Yeah, I grew up right outside of Rochester.*
>
>   *Therapist*   *So how long did you live there? When did you move to Minneapolis?*

This response conveys interest without being familiar.

Making an assessment

While you're creating a safe place, you're also making an assessment. Although you don't want to shoot rapid-fire questions, in the first few sessions you do want to get the details of the present illness, past illness, and personal/developmental history. Prescribing psychotherapy is just like prescribing anything else – you can't decide if it's the right treatment before you take a history and make a diagnosis. Doing a thorough assessment also fosters the therapeutic alliance because it assures patients that you are a careful clinician who wants to thoroughly understand them and the nature of their problems (see Chapter 9).

In the first session, be very explicit about how you're going to begin the assessment. Usually, it's the first thing you say:

>   *Can you tell me what brings you here to see me today?*

That tells patients that you are interested in what brought them to see you. If patients are in distress, you can then move on to explore the pressing problem. If things are less urgent, you can say a bit more to set up the framework for the assessment phase:

>   *Mr E, let's start today by talking about what's brought you to see me. We'll spend a few sessions talking about that and about things that will help me learn more about you. Then, we'll try to pull things together to get a sense of what the main problems are, and finally we can talk about treatment options.*

This framework helps patients understand how the first few sessions will proceed, how best to participate, and when to expect your recommendations. Notice that it does not promise that you will treat them. Since you have not yet completed your evaluation, you should not promise any sort of treatment at this point.

Using open-ended questions during the assessment helps patients tell their story. Consider the difference between these two questions:

>   *Have you been depressed?*

>   *Can you tell me more about how you were feeling?*

The first question could be answered with a simple "yes" or "no," while the second encourages the patient to be descriptive. Open-ended questions allow patients to talk about what's troubling them in their own words. This gives you an opportunity to begin to get a sense of how they see the world and interpret the events of their lives. As you will see, personal narratives are important in psychodynamic psychotherapy, and the story of what brought the person to see you is a critical first narrative to hear. This style of questioning is also likely to allow the person to express affect, which is essential for alliance building and may even be therapeutic. Although there is also a role for closed-ended questions, for example if you need to know details ("How many pills did you take?" "How many days ago was the accident?"), making sure that you ask open-ended questions during this phase is essential.

When we assess patients for psychotherapy we have to look at many things, including the following:

Chief complaint and current symptoms

Your first task is to assess the patient's chief complaint and current symptoms carefully. They are what brought the patient to see you, and so it's important to attend to them right up front. This will help you to get a sense of the immediate goals and recommendations, for example an urgent need for medication or hospitalization. Talking first about the patient's immediate concerns also helps to build an alliance. As you assess the current symptoms, make sure to be thorough about determining whether there are any DSM diagnoses [3]. Mood and anxiety disorders are very common among patients seeking psychotherapy. Don't forget to ask about substance abuse, as well as medical problems that might be contributing to the patient's difficulties. Your diagnosis will help you decide whether psychodynamic psychotherapy or any other type of treatment is indicated. Psychodynamic psychotherapy is indicated for many mood and anxiety disorders (see Chapter 6), but the presence of a DSM diagnosis might mean that another treatment, such as medication, might be indicated as well. Severe symptoms that have an impact on a person's capacity to function adaptively might also suggest the need for a more supportive stance, at least at first.

The history

This includes:

- **the history of the present illness** – which begins with the last time the person was at his/her usual state of mental and emotional functioning
- **the past history of symptoms** – which details past episodes of symptomatology
- **the developmental/personal history** – which includes assessment of early temperament; childhood symptoms; the quality of early relationships and attachments; and the person's educational, vocational, and relational history to the present day

In order to make the best formulation and recommendation possible, you should ask explicitly about the history at the beginning of the treatment. Of course, be alert to the fact that material about the history will continue to emerge throughout the treatment, and allow yourself to let new findings alter your initial impressions.

Domains of function

As we'll discuss more extensively in Chapter 4, assessing the patient's characteristic ways of thinking, feeling, and behaving (previously referred to as **ego functions**) is also essential for making decisions about treatment. We have to know whether the patient can make a relationship with the therapist, manage emotions, accurately perceive reality, control impulses, and delay gratification. This will also include an assessment of **ethical judgment** – the patient's capacity to distinguish right from wrong (see Chapter 4). Remember to assess both strengths and difficulties. While we're interested in helping people with difficulties, it is the areas of strength that will help us during the treatment. If psychodynamic psychotherapy is indicated, assessment of these domains of function will guide our decisions about whether we want to take a predominantly uncovering or supporting stance.

Reflective capacity

In order to begin to think about their behaviors, fantasies, and relationships, people have to be able to "step outside" their immediate thoughts to look at them critically. This **reflective capacity** is also important to learn about during the assessment phase. Questions that ask patients to think critically about themselves and their behavior will help you to gauge their capacity for reflection. Here are some examples:

> How would you describe yourself to another person?
>
> How do you think your partner would describe you?
>
> What kinds of things do you think are the easiest/most difficult for you in your relationships?

If this follows organically from what people tell you spontaneously, all the better. Consider this example:

> Ms F presents for psychotherapy saying that she has been fighting with her husband. She says that he is unemotional and unsupportive; for example, he did not come to a recent amateur concert that she gave that was very important to her. As you listen, you wonder whether she is doing anything to contribute to the couple's difficulties. You decide to ask about this to assess Ms F's capacity for self-reflection. You say:
>
> It really does sound like you and your husband are having a difficult time and that you are very upset about his lack of support. In order to best understand your relationship, I wonder if you could reflect on any possible ways in which you might be contributing to the difficulties that you're having.

A person with limited capacity for reflection might say:

> No way, it's all him. He's a jerk.

While a person with some capacity for reflection might say:

> Let me think about that . . . I suppose that I'm so angry that I'm pulling back and being very cold. I think that's definitely making him even less supportive.

The capacity to reflect is also critical for the ability to think about the treatment and the relationship with the therapist. This is important to know when making a treatment recommendation, since discussion of the therapeutic relationship is an important part of many uncovering techniques. You can begin to assess this from the beginning by asking simple, straightforward questions like:

What was your experience of being here today?

Did you have any thoughts or expectations about what I'd be like before you came?

How did your experience compare to what you thought it might be like?

If patients were previously in psychotherapy, don't hesitate to ask about their former therapists and about how talking to you is similar or different from what they experienced before.

Psychological mindedness

A particular aspect of reflective capacity that is important to understand when assessing someone for psychodynamic psychotherapy is **psychological mindedness**. Some people conceptualize their mind as having unconscious elements and some don't. Some people can learn to think this way and some can't. Assessing the way in which patients think about their mind is essential for deciding what type of psychotherapy is most appropriate. Making **trial interpretations** during the assessment phase can be very helpful in assessing this:

A 34-year-old man presents with difficulties committing to a relationship with a woman. In the course of the assessment, he reveals that his parents divorced when he was 8 years old. After more discussion, the therapist asks the patient whether he thinks that what happened in his family affected his adult relationships.

A psychologically minded person might say something like:

Oh yes, I've always known that though I don't know what to do about it.

or

Huh – I've never put the two together, but that's interesting.

or even

I could see how that might be true for someone, but I don't think that it's true for me.

Uncovering techniques are likely to help this patient further understand the way his feelings about his parents' relationship are affecting his capacity to commit to a relationship of his own. On the other hand, a non-psychologically minded person might say:

Why would their problems contribute to mine? I just can't find the right woman.

or

They just had a bad relationship. I don't think that that's relevant to my situation.

Supportive techniques may help this person understand his frustration with his situation in order to use new methods for meeting people.

Learning about psychological mindedness during the assessment is essential for determining what type of technique will help the patient most.

Prioritization of problems

Like a triage nurse in an emergency room, the therapist has to know not only what the patient's problems are, but also which are most pressing. For example, a patient might have panic disorder, but if he is suicidal, the safety issue takes priority. In general, potential violence (toward self or others) trumps all other problems. It is also critical to assess what patients feel are their most important problems. We'll discuss goal setting more extensively in Chapter 7.

Motivation for treatment

We might think that psychodynamic psychotherapy is the best treatment for a given patient, but if he or she has another idea, it won't fly. We can gauge motivation for treatment by asking patients questions designed to assess their ideas about therapy:

What did you imagine psychotherapy would be like?

Did you have any idea about how often you'd be coming here?

Do you have the feeling that psychotherapy could be helpful to you?

Resources and social matrix

Therapists must assess not only their patients' problems and inner resources, but also their external resources and social context. For example, a patient who is only in the country for two more months is not a good candidate for long-term psychodynamic psychotherapy, a student on a work/study stipend should probably be seen in a sliding-scale clinic.

More than one treatment might be appropriate for any given patient. For example, patients might need psychodynamic psychotherapy *and* medication. Sometimes these treatments are conducted one after another and sometimes they are conducted at the same time. We will review these options in Chapter 15.

Now that we've set the stage for the assessment, let's move on to **assessing function** in Chapter 4.

The assessment

- chief complaint and current symptoms (including any DSM diagnoses)
- the history
- domains of function – strengths and difficulties
- reflective capacity and psychological mindedness
- motivation and resources

Suggested activity

How would you assess the following patients' reflective capacity? What might that say about their ability to benefit from psychodynamic psychotherapy? What might you say to try to engage them in treatment?

1. Ms A

How long is this evaluation going to take? My husband made me come in – he said that it was this or lawyers. He makes it seem like it's all my fault – like I'm ruining our relationship. But he's the one who had the affair. OK, I'm not easy to live with, but he isn't either. I guess we stayed together for the children – now that they're gone we're like strangers. What kind of therapy is this, anyway? I'm not crazy – anxious, yes, I'm anxious – but so was my mother and she and my father had a fine relationship because he loved her and dealt with her anxiety. My husband doesn't love me. Go ahead, ask me questions.

Comment

Ms A has trouble with reflective function. She sees the difficulties in her life as arising almost exclusively from problems in her environment. She does not see herself as an agent of change in her life. Although she does have some awareness of her own anxiety and thinks that she might have inherited this from her mother, she believes that it is the way that others respond to anxiety that makes the difference. It would be challenging, but not impossible, to engage Ms A in psychodynamic psychotherapy. The best tack might be to empathize with her current difficulties and explore whether support for her current stress might be helpful. A question like "You mentioned that you are anxious – is that causing any difficulties for you now?" might open up potential goals for the initial treatment without challenging her assumptions about the etiology of her marital difficulties.

2. Mr B

I don't really know why I'm having such a tough time writing this job application. I keep sitting down at my desk to do it and staring at the screen – and all the ideas I had in the shower about what to write seem to fly out of my head. This is exactly what happened to me when I applied to college. That time, my mother was breathing down my neck – it was excruciating. She's 2,000 miles away now, but it's like she's in my head. It's like it's become part of me – this need to have it be perfect that stymies me every time. Can you help me with that?

Comment

Mr B's reflective capacity is quite good. Even though he doesn't know why he is having trouble, he locates the source of the problem in his own mind. And although he has a sense that his difficulty may stem from his relationship with his mother, he believes that it is now part of himself. He also connects two different situations, noting that his behavior in each may have common elements. He is likely to engage well in psychodynamic psychotherapy. Acknowledging Mr B's reflective capacity might sound something like this: "You have a real sense that looking inside of yourself will help you overcome this problem. I think that's right. And I also agree that while the difficulty might be related to your early relationships, you have the ability to change things by thinking about them differently. That's what we'll be doing in this treatment."

Chapter 3: References

1. Winnicott, D.W. (1965) Psychiatric disorders in terms of infantile maturational processes, in *The Maturational Processes and the Facilitating Environment: Studies in the Theory of Emotional Development*, International Universities Press, New York, p. 30–41.
2. Winnicott, D.W. (1963) Dependence in infant care, in child care, and in the psycho-analytic setting. *International Journal of Psychoanalysis*, **44**, 339–344.
3. American Psychiatric Association (2000) *Diagnostic and Statistical Manual of Mental Disorders: DSM-IV-TR*, 4th ed., Text Revision, American Psychiatric Association, Washington, DC.

4 Assessing Domains of Function

Key concepts

The processes people use to manage their inner mental life and relationship to the world can be organized into five basic domains of function:

- Self
- Relationships
- Adapting
- Cognition
- Work and Play

These functions may be both conscious and unconscious.

People are generally **mosaics**, with strengths in some areas of function and difficulties in others.

Defenses are unconscious mechanisms that people use to cope with thoughts and feelings that might otherwise overwhelm them or cause intolerable anxiety.

Assessing domains of function is essential for determining:

- what kind of psychotherapy will be most beneficial
- whether patients will benefit most from uncovering or supporting techniques

In order to benefit from uncovering techniques, patients must have enough functional strength to buoy them during the treatment, limit regression, support reality testing, and allow them to function in their outside lives. Difficulty in multiple domains of function is an important indication for supportive techniques.

Assessing domains of function

It's easy for us to maintain our equilibrium when things are calm – but how do we do it when the going gets rough? For this, we have a variety of functions that help us do everything from regulating self-esteem to managing emotions [1–7]. These were formerly called **ego functions**, based on Freud's division of the mind into three parts, **id**, **ego**, and **super-ego**. According to Freud's model, the id was thought of as consisting of wishes and desires, the super-ego contained conscience and personal ideals, and the ego managed the person's inner mental life and relationship to the world. These parts

Psychodynamic Psychotherapy: A Clinical Manual, Second Edition. Deborah L. Cabaniss, Sabrina Cherry, Carolyn J. Douglas and Anna Schwartz.
© 2017 John Wiley & Sons, Ltd. Published 2017 by John Wiley & Sons, Ltd.

were not thought of literally as divisions of the mind, nor were they considered to be located in any particular area of the brain; rather, they were conceptualized as clusters of functions. Interestingly, as we learn more about the way the brain creates the mind, it may be that Freud's structures have some neurobiological correlates. For example, there are similarities between the id, as Freud described it, and the limbic system of the brain, while higher-level neocortical structures, particularly in the frontal lobe, are likely to coordinate and regulate a number of mental activities that roughly correspond to what were called ego functions [1].

Today we no longer think of the mind as divided according to Freud's model, and therefore it is useful to think about these functions in a new way. As we discussed in Chapter 2, we will organize these functions into five basic domains:

- Self
- Relationships
- Adapting
- Cognition
- Work and Play

How do these functions come into being? Are they hard wired? Are they learned? Our hypothesis is that the answer involves some combination of nature and nurture, and that genetics and temperament, as well as early trauma and/or psychopathology, must affect their development. This is important to consider as you assess these crucial functions, take a developmental history, and begin to think about how they might be connected.

Ideally, you'll be able to learn about these domains of function from your patients' stories. If you keep these functions in mind, you'll be able to look for opportunities to ask about them, as in this example from a first session:

> Therapist   So glad that you could make this appointment. What brings you to see me today?
>
> Patient   I'm beside myself – can't sleep – don't know what to do – I was offered a new job a month ago and I don't know whether to take it. I flip-flop about it every day. See – even now I'm having trouble breathing as I talk about it.
>
> Therapist   That sounds very stressful. How have you been going about trying to make the decision?

Difficulty with decision making is front and center here, and this is a good opportunity to assess this important cognitive function. However, problems with function are not always so evident at the outset, so you'll need to ask about them. In this chapter, we'll outline each of these domains and suggest sample questions to help you learn about your patients' characteristic ways of managing their inner life and relationship to the world.

Self

By the time they reach adulthood, people develop characteristic patterns of experiencing themselves. This involves both **self-perception** and **self-esteem regulation**.

Self-perception

How we see ourselves is critical to how we function in the world. Our self-perceptions relate both to our sense of **identity** and to our **self-appraisal**.

- *Identity* is our sense of who we are. This includes our likes and dislikes, as well as our talents and limitations. Identity is often consolidated during the teen years.
- *Self-appraisal* relates to how well our subjective sense of our abilities matches up with what we are actually able to do. People who overinflate their abilities risk "biting off more they can chew" and setting themselves up for failure, while those who underestimate themselves often suffer from low self-esteem. Realistic self-appraisal generally leads people to set appropriate goals and perform effectively to get what they need from the world.

Self-appraisal also includes **ideals** for ourselves (previously referred to as the **ego-ideal**). This refers to inner images, or fantasies, of ourselves as we wish to be. Each of us has our own unique vision of an ideal self that is personally meaningful. Thinking and acting in concert with our inner ideals makes us feel proud and accomplished, while not living up to them can produce feelings of guilt, unworthiness, and failure.

Self-esteem regulation

It's easy to feel good about ourselves when things go well – but it's our ability to bounce back from self-esteem blows that is the measure of self-esteem regulation. While we're all vulnerable to temporary self-esteem fluctuations, it's harder for some people than others to buoy their sense of self when things aren't going their way. We need to think both about how vulnerable people are to self-esteem threats, as well as about the way they respond to them. One person might react by feeling depressed, while another might take things out on a loved one.

Sample questions for assessing Self

Self-perception

> *How would you describe yourself?*
>
> *Do you feel that you have a good sense of things you like and things you don't like? People you like and people you don't like? Your goals for the future?*
>
> *Do your ideas about yourself generally match the way others think about you?*

Self-esteem regulation

> *Do you think of yourself as "thin-skinned"? Would you describe yourself as sensitive to criticism or feedback?*
>
> *How do you handle it when things don't go your way?*
>
> *Do you tend to think that things that go wrong are your fault?*

Relationships

The capacity to have relationships is central to the way people develop and function. This is more than just the ability to form and maintain relationships; rather, it is the ability to sustain relationships that are stable, trusting, intimate, loving, and mutually gratifying, in which others are viewed as whole, separate, and three-dimensional. When we say three-dimensional, we mean that people can think about themselves and others as having:

- both good and bad qualities
- separate and unique feelings, beliefs, needs, and motivations
- generally consistent feelings about self and others from past to present

The abilities to **empathize** and **mentalize** are key for good functioning in this domain and need to be carefully assessed. Empathy is the ability to appreciate the way that others experience the world, while mentalization is the ability to think about others as having thoughts and feelings that are distinct from one's own [8]. Examples of people with impairment in this area include the person who lives as a recluse and needs a great deal of interpersonal distance, the person who is unable to tolerate separation and needs constant reassurance, and the person who lacks empathy and manipulates others without regard for their feelings.

Assessing this domain of function means understanding not only the relationships people actually have, but also their conscious and unconscious expectations of others and fantasies about relationships. For example, one person might always expect that others will abandon him, while another person might fantasize about being in a relationship in which she is prized and adored.

Sample questions for assessing **Relationships**

> *Who is important to you in your life? How long have you known them?*
>
> *Is there someone in your life you could call in an emergency? Tell me about him/her.*
>
> *Are you satisfied with your relationships? How would you like them to be different?*
>
> *Do you often have expectations of others that don't match up to what they can offer?*
>
> *Have people in your life complained about their relationship with you?*
>
> *How do you think your sister feels about that situation? (mentalization)*

Adapting

Adapting means adjusting. There are many types of internal and external stress that we need to adjust to on a daily basis. *Internal stress* includes thoughts and fantasies, feelings and anxiety, pain and other physical sensations. *External stress* includes relationships with others, economic and work-related pressures, trauma, and other environmental events. People can have trouble adapting to stress in two situations:

- when there is actually a lot of external or internal stress
- when the person has difficulty dealing with stress

Both have to be considered in the assessment of a person's capacity for adapting.

People have their own thresholds for tolerating stimulation. Some people can tolerate high levels of affect, anxiety, and environmental stress, while others develop difficulties at much lower levels.

Defenses

Defenses are the *unconscious* and *automatic* ways in which the mind responds to internal and external stress and emotional conflict [9]. They are coping mechanisms that limit a person's awareness of painful affects like anxiety, depression, or envy, and resolve internal emotional conflicts. We all need them, but some defenses are more adaptive than others [5,9–14]. For example, it is more adaptive to read a book about one's problems than to ignore them. More adaptive defenses are generally based on **repression**; less adaptive defenses are generally based on **splitting**. Whether people's defenses are based primarily on repression or splitting is related to whether they have achieved **object constancy**. (Note: **object permanence** is knowing that something that is out of sight is still there; object constancy is knowing that bad and good can exist in the same person [15].) If they can tolerate the idea that bad and good feelings can co-exist in themselves or others, they can deal with painful or anxiety-provoking thoughts and affects by keeping them within themselves but making them unconscious (repression). However, if they cannot tolerate the idea that anything bad exists in a good person, or vice versa, they need to separate the bad from the good. In order to do this, they have to experience some of their feelings as if they are coming from outside the self (splitting). Developmentally, splitting is normal in small children, but may persist (leading to lack of object constancy) when people need to protect their good image of an abusive or neglectful parent or caregiver. Here is a list of the major defenses, grouped according to how adaptive they are:

Less adaptive defenses

As already discussed, splitting-based defenses tend to be less adaptive because they protect people from negative feelings and thoughts at a very high cost [16]. Splitting-based defenses predominate when object constancy has not been achieved. While they help preserve good feelings, this comes at the cost of consolidating a three-dimensional view of the self and others. A predominance of splitting-based defenses is a good indicator of functional weakness and leaves the individual with less ability to have healthy relationships. Splitting-based defenses are sometimes called immature, primitive, or borderline. They are the following:

- **Splitting** preserves good feelings and avoids bad feelings by separating them into different people [13]:

    Although Ms A's mother never kept food in the house and was harshly critical, she idealizes her mother and vilifies her father. As an adult, Ms A is unable to see men as having any good qualities despite her desperate wish to be in a heterosexual relationship.

- **Projection** protects by perceiving unacceptable thoughts, feelings, and fantasies as originating outside the self:

    Mr B's girlfriend cheated on him. He did not experience any anger at her, but became paranoid that she was spreading unflattering rumors about him.

- **Projective identification** occurs when one person projects a thought or feeling into another person and then behaves in a way to make the second person experience the projected feeling. We say that in this way, the first person maintains an **identification** with the projected feeling:

    Mr C is passed over for a promotion by his boss. Although he says that this is fine with him, his unconscious rage is so overwhelming that he comes in two hours late for a week until his boss is so enraged that he fires him.

- **Pathological idealization and devaluation** are natural results of splitting. Remember that the person who is idealized today may easily be devalued tomorrow:

    One week, Ms D thought that her therapist completely understood her while her husband was an idiot; the next week it was the reverse.

The following are less adaptive defenses, although they are not linked as clearly to splitting. As with splitting, though, they "work" but at great cost to functioning:

- **Denial** protects people from unacceptable feelings by disavowing their existence. Note that denial can be a more or less adaptive defense based on how much reality is disavowed:

    Mr E presented to the dermatologist complaining of acne and was found to have an enormous tumor protruding from his cheek.

- **Dissociation** avoids unacceptable thoughts and affects by disconnecting the self from aspects of current reality. This can involve losing one's consistent sense of identity, memory, and ability to perceive sensations or current sense of reality. This is the quintessential "high-cost" defense, since major cognitive functions are sacrificed to avoid the experience or memory of massive trauma:

    When her mother was hitting her, Ms F retreated into a state in which she did not feel pain. This happened to her later in her life whenever her husband yelled at her.

- **Acting out** avoids painful or uncomfortable feelings by enacting the feeling without becoming consciously aware of it:

  Ms G was so upset after she failed her French final that she went out drinking with her friend and ended up blacking out in the apartment of a man she did not know.

  Classically, acting out referred to enacting feelings generated within therapy:

  Although Ms H said that she did not have any feelings about her therapist going on maternity leave, she signed up for several yoga classes during that time that prevented her from being able to return to her regular session times.

- **Regression** occurs when people go back to earlier ways of functioning to avoid anxiety-provoking feelings. People who generally function at a very high level may use this defense during periods of stress:

  Up against four medical school exams, Ms I retreated to her parents' home, where they made her meals and did her laundry.

More adaptive defenses

The more adaptive defenses tend to be based on repression. In repression-based defenses, all or part of an unacceptable thought or feeling is unconscious. We can think of thoughts and feelings as being linked in one unit (thought-feeling), as in the following example:

Mr J felt sad (affect) when he thought about his mother's death (thought, memory).

Here, sadness is linked to the memory of the mother's death. If this is unacceptable to Mr J, his mind will try to keep it unconscious. There are three options for repression here:

1. The mind represses both the affect and the thought – then Mr J never thinks about his mother's death.

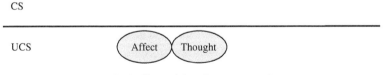

Both affect and thought are repressed

2. The mind represses the thought and leaves the affect conscious – then Mr J feels sad but doesn't know why.

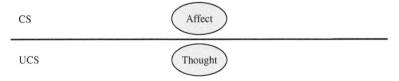

Affect remains conscious; thought is repressed

3. The mind represses the affect and leaves the thought conscious – then Mr J remembers his mother's death but has no feelings about it.

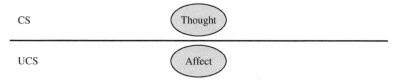

Thought remains conscious – affect is repressed

Different defenses repress different elements. The mind can also transform unacceptable unconscious elements by changing their object and reversing their affect. Here are some repression-based defenses:

- **Isolation of affect** occurs when the mind represses the affect but the thought remains conscious (#3 above). This makes the person seem devoid of feeling:

  Mr K said that he had no feelings about having just been left by his wife.

- **Intellectualization** uses substitution of excessive thinking to take the place of painful or uncomfortable feelings:

  Unable to process feelings of anxiety about beginning therapy, Mr L read ten books about Freud and began by engaging his new therapist in a discussion of the neurobiology of transference.

- **Rationalization** deals with unacceptable feelings by coming up with good reasons or justifications for problematic situations/feelings:

  Mr M is fired but tells his wife that it is for the best because he'd been unhappy at work for years.

- **Displacement** exchanges the object of a wish or feeling for one that feels more acceptable:

  Nate is afraid of his father, but instead feels afraid of the school principal.

- **Somatization** causes thoughts or feelings to be experienced as bodily sensations:

  Mr O began to experience stomach cramps in October. When his therapist wondered if this could be related to the upcoming second anniversary of his wife's death, he realized that he had completely forgotten that this was imminent.

- **Undoing** is the mind's "do-over" – it reverses something that feels unacceptable or uncomfortable:

  Ms P cheated people all day long in her work and then gave a dollar to a beggar on the street.

- **Reaction formation** turns unacceptable feelings into their opposite:

  Ms Q was excessively overprotective of her infant son in an effort to protect herself from her rage at his inability to sleep through the night.

- **Identification** is the "if you can't beat 'em, join 'em" defense. Feelings such as jealousy and competitiveness are dealt with by internalizing aspects of the other person. In many cases, identification is quite adaptive, for example when someone works in a productive way with a mentor. It is a normal and important part of adolescent development.

  Reina said that she didn't miss her sister who went to college, but began wearing the clothes her sister had left at home.

  Dr S noticed that her patient's new haircut resembled her own.

- **Excessive emotionality** represses thoughts while affect remains conscious. In some ways, this is the opposite of defenses such as intellectualization and isolation of affect:

  Ms T seemed unaffected by the fact that her divorce was final today, but became hysterical when she was told that her grocery order was delayed.

- **Externalization** leads people to perceive internal conflicts as if they were external conflicts. Note that this is *not* a splitting-based defense mechanism, because the feelings are still perceived as coming from within the self:

  Ms U consulted a therapist to talk about whether she should stay with her fiancé or begin to date an old boyfriend who had contacted her. Months into therapy, she realized that she was ambivalent about getting married at all.

- **Sexualization** takes issues that are not sexual and makes them sexual to avoid deeper uncomfortable feelings:

  Adrift during her mother's depression, 14-year-old Vanna began to flirt with her male gym teacher.

- **Repression** hides thoughts, feelings, and fantasies from consciousness, leading to forgetting, denial, and inhibited sexuality:

  After her divorce, Ms W was so anxious about paying taxes herself for the first time in 20 years that she completely forgot the tax deadline.

- **Turning against the self** substitutes the self for the object, particularly when it comes to negative affects:

  Mr X was angry with his father for buying a new house rather than paying for a year of his college education; however, he experienced this rage as self-criticism for not doing as well as he could have during his first semester.

Note that well-functioning people use these "repression-based" defense mechanisms *every day*, and, when under stress, they may regress and transiently use splitting-based defense mechanisms. Thus, it is not the presence of splitting-based defenses, but rather the predominance of them, that really makes it difficult for people to function well in love, work, and play.

Most adaptive defenses

Well-functioning people have several other mechanisms at their disposal to help buoy self-esteem and contain painful affects [17,18]. These may or may not be conscious and thus are not all classical defense mechanisms. Although they are very adaptive, they can also be problematic if used persistently and inflexibly.

- **Humor** makes light of uncomfortable thoughts and feelings:

  Adaptive – Mr Y made an uncomfortable slip during a sales pitch and then joked about it to his clients.

  Less adaptive – Ms Z complains that her boyfriend can never talk seriously about anything regarding their relationship and makes a joke of everything.

- **Altruism** involves doing things for others as a way of dealing with painful affects:

  Adaptive – After his father died of cancer, Mr AA started a foundation to raise money for cancer research.

  Less adaptive – Rather than care for herself, Ms BB spends all of her time caring for wounded animals.

- **Sublimation** occurs in physical science when an element goes directly from a solid to a gas. In psychodynamics, sublimation occurs when an uncomfortable thought or affect goes straight from the unconscious to consciousness in a useful form. Thus, when people discharge their anger by writing poems or going to the gym, the affect is completely discharged without having to launch a frank "defense." Sublimation often implies that the result is something that is useful or positive:

  Ms CC made sure that whenever she was frustrated with work she had time for a long run after she got home.

- **Suppression**, unlike repression, involves a conscious decision to put a thought or affect out of one's mind. "I won't think of that now," says Scarlett O'Hara in *Gone with the Wind*, "If I think of it now it will upset me" [19]. That's a classic example of suppression. Once again, suppression can be adaptive or non-adaptive. Putting one's bills out of mind for too many months leads to debt; however, the ability to put one's worries on the "back burner" is essential for mental health.

  Mr DD was worried about his mother who was developing Alzheimer's disease, but he was able to put this out of his mind while he was enjoying time with his friends.

Sample questions for assessing Adapting

You're telling me a very sad story without showing much emotion. Is that typical for you?

You've really subsumed your own needs in order to care for your mother during the past year. Has that happened to you before?

Defense mechanisms (adapted from Gabbard [13])

Less adaptive	More adaptive	Most adaptive
• Splitting	• Isolation of affect	• Humor
• Projection	• Intellectualization	• Altruism
• Pathological idealization and devaluation	• Rationalization	• Sublimation
	• Displacement	• Suppression
• Projective identification	• Somatization	
• Denial	• Undoing	
• Dissociation	• Reaction formation	
• Acting out	• Identification	
• Regression	• Excessive emotionality	
	• Externalization	
	• Sexualization	
	• Repression	
	• Turning against the self	

Cognition

Assessing cognition is critical for understanding how someone functions in the world. Cognitive function includes:

- general cognitive abilities (intelligence, memory, attention, speech, and language)
- reflective capacity (including reality testing)
- judgment (including ethical judgment) and impulse control
- managing emotions
- sensory stimulus regulation
- organizing, planning, and problem solving

Many of these are often called **executive functions** because, like an executive coordinating the activities of a company, they help coordinate the activities of the mind [20]. People vary widely in these functions, they cause tremendous difficulties in work and relationships, and they may have an impact on people's ability to use therapy.

General cognitive function

This is a person's built-in cognitive apparatus, including intelligence, memory, speech, and language, and the capacity for linear thinking. Gross impairments in this area make it difficult to benefit from psychotherapy, as these functions are vital for communicating, understanding, and making connections.

Reflective capacity

This refers to the ability to examine one's own thoughts and behaviors, to connect different aspects of experience, to recognize patterns, and to reconcile inconsistent attitudes and feelings [8]. At least some reflective capacity is necessary to be able to benefit from uncovering techniques. Two other aspects of reflective capacity are:

- **Psychological mindedness**, which is the ability to think about possible unconscious motivations for one's thoughts, feelings and behavior.
- **Reality testing**, which is the ability to differentiate reality from fantasy. This includes the ability to discriminate between perceptions that are real and those that are not (such as hallucinations, delusions, illusions, or grossly distorted perceptions of events). Having an intact **sense of reality** means that external events as well as one's own body are experienced as real and familiar (as opposed to having feelings of derealization and depersonalization, déjà vu experiences, dream-like states, out-of-body experiences, feelings of merger with others, or a grossly distorted body image).

Judgment/impulse control

Having intact **judgment** means that the person

- is aware of the appropriateness and likely consequences of an intended behavior (including the probable dangers, social consequences, and legal ramifications), and
- behaves in a way that reflects this awareness

Thus, knowledge of consequences does not in itself constitute good judgment. For example, patients may know that having unprotected sex is dangerous, but if they don't also practice safe sex, their judgment is impaired.

An important aspect of this function is **ethical judgment (conscience)** or the ability to distinguish right from wrong (previously called **super-ego function**). As we will explore more fully in Chapter 25, an overly harsh conscience can lead someone to feel too guilty about something very minor, as in this example:

> *Mr EE, who was caring for his elderly mother, thought that he was a terrible person for occasionally having the wish that she would die.*

Mr EE has done nothing wrong – he has just had a thought. Nevertheless, he is quite self-punishing, which can lead to symptoms of anxiety and depression. It can also affect how people think about themselves and have relationships. On the other hand, people with an underdeveloped sense of right and wrong do not feel guilty when they do things to hurt others:

> *Ms FF routinely hits her children with a brush when they misbehave. When asked about this, she says, "Feel bad about it? Are you kidding? They had it coming and will get more if they don't listen."*

Here, Ms FF has no remorse for actions that would make most people feel bad. A healthy conscience allows someone to have a sense of right and wrong and to experience enough guilt to be kind to themselves and others. It is important to remember that people can feel guilty about thoughts, feelings, and fantasies, as well as about actions and omissions. As with the assessment of other domains of function, any story can help you to assess ethical judgment – whenever you hear something related to guilt or absence of guilt, you can use the opportunity to learn about this important aspect of emotional functioning.

Closely related to judgment, **impulse control** refers to people's ability to act on or channel their feelings, urges, or wishes in a controlled way. People with poor impulse control act on feelings and urges in uncontrolled and maladaptive ways such as constantly needing to be in motion, throwing temper tantrums, binging on food, overusing alcohol and other substances, engaging in impulsive sexual activity, and self-mutilating. Also related to this are frustration tolerance and the capacity to delay gratification.

Managing emotions

This refers to the ability to tolerate and regulate anxiety and other intense positive and negative emotions (such as anger, envy, despair, longing, or love). Some people are more able to experience, tolerate, and express a wide range of feelings than others. People with a poor ability to manage emotions feel easily disorganized and unmoored by their own feelings, or may have rapid and dramatic swings from one mood state to another.

Sensory stimulus regulation

People with intact stimulus regulation automatically tune out insignificant stimuli (such as traffic noise outside a classroom) so that these do not divert attention from other important aspects of the environment (such as the teacher's lecture). Without this function, people can feel flooded by noises, smells, and visual stimuli. For example, some people with impaired stimulus regulation cannot tolerate crowds because of the heat/noise/smells; others are bothered if they are not in a perfectly quiet room. Too much environmental stimulation makes them shrink away, withdraw, or feel overwhelmed.

Organizing, planning, problem solving, and decision making

Part of the executive function group, these functions are essential for working, loving, and playing. Often, the presenting problem will tell you something about them, such as when the chief complaint involves making a decision or solving a problem. If not, the following questions can give you an idea of how to assess these critical functions.

Sample questions for assessing Cognition

General cognitive function

> Tell me the story of the last few weeks. Can you tell it in the order that it happened?
>
> Do you ever have difficulty concentrating or find your mind wandering? Has this been a problem?
>
> (Consider formal memory testing when appropriate, as well as assessment of attention using standardized instruments)

Reflective capacity

> How do you understand what led to this difficulty? What do you think your role has been?
>
> Does this pattern feel familiar to you? How do you think it started?
>
> Have you ever wondered if it might have to do with thoughts and feelings that are out of your awareness? (psychological mindedness)
>
> Are you sure that your husband feels that way about you, or is it just the way you are looking at things? (reality testing)

Judgment

> What are your thoughts about having stopped your medication?
>
> How did you feel after you did/thought that? Did you think that you had done something wrong? Did you think that you should be punished for that? How did doing that/thinking that make you feel about yourself? (ethical judgment)

Impulse control

> How much alcohol do you generally drink in a week? During a night out? How do you limit yourself?
>
> Do you have trouble keeping yourself from doing something – even if you think you shouldn't do it?

Managing emotions

> Everyone has really strong feelings from time to time. How do you deal with yours?
>
> Have people ever complained to you that you get too angry? Anxious? Have strong feelings ever gotten in the way of your work or your relationships?

Sensory regulation

> Do you find that you are really sensitive to sounds/smells/textures? Does this limit your ability to do things that you want to do? How do you deal with it?

Organizing, planning, problem solving, decision making

> Tell me about a big decision you made recently – how did you make it?
>
> Have organizational or time management issues ever been problems for you?

Capacity for work and play

Freud is reputed to have said that mental health depends on the ability to "love and work," and to this many have added "play." As mental health professionals, we don't have preconceived notions about what people *should* do in life, but are interested in assessing whether what they *choose* to do is well matched to their developmental level/talents/limitations, satisfying for them, and well suited for their lives as individuals and members of society. The capacity for play includes the ability to relax, drift into fantasies and daydreams, and experience deeply seated emotions and urges without feeling anxious or overstimulated. The capacity for play is also important for psychotherapy – it allows patients to retrieve and experience unconscious thoughts and feelings, and it facilitates empathy in therapists.

Sample questions for assessing Work and Play

What to you like to do for fun? How do you relax?

Tell me about your work. Is it what you hoped you'd be doing? Is it what you are trained to do? Does it feel enjoyable and satisfying?

Why is the assessment of functional domains important when we assess people for psychodynamic psychotherapy?

People with good mental and emotional functioning can tolerate internal and external stimuli well without being overwhelmed. Since they don't have to expend a tremendous amount of energy simply staving off stimulation, they can spend energy on other things, such as thinking, loving, and playing. Conversely, people with difficulty in these domains of function spend much of their energy just dealing with what feels like overwhelming levels of internal and external stimulation. How much energy is left over?

To get a better sense of this, think of two towns: one next to a river that constantly floods, and one that is well positioned on a hill. The town near the river has to spend most of its resources just dealing with the river – anticipating floods, dealing with floods, and cleaning up after floods – while the town on the hill can relax, play, and develop cultural activities. If you want to help the people in the town by the river, you have to help them with flood issues. On the other hand, helping the people in the town on the hill can take other forms, since they are not preoccupied only with survival. Using this analogy, people who grapple on a daily basis with problems like impulse control and managing emotions need a therapy that regularly and directly helps them to strengthen these functions, while people who do not have to struggle with these functions can concentrate on difficulties that relate to unconscious thoughts, feelings, and fantasies.

In order to benefit most from uncovering techniques, patients need strengths in several important domains of function. As we discussed in Chapter 1, uncovering techniques often involve discussion of the therapeutic relationship (**transference**) in order to understand aspects of the patient's defenses, relationships with others, and self-perceptions (see Chapters 12 and 21). In order to utilize this technique effectively, patients have to understand that discussion of their feelings about the therapist *will not lead* to a relationship with the therapist outside of the therapeutic situation. This requires the capacity to think abstractly, control impulses, test reality, have a developed sense of right and wrong, and manage emotions. Other functions, such as the capacity for play (in order to make connections and to associate to dreams and fantasies) and the ability to delay gratification (in order to stay with what can be a lengthy treatment), are also helpful for the uncovering process.

For all of these reasons, *people with problematic functioning generally need support, while people with healthier functioning can tolerate and benefit from the uncovering of unconscious thoughts and fantasies.*

There are, of course, exceptions to every rule. For example, patients with difficulties in multiple domains of function, such as those with borderline personality disorder, have historically been considered less suitable for uncovering work. However, in recent studies these patients were found to respond well to uncovering treatments that emphasize transference interpretation [21–24]. We will discuss this further in Chapter 21.

Strengths and difficulties

In terms of function, people are generally **mosaics**, with strengths in some domains and difficulties in others. They may even have both strengths and difficulties within a single area of function. For example, a man with many close friends may never have experienced a long-term romantic relationship. Some patients have global problems in all dimensions, while others have good function in one area and more difficulty in another. When we assess someone's domains of function, it is important to remember that we are looking for points of strength as well as points of vulnerability. This is essential not only for our assessment, but also for the treatment, since we will utilize areas of strength throughout the work.

> *Mr GG avoids socializing in order to deal with his extreme anxiety. In his isolation, he has become an excellent carpenter, spending many hours carefully constructing beautiful furniture.*

Although Mr GG's difficulty with relationships is an area of vulnerability, his talent for and love of his craft are strengths. His ability to concentrate and persevere could become important to his capacity to work in therapy.

Ever-changing patterns of function

It is also important to remember that functioning is not static, and thus a person's need to have support supplied from the outside waxes and wanes. Stress caused by medical and psychiatric illness, bereavement, role transitions, and blows to self-esteem can temporarily weaken function. For example, a woman who generally manages emotions well may be more labile after giving birth to a child, due to a combination of hormonal changes, sleep deprivation, or the stress of becoming a new parent. Function can also be affected in a moment-to-moment way, for example when a patient feels misunderstood or criticized by the therapist. Drugs and alcohol can alter multiple areas of function, including impulse control and judgment. These changes require us to be flexible in the use of uncovering and supporting techniques and to keep asking ourselves:

- What are the goals at this moment in the treatment?
- What is the patient's function at this moment in the treatment?

Now that you've done a thorough assessment of the patient, let's move on to Chapter 5 to consider how to use the information you've collected to generate a **formulation**.

Suggested activities

Here are some exercises that will help you to assess domains of function.

Activity 1: Assessing domains of function

What functions are impaired in these patients?

1. *Ms A only feels good about herself on days that she gets a call or text from her boyfriend.*
2. *Mr B drinks excessively after he fights with his wife.*
3. *Ms C can't stop herself from going home with random men she meets at bars.*
4. *Ms D says that she has many friends, but no one she could call in an emergency.*
5. *Mr E thinks his therapist is trying to get rid of him as a patient by charging for missed sessions.*
6. *After a hard day at work, Ms F comes home and yells at her children.*

Comment

1. Ms A has a tenuous ability to regulate her self-esteem.
2. Mr B has difficulty managing emotions – he can only calm himself down by drinking.
3. Ms C has poor impulse control and impaired judgment.
4. Ms D has poor relationships with others – all of her friendships are superficial.
5. Mr E has poor reality testing.
6. Ms F has difficulty managing emotions.

Activity 2: Assessing defenses

What defenses do you think that these people are using? Are they repression based or splitting based?

1. *Ms A has a three-month-old baby boy who cries day and night. Her husband never gets up to help her during the night. She has dark circles under her eyes and is exhausted. She will not leave the baby with anyone, including her mother, for fear that something will happen to him.*

2. *While studying for his bar exam, Mr B, a healthy 25-year-old law student, becomes panicked that he is going to have a heart attack. He begins to feel odd sensations in his chest and worries that he is winded when he walks up the stairs.*

3. *After failing his orals, Mr C tells his roommate that it's all for the best because it will force him to bone up on ancient Chinese history.*

4. *When Ms D's roommate begins dating their mutual friend, she becomes convinced that her roommate hates her and is trying to steal all of their other friends.*

5. *Mr E completely forgot that he had to pay his taxes until he received a warning note from the Internal Revenue Service.*

6. *When Ms F was late for her session, she berated her therapist for not giving her extra time at the end. The therapist left feeling guilty.*

7. *Mr G consulted a therapist after he was fired from his job, but in the first session he explained the situation in a near monotone. When the therapist asked him if he was upset about this, he said, "Why should I be? It's all part of the job."*

Comment

1. **Reaction formation**: It is likely that Ms A's overprotectiveness is covering repressed aggression toward her inconsolable child. This is repression based because the aggression remains within Ms A, but is experienced consciously as its opposite.

2. **Somatization**: Mr B is experiencing his anxiety as if it is originating in physical symptoms. This is repression based because the anxiety remains within Mr B, but is experienced as physical symptoms.

3. **Rationalization**: Mr C deals with his disappointment by finding a good reason for his failure. This is repression based because the disappointment of the failure remains within Mr C, but is experienced without the affect.

4. **Projection**: Ms D deals with her rage by experiencing it as originating in her roommate. This is splitting based since she cannot deal with the affect by keeping it within herself.

5. **Repression**: Mr E deals with the anxiety of paying taxes by completely putting it out of his mind. This is repression based because it remains within him but is not conscious.

6. **Projective identification**: Ms F deals with her feelings by projecting them into the therapist and then behaving in such a way that the therapist experiences those feelings herself. This is splitting based because Ms F cannot keep the feelings contained within herself.

7. **Isolation of affect and rationalization**: Mr G knows what happened, but has repressed the affect. This is repression based because the affect remains within Mr G and is just out of his awareness. Further, he uses rationalization because he gives a justification for being fired; this is also repression based.

Activity 3: Strengths and difficulties

Think about the areas of both strength and difficulty in these patients:

1. *Mr H is a 45-year-old man who presents for therapy saying that he is conflicted about an extra-marital affair. He worked for many years as a contractor, but was recently laid off. When he meets his union buddies each evening at the local bar, he confides to them that he is bickering daily with*

his wife. He is listless during the day and having difficulty curbing his appetite for internet pornography. He says that the only thing that has made him feel like a "man" recently is "hooking up" with a waitress from the bar – she is "young and pretty," but he's sure that she'll "dump him."

2. *Ms I is a 65-year-old woman whose husband of 40 years has just died. She feels lonely and isolated, as many of her friends no longer live in her neighborhood and her children live in far-away states. She has kept up her daily schedule of swimming, reading, gardening, and cleaning the house, but says it feels "empty." She says that she has always been shy and that her husband helped her have an active social life. She wonders what the next phase of her life will be like and asks you for help.*

Comment

1. During this period, Mr H is having difficulty with self-esteem regulation, impulse control, and managing emotions. He is aided by having friends and a long-term relationship. He has some reflective capacity, as evidenced by his decision to seek out psychotherapy.

2. Ms I is using her patterns of work and play to get her through this period of mourning. Although early in her life she had difficulty with relationships (shyness), with her husband's help she had a life full of people. Now that her husband has died, she has lost her "relationship helper" and may need assistance overcoming this difficulty in a new way. Her reflective capacity and interest in collaborating with you are strengths.

Chapter 4: References

1. Lacy, T.J., and Hughes, J.D. (2006) A systems approach to behavioral neurobiology: Integrating psychodynamics and neuroscience in a psychiatric curriculum. *Journal of the American Academy of Psychoanalysis and Dynamic Psychiatry*, **34** (1): 43–74.
2. Bellak. L., and Goldsmith, L.A. (eds.) (1984) *The Broad Scope of Ego Function Assessment*, John Wiley & Sons, New York.
3. Bellak, L., and Meyers, B. (1975) Ego function assessment and analyzability. *Journal of the American Psychoanalytic Association*, **2**, 413–427.
4. Bellak, L. (1975) *Ego Function Assessment (EFA): A Manual*. CPS, Larchmont, NY.
5. Vaillant, G.E. (1992) *Ego Mechanisms of Defense: A Guide for Clinicians and Researchers*, American Psychiatric Press, Washington, DC.
6. Pine, F. (1990) The concept of ego defect, in *Drive, Ego, Object, and Self: A Synthesis for Clinical Work*, Basic Books, New York, p. 198–231.
7. MacKinnon, R.A., and Yudofsky, S.C. (1986) *The Psychiatric Evaluation in Clinical Practice*, Lippincott, Williams & Wilkins, Philadelphia.
8. Auchincloss, E.L., and Samberg, S. (2012) *Psychoanalytic Terms and Concepts*, Yale University Press, New Haven, p. 151–153.
9. Freud, A. (1937) *The Ego and the Mechanisms of Defence*, Hogarth Press and the Institute of Psychoanalysis, London.
10. Perry, C.J., Beck, S.M., Constantinides, P., *et al.* (2009) Studying change in defensive functioning in psychotherapy using the defense mechanism rating scales: Four hypotheses, four cases, in *The Handbook of Evidence-Based Psychodynamic Psychotherapy* (eds R.A. Levy and J. S. Ablon), Humana Press, New York, p. 121–153.
11. Freud, S. (1894) The neuro-psychoses of defense, in *The Standard Edition of the Complete Psychological Works of Sigmund Freud (1893–1899): Early Psycho-Analytic Publications*, Vol. **III**, Hogarth Press, London, p. 41–61.

12. Kernberg, O.F. (1976) *Object-Relations Theory and Clinical Psychoanalysis*, Aronson, New York.
13. Gabbard, G.O. (2005) *Psychodynamic Psychiatry in Clinical Practice*, 4th ed., American Psychiatric Publishing, Washington, DC.
14. Perry, J.C., and Bond, M. (2005) Defensive functioning, in *The American Psychiatric Publishing Textbook of Personality Disorders* (eds J.M. Oldham, A.E. Skodol, and D.S. Bender), American Psychiatric Publishing, Washington, DC, p. 523–540.
15. Caligor, E., Kernberg, O.F., and Clarkin, J.F. (2007) *Handbook of Dynamic Psychotherapy for Higher Level Personality Pathology*, American Psychiatric Publishing, Washington, DC.
16. Kernberg, O.F., Selzer, M.A., Koenigsberg, H.W., *et al.* (1989) *Psychodynamic Psychotherapy of Borderline Patients*, Basic Books, New York.
17. Vaillant, G.E. (1977) A glossary of defenses, in *Adaptation to Life: How the Best and the Brightest Came of Age*, Little, Brown, Boston, p. 383–386.
18. American Psychiatric Association (2000) Defensive functioning scale, in *Diagnostic and Statistical Manual of Mental Disorders: DSM-IV-R*, American Psychiatric Association, Washington, DC, p. 807–813.
19. Mitchell, M. (1993) *Gone with the Wind*, Warner Books, New York, p. 76.
20. Loring, D.W. (ed.) (1999) *INS Dictionary of Neuropsychology*, Oxford University Press, New York, p. 1–2.
21. Clarkin J.F., Yoemans, F.E., and Kernberg, O.F. (2006) *Psychotherapy for Borderline Personality Disorder Focusing on Object Relations*, American Psychiatric Association, Washington, DC.
22. Clarkin, J.F., Levy, K.N., Lenzenweger, M.F., and Kernberg, O.F. (2007) Evaluating three treatments for borderline personality disorder: A multiwave study. *American Journal of Psychiatry*, **164**, 922–928.
23. Levy, K.N., Meehan, K.B., Kelly, K.M., *et al.* (2006) Change in attachment patterns and reflective function in a randomized control trial of transference-focused psychotherapy for borderline personality disorder. *Journal of Consulting and Clinical Psychology*, **74** (6), 1027–1040.
24. Hoglend, P. (2014) Exploration of the patient-therapist relationship in psychotherapy. *American Journal of Psychiatry*, **171**, 1056–1066.

5 The Initial Formulation

Key concepts

After conducting an assessment, we need to create an **initial formulation** in order to recommend treatment.

A formulation is a hypothesis. In mental health fields, formulations are hypotheses about how and why patients are having the difficulties that brought them to treatment. A **psychodynamic formulation** is one that considers the role of unconscious processes and development in the etiology of those difficulties.

We can create a formulation by

- **Describing** the person's problems and patterns of function
- **Reviewing** the history
- **Linking** the history to what we have described to answer the questions:
  - Why is this person having difficulty now?
  - What can we do to help?

Formulations are critical for setting goals.

Our formulations change throughout treatment.

Two people present to a primary care doctor with shortness of breath. Do they get the same treatment? Not necessarily – the treatment will depend on the etiology of the problem. The doctor will take histories and perform physical examinations in order to form hypotheses about what is causing the problem for each person. Those hypotheses are **formulations**, and they guide decisions about treatment. In mental health fields, formulations are hypotheses about how and why people develop the problems that bring them to treatment. At the beginning, formulations guide treatment recommendations, sometimes called **treatment plans**. As treatment progresses, they guide everything the therapist does, from making interventions to deciding when to end therapy. There are many kinds of formulations – psychopharmacologic formulations, CBT (cognitive behavioral therapy) formulations, and family systems formulations, to name just a few. What makes a formulation **psychodynamic** is the inclusion of ideas about the way in which unconscious thoughts and feelings contribute to the development of difficulties.

Students need not feel intimidated about creating psychodynamic formulations. Formulating is quite straightforward and involves three basic steps: Describing,

Psychodynamic Psychotherapy: A Clinical Manual, Second Edition. Deborah L. Cabaniss, Sabrina Cherry, Carolyn J. Douglas and Anna Schwartz.
© 2017 John Wiley & Sons, Ltd. Published 2017 by John Wiley & Sons, Ltd.

Reviewing, and Linking. In this chapter, you will learn how to use this model to make the best treatment recommendation for your patient. It will help you to decide whether

- psychodynamic psychotherapy is indicated
- uncovering or supporting will be more helpful

We will briefly review this model here, but for much more on this topic refer to our companion book, *Psychodynamic Formulation*.

Describe

Before you can make a hypothesis about etiology and recommend treatment, you have to have a good idea about what the difficulty is. There are two parts to this – describing the **problem** and describing the **person**. Let's first consider the difference between these two. The problem refers to the difficulty that brings patients to treatment *now*, while the person refers to general aspects of their baseline functioning, including areas of strength and difficulty. We need to know both in order to recommend the appropriate treatment. Two people might present with similar problems; however, if they have different patterns of function they will benefit from different types of therapy. Consider the following:

> *A 35-year-old woman presents to a therapist with the chief complaint that she is confused about her career. She states that she is conflicted about whether to stay at her present job, which she has held for six months and which offers her stability, or whether to leave to pursue a PhD in art history.*

This is a fairly typical chief complaint for someone to bring to a psychotherapist. She is confused about life choices – we hypothesize that she has a conflict. But let's consider two different people who both present with the same chief complaint:

> *Ms A is a 35-year-old woman who presents with the chief complaint that she is confused about her career. She states that she is conflicted about whether to stay at her present job, which she has held for six months and which offers her stability, or leave to pursue a PhD in art history. She says that she wants a job that is "more like the ones my friends have." Ms A states that she has had eight jobs in the last five years. She initially says that she left each job because the people were "so stupid," but further discussion reveals that she might have been fired for clashes with superiors. The "friends" that she mentioned are a group of people she met three months ago at a self-realization retreat. The anxiety produced by her current job situation has prompted her to binge drink on weekends. When you ask her why she'd like to pursue a PhD in art history, she has only a vague idea of what it would entail and confesses that she knows very little about art. "One of my friends is doing it and it seems really cool," she says. "I went to a party at her house with a lot of people from her program and they were really smart – that's where I should be."*

> *Ms B is a 35-year-old woman who presents with the chief complaint that she is confused about her career. She states that she is conflicted about whether to stay at her present job, which she has held for six months and which offers her stability, or leave to pursue a PhD in art history. In college, Ms B loved Italian Renaissance art, but was told by her parents, both of whom are successful attorneys, that anything less than a "profession" (medicine or law) was a waste of time. At the end of college, she and*

several of her close friends studied for their law school entrance exams. She was accepted to several good law schools, but developed a "mono-like" illness prior to matriculation and never began a program. She is still very close to most of her college friends, many of whom are now unhappy lawyers. Ms B floundered for a while and found success working for a non-profit company. She was just hired to a high-level administrative position at another non-profit, but realizes that it's "now or never" for her dream of becoming an art history professor. She has been dealing with her frustration by immersing herself in the art world again, attending lectures at a local museum and reading new books about Renaissance art.

Although Ms A and Ms B present with similar problems, they have very different patterns of thought, feeling, and behavior, in particular their

- self-experience and ability to regulate self-esteem
- relationships with others
- characteristic ways of adapting to stress
- decision making
- work patterns

Thus, although their *problems* sound similar, Ms A and Ms B are very different *people*. Ms A is conflicted, but has great difficulty containing her anxiety without acting out in a variety of self-destructive ways. Her conflict about her job status is the latest manifestation of a chaotic work history and her quest for a PhD seems superficial. In contrast, Ms B has a longstanding interest in art history that she did not pursue because her parents wanted her to be a doctor or a lawyer. She has dealt with her frustration by satisfying her hunger for immersion in the art world.

Undergoing psychodynamic psychotherapy is often very difficult. When we use a more uncovering mode, we try to unearth feelings, conflicts, and fantasies that are experienced as terrifying or shameful, change automatic defenses that have become habitual, and alter behaviors that "protect" people from overwhelming anxiety. In order to do this, people need **strengths** to help them. Thus, having a full understanding of a person's underlying strengths and difficulties – apart from the presenting problem – is essential for deciding what type of psychotherapy or technical stance will be most helpful to a given person at a given time. In sum, understanding the *person* involves identifying not just observable symptoms and behaviors, but also lifelong patterns in all of the major domains of function.

Problem

So let's begin with the *problem*. Defining the patient's problem often sounds easier than it is. Patients might not be aware of what their problems are, or the most pressing problem might not be their chief complaint. During the assessment phase, one of the therapist's main jobs is to determine what we think the patient's problem is – and, if there are numerous problems, to prioritize them.

Ms C presents for psychotherapy saying that she is lonely and has heard that psychotherapy could be helpful with commitment problems. In the course of the evaluation, you learn that Ms C has been drinking a bottle of wine per night.

In this example, Ms C says that she has a problem with relationships, but it becomes rapidly evident that she has a problem with alcohol. Thus, her chief complaint may not be her most pressing problem. What is important is to prioritize patients' problems without dismissing their subjective experience of what they think is most important. Continuing with Ms C, let's fast-forward to how a therapist might discuss this:

> Ms C, I'm so glad you learned about this treatment and that you are interested in exploring it. You've really been unhappy about your relationships and I think that I can help you with that. It also sounds like you're drinking more than you had been and that this might be exacerbating some of your difficulties. Let's see if we can create a plan that addresses both of these issues.

We have to remember that just because we're assessing the patient for psychotherapy doesn't mean that some other form of treatment might not be indicated. Patients who present for psychotherapy have many different types of problems, including mood, anxiety, eating, and substance abuse disorders. The presence of a disorder requiring medication doesn't preclude the use of psychodynamic psychotherapy, but, depending on the situation, patients might need to be stabilized with medication before beginning. For example, a very depressed patient with psychomotor retardation might have difficulty speaking in sessions, but might benefit from psychotherapy once her symptoms improve. On the other hand, a patient with dysthymia and relationship issues might begin medication and psychotherapy at the same time (see Chapter 15 for further discussion of medication and psychotherapy).

Person

As discussed in Chapter 4, people have characteristic ways of dealing with their internal and external environments in five major domains of function. These develop throughout life and form the basis of their characteristic patterns of functioning. To come up with the best treatment plan, we need to consider the current problem that brings patients to see us, as well as their underlying ways of thinking, feeling, and behaving. We call this understanding the *person*. This includes the assessment of strengths and difficulties in the five major domains of function described in Chapter 4:

- Self
- Relationships
- Adapting
- Cognition
- Work and Play

Review

Once we have described the problems and the person, we are ready to **review** the developmental history. Often, experiences that people have early in life contribute to their current problems and patterns – even they are not aware of the connection. Thus, in order to form a hypothesis about the question "Why does this person have this difficulty now?" we need to be able to review their lifelong, developmental history. This is much more than a typical "history of present illness" – it is the history from childhood to the present.

Developmental phases (adapted from Erikson [1])		
Developmental phase	**Age**	**Important historical elements**
Prenatal development	Conception to birth	Heredity, prenatal development, peripartum events
Earliest years	0–3 years	Temperament, attachment, environment into which child was born, quality of relationships with primary caregivers
Middle childhood	4–6 years	Caregivers' response to child's early sexuality, jealousy/rivalry among family members
Later childhood	7–12 years	Peer relationships, school experiences, skill building
Adolescence	13–18 years	Identity formation
Young adulthood	19–23 years	Formation of intimate relationships, assuming responsibility for oneself in the world
Adulthood	24–65 years	Family life, career development, successes and disappointments
Later adulthood	66 years and on	Losses, physical difficulties, response to aging

Each period of life has characteristic developmental issues that should be explored, with particular attention to a history of trauma, and mental and emotional difficulties during any phase. (See the box above for a list of the important developmental phases, and see our companion text, *Psychodynamic Formulation*, for a more thorough treatment of each developmental phase, taking a developmental history, and how early life experiences contribute to adult problems/patterns.) Although we try to obtain a full history early in the treatment, the circumstances of the assessment do not always make this possible – for example, if the treatment is in the context of a brief hospitalization. In addition, at the beginning of treatment patients may not be able to remember aspects of their history that may be more accessible to them as the therapy proceeds. Nevertheless, trying to get at least some sense of each period of the patient's life is important for creating an initial formulation.

Link

After describing the problem and the person, and taking a developmental history, we can **link** these to construct an initial formulation. Linking involves forming hypotheses about how a person's history might have led to the development of their problems and patterns. We do this in order to answer two questions:

- *Why is this person having difficulty now?*
- *What can we do to help?*

A sample initial formulation

Let's look at how to use the Describe/Review/Link method to construct an initial formulation for Mr D:

> *Mr D is a 65-year-old man who presents with the chief complaint: "I'm not getting along with my wife."*

DESCRIBE

Problem: Marital discord

> *Mr D says that for the past six months, he and his wife have been arguing more than usual. This is in the context of Mr D's mother-in-law coming to live with them so that his wife can nurse her while she recovers from a major illness. There is no evidence of mood or anxiety disorder.*

Person

Domains of function

Self	*Mr D has a consolidated identity and is able to modulate self-esteem well.*
Relationships	*Mr D has many long-term relationships. He has a nuanced view of others and perceives them as having both good and bad qualities.*
Adapting	*Mr D generally uses adaptive defenses that are repression based. He sublimates anxiety and aggression by excelling in athletics and pursuing hobbies such as woodworking. He habitually keeps strong feelings out of awareness, suggesting a prominent reliance on defenses that isolate affect. He often intellectualizes; for example, he is currently reading books about marriage in mid-life.*
Cognition	*Mr D uses very good judgment and is generally able to manage emotions. This is part of why his recent anger stands out as a problem. He is fairly psychologically minded, expressing a sense that his anger toward his wife might relate to feelings about his mother-in-law. He has close, personal relationships that help him cope with anxiety and stress. Mr D also has a developed sense of right and wrong. His guilt regulation tends to be appropriate, as evidenced by his consultation for this problem*
Work and Play	*Mr D has worked consistently at a job at which he excels and which he enjoys. He has hobbies, but often has difficulty relaxing on weekends and during vacations.*

REVIEW

Mr D is the first of two sons born to married parents. He recalls feeling close to both his mother and father early in his life and generally having had his needs met. When he was 5 years old, his mother died precipitously of a brain aneurysm. He recalls being praised for being a "strong little boy" and was told that he was a "quiet, determined" child. He did well in school, excelling in academic subjects and sports. His father remarried two years after his mother's death. Mr D was sent to boarding school after sixth grade. He had friends and often stayed to study over breaks. He met his wife at 21 and says, "marrying her was the best thing I ever did – she has spent her life running mine." Mr D works hard in a career he enjoys. He has never had depression or anxiety, but from age 35 to 55 had 3–4 drinks on weeknights and more on the weekends. He and his wife have two children, both of whom are doing well and are now living on their own.

LINK

Mr D identifies his main problem as interpersonal conflict with his wife. Although he has many strengths, including a generally well-developed sense of self, good relationships, many adaptive ways of dealing with stress, good cognitive function, and a fair degree of psychological mindedness, his major challenge is his tendency to keep strong feelings out of awareness. His history suggests that he may have unresolved feelings about his mother's death, and that his wife has served a maternal role in his life. It is likely that he is anxious that his mother-in-law's presence and needs will interfere with the care that he generally gets from his wife, and that he is experiencing this anxiety as irritability and anger.

This formulation brings together what we have learned to form an initial hypothesis about the etiology of Mr D's current problems. It suggests that Mr D's present difficulties may stem from early, unconscious fears about abandonment that are being stirred up in the context of having to share his wife with her mother. As you will see in Chapter 6, we can use what we learn from the formulation to help decide whether psychodynamic psychotherapy is indicated.

Formulating is key to goal setting

Since your formulation is your hypothesis about what is causing the patient's problems, it is key for setting treatment goals. For example, in the case of Mr D, his chief complaint is interpersonal conflict with his wife, but our formulation suggests that underlying anxiety and unresolved grief may be at the heart of his problems. Therefore, our goals will be to help him become more aware of his feelings, particularly those related to his wife and his mother, and to understand the way in which his characteristic ways of adapting lead him to keep a distance from his emotions. Your formulation is critical to your ability to set goals.

Formulating throughout the treatment

As we work with patients over time and get to know them better, our formulations grow and change. At the beginning of treatment, the formulation helps us to make a treatment recommendation, but we need to understand how and why our patients are thinking, feeling, and behaving the way they are in order to conduct every aspect of the treatment. Our formulations guide our moment-to-moment therapeutic strategy, choices about interventions, and decisions about ending. As therapists, we don't construct formulations ourselves – we co-construct them with our patients as we learn together about their lives and their minds. For more on constructing psychodynamic formulations throughout the treatment, refer to our companion text, *Psychodynamic Formulation*. In the next chapter, we will review the **indications** for psychodynamic psychotherapy so that you can use your formulation to make the best treatment plan with your patient.

Suggested activities

Activity 1

For each patient, name two things that are *problems* and two things that characterize the *person*.

> *Mr A is a 45-year-old man who presents with new-onset anxiety related to problems with his 16-year-old daughter. A single parent since his wife died five years ago, he says that he doesn't know how to deal with his daughter's promiscuity and marijuana use. "I just can't talk to her like my wife did," he laments, telling you that he often withdraws and doesn't confront her about her behavior. He says that this pattern reminds him of how he dealt with his "spirited" wife as well. His worry that his daughter is on the "wrong track" has led him to have insomnia, daily ruminations, and "one too many" beers at night.*

> *Ms B is a 35-year-old woman who presents because her boyfriend has broken up with her. She says that she is tearful at work and that for the last week it has been difficult to concentrate. She explains that although her boyfriend is married, she knows that he was closer to her than he was to his wife and she can't understand why he has made this choice. She says that she has dated married men before, but that this was "different" because she was "sure" that he was going to leave his wife.*

Comment

Mr A

Problem:

- Anxiety symptoms
- Difficulty communicating with his daughter
- Increased drinking

Person:

- Tends to withdraw rather than confront
- Single parent
- Moderate reflective capacity

Ms B

Problem:

- Depressive symptoms
- Recent break-up

Person:

- Pattern of dating unavailable men
- Tends to use denial to deal with difficulties
- Limited reflective capacity

Activity 2

How might you link the description of Ms C's problems and person with her developmental history to create a formulation?

DESCRIBE

Problem

Ms C is a 30-year-old woman who reports low mood and listlessness for the past two months. There are no other neurovegetative symptoms of depression. She is also ruminating about whether to accept a promotion in her firm's overseas office.

Person

Five domains of function

self	*Despite doing very well in school and having attained a very responsible position at work, Ms C reports a lifetime of low self-esteem.*
Relationships	*She has very close friends, for whom she is almost too available, often babysitting for them and anticipating their needs.*
Adapting	*Ms C often blames herself for things that might have been caused by others. She is often unaware of her feelings, always trying to "put on a good face" for friends and family.*
Cognition	*She has good judgment and impulse control, but has difficulty relaxing on weekends. She tends to make decisions in an overly careful way, continually weighing pros and cons. She is capable of self-reflection. She has a well-developed sense of right and wrong, but is often overly hard on herself.*
Work and Play	*Ms C has excelled at her job, but has difficulty relaxing.*

REVIEW

Ms C grew up in a lower-middle-class family, with parents who had been high-level academics in another country before emigrating for political reasons. She describes her father as a resilient and generally happy person, who made the most of his new and altered circumstances. He spent his life working in a technical position before retiring early due to congestive heart failure. She describes her mother as extremely brilliant and exacting, always pushing Ms C to excel academically and pursue a university career. She reports, "I felt so bad for my mother – she tried and tried to get work as a professor here but never did. She ended up teaching high school to kids who really never appreciated her brilliance." Ms C says that she took on many of the household chores so that her mother could continue her writing, though it never got published. She was well liked in school and always had friends, but was never part of a peer group. She attended excellent schools and pursued a career in accounting, which she enjoys but which her mother thinks is "just a trade." She has had boyfriends, but tends to find men who, she says, "are not that into me." She has always lived near her parents, and continues to help around the house. Three months ago, she was offered a promotion in her firm's overseas office. She was excited about this offer, but continues to ruminate about whether to accept it.

LINK

How can you link the review of Ms C's developmental history to what has been described of her problems/person/goals and resources to answer the questions:

- *Why is Ms. C having this problem now? and*
- *What can we do to help her?*

Comment

Ms C has a lifetime history of self-esteem issues and a tendency to prioritize helping others over helping herself. Currently, she has low mood and listlessness. This may be linked to her recent job offer. It is likely that Ms C has unconscious feelings toward her mother, who devalued her career choice and for whom Ms C continues to make personal sacrifices. She may be conflicted about whether to pursue her own career at the expense of no longer being available to help her chronically disappointed mother. She may keep negative feelings about her mother out of awareness by tending generally to repress her feelings. She is bright, interested in her mind, and able to pursue psychotherapy. Because it is likely that this problem is linked to unconscious thoughts and feelings, psychodynamic psychotherapy is indicated (see Chapter 6).

Chapter 5: Reference

1. Erikson, E. (1993) *Childhood and Society*, 2nd ed., Norton, New York, p. 247–274.

6 Indications for Psychodynamic Psychotherapy

Key concepts

The **psychodynamic formulation** helps us determine when to recommend psychodynamic psychotherapy.

We think of psychodynamic psychotherapy as the treatment of choice when we hypothesize that our patients' **problems** are linked to

- unconscious factors
- acute or persistent functional difficulties

A person's characteristic patterns of functioning help us decide whether to predominantly uncover or support.

Considering the patient's **goals** and **resources** is also key to making treatment recommendations.

Choosing psychodynamic psychotherapy

Psychodynamic psychotherapy is an evidence-based treatment. The results of nearly 40 randomized controlled trials (RCTs) support the efficacy of psychodynamic psychotherapy in many psychiatric disorders in the *Diagnostic and Statistical Manual of Mental Disorders* (DSM), including major depressive disorder (MDD), social anxiety disorder, somatoform pain disorder, anorexia nervosa, borderline personality disorder, and Cluster C personality disorders. There is also growing evidence that it is effective for dysthymia, panic disorder, generalized anxiety disorder (GAD), and complicated grief. Transference focused psychotherapy (TFP), which is based on psychodynamic principles and techniques, has been shown to be an effective treatment for borderline personality disorder. Data for psychodynamic psychotherapy conducted with a primarily supportive stance suggests that it is effective for a wide variety of problems, including personality disorders, medical illness, generalized anxiety disorder, social anxiety, depression, adjustment disorders, opiate addiction, and cocaine abuse. While further randomized controlled trials are needed for psychodynamic psychotherapy, the evidence base is clear [1–21].

Nevertheless, we think about more than just studies when deciding whether to recommend psychodynamic psychotherapy. As we've reviewed in the last few

---

Psychodynamic Psychotherapy: A Clinical Manual, Second Edition. Deborah L. Cabaniss, Sabrina Cherry, Carolyn J. Douglas and Anna Schwartz.
© 2017 John Wiley & Sons, Ltd. Published 2017 by John Wiley & Sons, Ltd.

chapters, we look not only at patients' acute problems, but also at their general functioning, reflective capacity, goals, and resources. When we assess all patients, we thoroughly explore their current/acute symptoms in order to determine whether they meet the criteria for any DSM diagnoses. Acute depression and anxiety often require initial or ongoing treatment with medication, and thus it is very important to diagnose these disorders carefully at the outset. Simultaneously, we listen for suggestions that unconscious processes might be involved and thus that psychodynamic psychotherapy might be indicated. Although no one knows what causes mood or anxiety problems, as psychodynamic psychotherapists we hypothesize that they may be linked to unconscious factors, such as conflicts, repressed feelings, difficulties with self-esteem, and maladaptive expectations of others. *When we hear clues that unconscious factors are involved, it suggests to us that psychodynamic psychotherapy might be indicated.* It is thus critical to be able to listen for those clues – this chapter will help you do just that.

We also listen for evidence that general function in the five domains – self, relationships, adapting, cognition, work/play – might be acutely or persistently weakened. *Weakened function is our second suggestion that psychodynamic psychotherapy might be indicated.* Thus we can say that **psychodynamic psychotherapy is indicated when our formulation suggests that our patients' problems are linked to**

- unconscious factors
- acute or persistent problems in domains of function

Let's turn now to how to identify these clinical situations:

Unconscious factors

Interpersonal difficulties, distorted self-perceptions, and maladaptive ways of dealing with stress are undoubtedly the complicated end products of myriad factors, including inborn temperamental factors, the impact of early attachments, traumatic experiences, mood and anxiety disorders, and cognitive strengths and difficulties. However, based on our clinical experience, there are certain kinds of problems that improve when unconscious elements are brought into conscious awareness.

As we discussed in Chapter 2, we can think about this using a developmental model. As people develop, certain affects, wishes, fantasies, fears, and conflicts threaten to cause us intolerable anxiety. According to this model, we keep these affects, fears, and wishes out of awareness to protect us, but we do so *at the expense of continued normal development.* Depending on what we repress, development is affected to a greater or lesser degree. Here are two examples:

> *Ms A is chronically abused by her mother. Keeping negative feelings about her mother out of awareness leads to global problems in the development of trust, self-esteem management, the capacity for attachment, and a host of other critical functions.*

> *Mr B has loving parents but competes with his younger brother for his mother's attention. Keeping his aggressive feelings toward his brother out of awareness impedes his ability to compete in a healthy way with male peers, affecting some aspects of his adult career advancement.*

Because of the extent of her abuse, Ms A's repression affects her functioning to a greater degree than Mr B's affects his.

When we assess patients for psychodynamic psychotherapy, we look for indicators that the problems we are seeing are linked to hidden, unconscious factors. But, once again, how can we find factors that are out of awareness? Sometimes, we can determine this from the history – in other words, patients give us clues at the outset that their problems are related to something in their past that is now inappropriately transposed onto a current situation. Here's an example:

> *Mr C is a 34-year-old heterosexual man who describes becoming anxious every time he is in a relationship with a woman that starts to become serious. You do a thorough assessment and find that he does not have an anxiety or mood disorder. He also has generally good functioning – he has good friends, is intelligent, functions well at work, and is able to manage his emotions. According to the DSM he's healthy – no problems at all. But he has come to you because he's very upset – he wants to have a long-term relationship and his inability to do so is greatly affecting his quality of life. When you take a **developmental history** you discover that his father had to forgo his wish to be a writer in order to support his wife and son. The patient says that his father became persistently withdrawn from the family and that his mother relied on the patient for emotional support.*

Once you hear the developmental history, you hypothesize that the patient's fears about long-term relationships have more to do with his thoughts, feelings, and fantasies about his parents than with the actual women in his current life. Psycho-dynamic psychotherapy can help to make the patient aware of this and can help him to move forward as an adult.

But what if we don't explicitly hear this link to the person's past? How can we tell if the person's problems are linked to unconscious factors? In these cases, we're like geologists who need to rely on surface indicators when looking for subterranean formations. What kinds of clues can we use to help us know whether a person's problem may be linked to unconscious factors? Here are a few of the chief complaints that often signal that unconscious elements are at play:

"I'm stuck"

One of the most common chief complaints that psychodynamic psychotherapists hear from their patients is that, in some way, they feel stuck. Some are stuck in their careers, others are stuck in their romantic relationships – but whatever it is, they don't know how to move forward. Generally, patients presume that this indicates that things are not moving, but as therapists we know better. We know that the feeling of being stuck is usually caused by **conflict** that is out of awareness. If two horses are pulling a cart, and one is going due east and the other is going due west, there's plenty of force but the cart isn't going anywhere. It's stuck. That is what our patients feel. Here's an example:

> *Mr D is a 30-year-old writer who has published one novel and presents saying that he can't seem to start his second. He has hundreds of pages of notes, but freezes when he starts to write. He says that he wants to write; however, as you discuss this with him, it becomes clear that he is desperately afraid that he will get a bad review and that his earlier success will be seen as a "fluke."*

Mr D is stuck, but it's because he has two equal and opposite forces going on in his unconscious. One wish is to move ahead and write his second novel. Yet an equal and opposite force is the fear or shame involved in exposing himself to scrutiny. If he never writes, he can never be judged. If we can help him understand this, he can resolve this conflict and move forward in life.

"My life is great except for . . ."

A good indicator that some developmental trajectory has arrested is the situation that occurs when only one aspect of a person's life is problematic. Very often, people present who are moving ahead with their careers and have many friends, but have persistent difficulties with intimate, romantic relationships. Conversely, some people have no problems with relationships but have difficulty with assertion, ambition, or competitiveness that translates into career dissatisfaction. Of course, further investigation may reveal that there is more to the story, but this type of presentation is often a good clue that unconscious factors are involved.

"I don't know why I keep doing . . ."

Persistent patterns of maladaptive choices, particularly in someone who seems to have the capacity to make better ones, is often a good indicator that something unconscious is perpetuating the situation. Consider an attractive, intelligent young woman with very close female friends who repeatedly dates married men, or an earnest young father who keeps getting into dead-end business situations.

"I started to feel bad when . . ."

Listening to what triggers our patients' difficulties is key to picking up links to unconscious processes and early developmental experiences. Mood and anxiety symptoms related to interpersonal difficulties, such as break-ups, separations, losses, and relationship conflicts, suggest links to unconscious factors, as do symptoms related to self-esteem blows.

"I always feel bad"

Acute or persistent negative emotional states (such as sadness, anger, envy, and shame) that are enduring but not symptoms of underlying major psychiatric disorders (such as major depression or panic disorder) suggest links to unconscious factors [22–24]. These may be related to temperament and/or histories of trauma or insecure attachment. Consider Ms E:

> Ms E is a 40-year-old woman who presents complaining of frequently feeling angry and sad, and of a lack of closeness in relationships with other people. She notes, "People always disappoint me, and that makes me angry." She does not have any other mood or anxiety symptoms, and does not meet the criteria for any mood or other DSM disorder. Her mother was an alcoholic and often too drunk to take

care of Ms E and her siblings. Her father was preoccupied with work, and often made promises to Ms E that he didn't follow through on, such as taking her to the park on weekends or buying her things she needed.

Ms E internalized being let down by her parents, leading her to experience people in her adult life as disappointing or uncaring. Her persistent anger, while understandable and appropriate in response to her parents' behavior, may be disproportionate to current situations and may make others pull away from her, thus perpetuating negative affects. Helping Ms E become aware of these patterns may help her to feel less angry and sad and enable her to have more satisfying interactions with others.

Acute or persistent functional difficulties

Patients whose problems stem from acute (temporary) or persistent difficulties in the five domains of function (self, relationships, adapting, cognition, work/play) are likely to benefit from psychodynamic psychotherapy with a supporting stance. Here is an example:

A seemingly healthy and previously well-adjusted 21-year-old college senior presents to his student health center at a large university a few months before graduation. He says that he has just been dumped by the love of his life, feels depressed and overwhelmed, can't study, and feels panicked and suicidal because he is in danger of flunking his midterms. He admits he is also drinking more than he should, but can't find any other way to calm himself. He has always considered himself a "strong" person and is appalled and ashamed by his "total collapse." If he manages to graduate, he plans to go to medical school in the Caribbean, but he is beginning to doubt whether he has made the right career choice. His own dream was to study philosophy, but his parents thought this was "too impractical" and urged him to pursue medicine, despite his lack of aptitude in the pre-med courses and middling performance on his medical school entrance exams.

The therapist thinks that, in addition to this young man's acute grief over losing his girlfriend, he may be unconsciously "shooting himself in the foot" as a way of defying his parents' expectations, and might benefit from uncovering psychodynamic psychotherapy. However, at this moment he is less interested in a deeper understanding of his difficulties than he is in rapid relief of his symptoms and a concrete plan for getting through his exams. His life circumstances (and perhaps the health center's policies) also dictate that the treatment will be brief. Is psychodynamic psychotherapy contraindicated? Not necessarily, but the patient's acute needs may dictate a supportive approach that takes into account – without necessarily exploring – some of the unconscious thoughts and feelings fueling his behavior.

Psychodynamic psychotherapy with a supporting stance may be indicated for the following:

People with generally good function who are experiencing temporary weakness in certain areas in the face of stress, such as:

- **Newly diagnosed medical illnesses**: Blows to our physical functioning frequently affect our emotional functioning. Support can often help patients who are newly physically ill manage feelings such as rage and loss, and develop coping mechanisms to deal with their altered level of physical function.

- **Social upheavals**: Events that acutely alter the way we relate to people in our environment can often dramatically affect function. Examples include divorce, death of a parent or spouse, break-ups and relationship loss, leaving home, getting married, becoming a parent, losing a job, and retiring.
- **Other crises**: Anything that acutely overwhelms our capacity to function at baseline has the potential to weaken function temporarily. This could include business reversals, financial problems, natural disasters, physical threats/trauma, and legal problems.
- **Stressful periods during uncovering psychotherapy**: Sometimes the emotional work of psychodynamic psychotherapy can temporarily overwhelm a person's function. This may require a period of support to deal with very strong affects or anxiety.

People with persistent difficulties with function, such as:

- **Lack of psychological mindedness and/or motivation for understanding**: People who persistently lack the ability and/or motivation for thinking about the way in which unconscious factors affect their lives will often benefit from therapy that more directly addresses their functioning.
- **Difficulty managing emotions and overwhelming anxiety around separations**: Some people have a harder time than others in tolerating their distress and may always need immediate relief from their symptoms. Support for function can provide this.
- **Lack of trust and/or a history of problematic relationships**: People with seriously impaired relationships and a tenuous ability to trust others often benefit from ongoing support to help them improve their relationships.
- **Poor impulse control**: People with poor impulse control are generally best treated, at least initially, with supporting techniques that help them control their feelings and impulses long enough to talk about them. Such patients may suffer from affect storms or tantrums; may binge on food, alcohol, or drugs; may self-mutilate; may engage in risky or dangerous sexual activity; or may generally act on feelings in an uncontrolled and maladaptive way.
- **Persistent psychotic, mood, or anxiety disorders**: People with persistent major psychiatric disorders may have persistently impaired reality testing, poor impulse control, and difficulty managing emotions. They often benefit from psychodynamic psychotherapy that focuses on actively supporting weakened function.
- **Persistent physical illness**: Ongoing physical illness can persistently weaken function. Reasons for this include the stress of treatments, permanent loss of mental and physical functioning, and ensuing changes in a person's ability to work, play, and have relationships. Support is often an essential component of the maintenance treatment of myriad illnesses such as cancer, diabetes, neurodegenerative disorders, and HIV-related conditions.

Assessing domains of function guides therapeutic strategy

The patient's baseline function – which we called the **person** in our formulation (Chapter 5) – will help us determine whether a predominantly uncovering or supporting stance will be more helpful. As we have discussed in previous chapters (and just now), patients with functional difficulties are best helped by support, while patients with stronger function are likely to benefit from uncovering techniques.

We also have to assess our patients' **motivation** and **psychological mindedness**. Although most people have unconscious factors that impede their adult function in some way, not everyone is interested in exploring these or thinks that they could be related to their current problems. For example, a patient could have a problem that we think might be helped by uncovering unconscious material, but might lack the motivation or resources to make this treatment feasible. Here's an example:

> *Mr F consults a therapist because he is having difficulty with his 16-year-old son. A generally patient and thoughtful man, he cannot understand why he and his son are constantly yelling at each other. When you take a history, you find that Mr F's father is a volatile, abusive man from whom Mr F has been estranged for many years. You think that Mr F might be unconsciously identifying with his father in his dealings with his son, and that uncovering this could be helpful to this relationship. However, when you begin to explore this with Mr F, he becomes upset and says that:*

- *he's nothing like his father, and*
- *he wants to clear up the whole situation in three weeks.*

Despite your hypothesis that Mr F has a problem that is caused by something in his unconscious, he is not motivated for this type of treatment and he is not interested in committing the resources needed for an in-depth, uncovering treatment.

This is not to say that patients cannot gain understanding and motivation over time. *Patients for psychodynamic psychotherapy are made, not born* – that is, we can teach our patients about psychodynamic principles, demonstrate to them that these principles work, and help them to develop the ability to benefit from this type of treatment.

Goals

Both long-term and short-term goals can be addressed by psychodynamic psychotherapy. When most people present for treatment, they are in some sort of crisis, and thus short-term goals are primary. Generally, we can help them with these fairly rapidly, either with psychotherapy alone or with some combination of medication and therapy. However, many people soon realize that their acute problem is part of a longer-term pattern that will continue to trip them up if it is not addressed. Sometimes, we can help our patients recognize this and reframe their short-term goals into long-term goals. Here are two examples:

Short-term goal	*I just want to be able to get married next month without calling the wedding off.*
Long-term goal	*I need to figure out why I keep doubting my relationships.*

Short-term goal   *I need to get my father off my back.*

Long-term goal   *I need to figure out how to have a more adult relationship with my parents.*

In general, appropriate goals for psychodynamic psychotherapy relate to improving

- self-perception and self-esteem management
- relationships with others
- characteristic ways of adapting to stress
- cognitive function

Even when the presenting problem is a mood or anxiety disorder, we don't think of directly addressing the symptoms; rather, we think of addressing the underlying unconscious factors and/or strengthening domains of function. For example, treating depression is often correlated with improving self-function [25], while treating panic is often correlated with improving tolerance of anger (adapting) and conflicts around dependency (relationships) [26]. Understanding the goals of treatment is essential for making an informed treatment recommendation, and, as we'll see in Chapter 7, is an important part of beginning the treatment.

Resources

Sometimes, psychodynamic psychotherapy is indicated but the resources are not available. Resources include:

- factors related to the system, including availability of therapists, types of treatment, and treatment hours
- factors related to the patient's resources, including financial situation, health insurance, family support, and time

Consider these situations:

Ms G is interested in undergoing psychodynamic psychotherapy, but there isn't a therapist in her part of the state who is familiar with this type of treatment.

Mr H has an assessment for psychotherapy but decides that he can't afford it.

Mr I is on a waiting list for an appointment for a psychotherapy intake.

Eight-year-old Javier would benefit from psychotherapy, but both parents work two jobs and aren't available to take him to appointments after school.

In a perfect world these things wouldn't matter – but in the real world they do. If we don't take them into consideration, we suggest treatment plans that are potentially unrealistic. Thus, thinking about resources is essential to deciding whether psychodynamic psychotherapy is indicated.

   We have now finished our initial assessment and are ready to **begin the treatment**, which is the topic of Part Three of this manual.

Suggested activity

For each of the following patients, would you begin psychodynamic psychotherapy with a predominantly uncovering or supporting stance? Give two reasons for your answer in each case.

1. *Ms A is a 29-year-old graduate student who presents with difficulty finishing her dissertation. She describes thinking obsessively about her topic all day long, but being unable to sit down to write. "The dissertation seems like an enormous blob," she tells you. "I don't know where to begin." She lives with roommates with whom she eats meals but does not socialize, and she says that there's "no one around whom I can count on." She says that her adviser "hates" her and may even be actively thwarting her academic efforts in order to kick her out of the program. She tells you that her father was a fairly prominent professor at a rival institution who has "very high expectations" of his children, but who "favors" her older brother. She denies symptoms of depression and, aside from obsessing, does not have other symptoms of anxiety. She says that "some teachers" thought that she might have had attention deficit disorder (ADD) as a child, and that despite her good performance in college, distraction did cause her to have problems in "less structured" courses.*

2. *Mr B is a 32-year-old man who is contemplating proposing to his girlfriend, Y. After dating different women for many years, he says that he "really loves" Y and that she's the first woman he could imagine "sharing his life with." His friends – many of whom have known him since college – really like Y and are encouraging him to "seal the deal." However, he is hesitating and this is causing him anxiety. He does not report any symptoms of depression or anxiety. The one person who is "not so hot" about Y is his mother, who worries that she's "not good enough" for him because she "doesn't have the graduate degrees" that he has. In the last few weeks he has found himself calling his mother more often, which feels a little "automatic" and he has "wondered why" he's doing it. Since his father died 10 years ago, he says that he has felt "responsible" for his mother, which makes him both "proud" and "resentful."*

Comment

1. **Begin with a supportive stance**: Ms A's isolation (problems with relationships with others), her inability to create a plan for writing her dissertation (cognitive problem), and perhaps some paranoia (problems with reality testing) suggest that she requires support at this point in her treatment. She seems to be intelligent (a strength) and there may be some unconscious factors at play (competition with her father), but she needs help with her weakened function first in order to improve her current situation.

2. **Begin with an uncovering stance**: Mr B is in the classic "stuck" position of someone who has an unconscious conflict. It is likely that two conflicting unconscious fantasies – "I love my girlfriend" and "I need to take care of my mother" – are colliding and leading him to feel that he can't move in any direction. The fact that his calls to his mother feel "automatic" and that he has "wondered" about this suggests that he is somewhat aware that unconscious factors are involved. There is no indication of difficulty functioning at this time – on the contrary, it sounds like he has very good friends in whom he is confiding. An uncovering approach is likely to help him to understand how these unconscious factors affect him, and to allow him more freedom to make decisions.

Chapter 6: References

1. Clarkin, J.F., Levy, K.N., Lenzenweger, M.F., and Kernberg, O.F. (2007) Evaluating three treatments for borderline personality disorder: A multiwave study. *American Journal of Psychiatry*, **164**, 922–928.
2. Levy, K.N., Meehan, K.B., Kelly, J.M., *et al*. (2006) Change in attachment patterns and reflective function in a randomized control trial of transference-focused psychotherapy for borderline personality disorder. *Journal of Consulting and Clinical Psychology*, **74** (6): 1027–1040.
3. Hoglend, P. (2014) Exploration of the patient-therapist relationship in psychotherapy. *American Journal of Psychiatry*, **171**, 1056–1066.
4. Shedler, J. (2010) The efficacy of psychodynamic psychotherapy. *American Psychologist*, **65** (2), 98–109.
5. Leichsenring, F., Rabung, S., and Leibing, E. (2004) The efficacy of short-term psychodynamic psychotherapy in specific psychiatric disorders: A meta-analysis. *Archives of General Psychiatry*, **61** (12), 1208–1216.
6. Leichsenring, F., and Rabung, S. (2008) Effectiveness of long-term psychodynamic psychotherapy: A meta-analysis. *Journal of the American Medical Association*, **300** (13), 1551–1565.
7. Leichsenring, F. (2009) Applications of psychodynamic psychotherapy to specific disorders, in *Textbook of Psychotherapeutic Treatments* (ed G. Gabbard), American Psychiatric Publishing, Washington, DC, p. 97–132.
8. Leichsenring, F., Salzer, S., Beutel, M.E., *et al*. (2014) Long-term outcome of psychodynamic therapy and cognitive-behavioral therapy in social anxiety disorder. *American Journal of Psychiatry*, **171** (10), 1074–1082.
9. Leichsenring, F., and Slein, S. (2014) Evidence for psychodynamic psychotherapy in specific mental disorders: A systematic review. *Psychoanalytic Psychotherapy*, **28** (1), 4–32.
10. Leichsenring, F., Leweke, F., Klein, S., and Steinert, C. (2015) The empirical status of psychodynamic psychotherapy, an update: Bambi's alive and kicking. *Psychotherapy and Psychosomatics*, **84**, 129–148.
11. Conte, H.R. (1994) Review of research in supportive psychotherapy: An update. *American Journal of Psychotherapy*, **48** (4), 494–504.
12. Milrod, B., Leon, A.C., Busch, F., *et al*. (2007) A randomized controlled clinical trial of psychoanalytic psychotherapy for panic disorder. *American Journal of Psychiatry*, **164** (2), 265–272.
13. Buckley, P. (2009) Applications of individual supportive psychotherapy to psychiatric disorders, in *Textbook of Psychotherapeutic Treatments* (ed G. O. Gabbard), American Psychiatric Publishing, Washington, DC, p. 447–463.
14. Winston, A., Rosenthal, R.N., and Pinsker, H. (2004) Assessment, case formulation, goal setting and outcome research, and applicability to special populations, in *Introduction to Supportive Psychotherapy* (eds A. Winston, R.N. Rosenthal, and H. Pinsker), American Psychiatric Publishing, Washington, DC, p. 115–132.
15. Gerber, A.J., Kocsis, J.H., Milrod, B.L., *et al*. (2011) A quality-based review of randomized controlled trials of psychodynamic psychotherapy. *American Journal of Psychiatry*, **168** (1), 19–28.
16. Driessen, E., Van, H.L., Don, F.J., *et al*. (2013) The efficacy of cognitive-behavioral therapy and psychodynamic therapy in the outpatient treatment of major depression: A randomized clinical trial. *American Journal of Psychiatry*, **170** (9): 1014–1050.
17. Driessen, E., Van, H.L., Peen, J., *et al*. (2015) Therapist-rated outcomes in a randomized clinical trial comparing cognitive-behavioral therapy and psychodynamic therapy for major depression. *Journal of Affective Disorders*, **170**, 112–118.

18. Town, J.M., Abbass, A., and Hardy, G. (2011) Short term psychodynamic psychotherapy for personality disorder: A critical review of randomized controlled trials. *Journal of Personality Disorders*, **25** (6), 723–740.

19. Barber, J.P., Muran, J.C., McCarthy, K., *et al.* (2013) Research on psychodynamic therapies, in *Bergin and Garfield's Handbook of Psychotherapy and Behavior Change*, 6th ed. (ed M. J. Lambert), John Wiley & Sons, Inc., New York, p. 443–494.

20. Doering, S., Horz, S., Rentrop, M., *et al.* (2010) Transference-focused psychotherapy v. treatment by community psychotherapists for borderline personality disorder: Randomised controlled trial. *British Journal of Psychiatry*, **196**, 389–395.

21. Giesen-Bloo, J., van Dyck, R., Spinhoven, P., *et al.* (2006) Outpatient psychotherapy for borderline personality disorder: Randomized trial of schema-focused therapy vs. transference-focused psychotherapy. *Archives of General Psychiatry*, **63**, 649–658.

22. Kohut, H. (1972) Thoughts on narcissism and narcissistic rage. *Psychoanalytic Study of the Child*, **XXVI**, 360–399.

23. Morrison, A.P. (1983) Shame, ideal self, and narcissism. *Contemporary Psychoanalysis*, **19**, 295–318.

24. Ornstein, P.H. (1999) Conceptualization and treatment of rage in self psychology. *Journal of Clinical Psychology*, **55**, 283–293.

25. Busch, F.N., Rudden, M., and Shapiro, T. (2004) *Psychodynamic Treatment of Depression*, American Psychiatric Press, Washington, DC.

26. Milrod, B., Busch, F., Cooper, A., and Shapiro, T. (1997) *Manual of Panic-Focused Psychodynamic Psychotherapy*, American Psychiatric Press, Washington, DC.

PART THREE: Beginning the Treatment

Introduction

Key concepts

The important goals of the beginning phase of psychodynamic psychotherapy are

- discussing treatment recommendations and alternatives in order to obtain informed consent
- collaborative goal setting for the treatment
- setting the frame
- establishing boundaries
- developing a therapeutic alliance

These techniques include many of the **common factors** that affect outcome in all types of psychotherapy.

During this phase, and throughout the treatment, empathic listening and attention to the patient's feelings about the therapist and the therapist's feelings about the patient are essential tools.

The beginning of a psychodynamic psychotherapy may also involve pharmacotherapy. Understanding the way in which the two treatments work together is important at the beginning and throughout the treatment.

Psychodynamic Psychotherapy: A Clinical Manual, Second Edition. Deborah L. Cabaniss, Sabrina Cherry, Carolyn J. Douglas and Anna Schwartz.
© 2017 John Wiley & Sons, Ltd. Published 2017 by John Wiley & Sons, Ltd.

Setting things up clearly from the beginning

With most things in life, a good beginning is critical for the rest of the project. Think about . . .

- writing an outline for a paper
- gathering the best ingredients for a recipe
- planning an itinerary for a trip
- digging a foundation for a building

In all of these cases, a solid beginning and good planning are keys to success.

The same is true with beginning a psychodynamic psychotherapy. Establishing a framework, engaging the patient, and setting goals are crucial to the potential success of the treatment. These techniques are central not only for psychodynamic psychotherapy, but also for any type of psychotherapy you conduct. In addition, they are closely linked to many of the **common factors** that have been shown to have a major role in psychotherapeutic treatment outcomes.

In the next chapters, we'll discuss essential elements for beginning a psychodynamic psychotherapy. Chapter 7 outlines how to talk to patients about informed consent and collaborative goal setting; you'll learn how to set the frame and establish boundaries in Chapter 8; and Chapter 9 will teach you how to make a strong alliance. In this part of the book you'll also learn about topics like empathic listening, conducting a psychotherapy session, and combined treatment – all of which are essential for beginning the treatment.

7 Informed Consent and Collaborative Goal Setting

Key concepts

Before beginning a psychodynamic psychotherapy, the therapist and patient should

- discuss treatment recommendations and alternatives in order to obtain informed consent
- discuss and collaboratively establish realistic goals for the treatment

Once you have completed your assessment, you need to discuss your recommendation with the patient and set goals. Even though psychodynamic psychotherapy can be an open-ended treatment, you and your patient still need to have some agreement about what the treatment will be like and what you're aiming to achieve. These discussions should be conducted in an open, collaborative way that engages the patient in the treatment and demonstrates the need for the patient's active participation.

Informed consent in psychodynamic psychotherapy

Talking to patients about why you're recommending psychodynamic psychotherapy while also discussing potential alternatives enables them to give their **informed consent** for beginning the treatment. We often think about informed consent as something surgeons or anesthesiologists need to get before undertaking procedures, but psychotherapy is a procedure, and we should treat it as such. There are different opinions about what should be included in informed consent. Rutherford *et al.* outline a "minimum" informed consent and a more "comprehensive" informed consent [1]. The minimum informed consent includes:

- statement of the problem
- description of the recommended treatment
- likely course with and without treatment
- common and serious side effects
- cost
- supervision (if applicable, as for a case conducted by a trainee)

Psychodynamic Psychotherapy: A Clinical Manual, Second Edition. Deborah L. Cabaniss, Sabrina Cherry, Carolyn J. Douglas and Anna Schwartz.
© 2017 John Wiley & Sons, Ltd. Published 2017 by John Wiley & Sons, Ltd.

The more comprehensive informed consent also includes:

- more extensive discussion of differential diagnostic possibilities and treatment options
- the expected duration of the treatment
- confidentiality issues
- information about the clinician's qualifications

Learning to talk about these elements in a clear, non-jargon-filled way will not only help the patient understand the treatment, but will also help you clarify your thinking about the recommendation.

As an example, let's think about Mr A and how we'd discuss informed consent with him at the beginning of his treatment. First, some information from Mr A's evaluation:

> *Mr A is a 45-year-old man who presents with vague feelings of dissatisfaction with his career and relationships. Your assessment reveals that he does not have a major psychiatric disorder, but that he has low self-esteem and frequently makes self-defeating decisions. You also determine that his general functioning is good – he has many friends, manages emotion well, and has good impulse control. You decide that psychodynamic psychotherapy is the treatment of choice.*

Now, here's a conversation from Mr A's third session:

Therapist	*Now that we've talked about some of the things that have been troubling you, let's try to pull things together so that we can talk about what might help you most.*
Mr A	*So what do you think is wrong?*
Therapist	*Well, many of the things we've discussed point to the idea that you're having difficulty feeling good about yourself, despite the fact that things are going well. When that happens, it often means that feelings you're not even aware of are affecting your self-esteem. I have a feeling that that might be what's going on with you (**statement of problem**).*
Mr A	*Yeah, I know – it looks like things are going well but I still feel bad. But what can I do about that?*
Therapist	*This kind of problem is often very well treated with a psychotherapy that helps you to look into yourself to learn about things that might be affecting your self-esteem even though you're not aware of them (**description of the recommended treatment**).*
Mr A	*That sounds hard. Is that the only choice?*
Therapist	*Some people might also recommend other forms of psychotherapy, such as cognitive-behavioral therapy and interpersonal therapy, but my feeling is that your long-standing difficulty with this is best treated by trying to look at what's under the surface (**differential discussion of therapeutics**).*
Mr A	*How long will that take?*
Therapist	*This type of treatment typically takes a while – it's taken 45 years for these patterns to develop, so it makes sense that it will take months or possibly even a few years to help change them (**expected duration of treatment**). It's great that you're coming for this*

treatment now, because my sense is that this has been a problem for you in the past and will likely continue to be in the future (**likely course without treatment**).

Mr A   *That makes sense. I hate to think it will take a long time, but I understand what you're saying. One thing that's worrying me is the cost.*

Therapist   *We can offer this treatment to you at a sliding scale at our clinic* (**cost**). *I will be your therapist. I'm a third-year resident in psychiatry – that means that I'm a physician training to be a psychiatrist. I will only discuss this case with my supervisor, who is a senior psychiatrist here* (**confidentiality and supervision**).

Honesty, as usual, is the best policy. If you're a trainee, you have to let your patients know. Understandably, people may be wary about putting themselves in the hands of someone who seems inexperienced, but your willingness to discuss their concerns in an open and non-defensive way will generally be enough to allay their worries. As you can see from the example, there are ways to do this that make the patient feel comfortable and well cared for. Although some therapists have patients sign an informed consent form, documenting the process in your notes will usually suffice.

Giving patients a clear description of the recommended treatment means more than telling them how many sessions per week there will be (see Chapter 11 for more on session frequency). It means giving them a real sense of how we think psychodynamic psychotherapy works. Offering a cogent explanation or **rationale** for treatment is one of the **common factors** that predict a good outcome [2]. This is often difficult for trainees who have not yet seen a treatment through to the end or who may still be grappling with understanding how *they* think psychodynamic psychotherapy works. Trainees and practicing clinicians may benefit from using brief, psychoeducational materials, such as the Post-evaluation Psychodynamic Psychotherapy Educational Resource (the PEPPER – see Appendix 3) that they can give to patients and discuss with them. We suggest using this during the informed consent process to help patients better understand the treatment recommendation.

> **Common factor** – explaining treatment rationale

Collaborative goal setting

Once patients give their informed consent to begin treatment, the next step is to set goals. Collaborative goal setting is another common factor critical for the outcome. Studies indicate that patients are much more likely to return for a second appointment if their sources of distress have been heard, understood, and clarified *and* some consensus has been reached about reasonable goals for treatment [3].

> **Common factor** – collaborative goal setting

The ability to set goals is as important for the therapist as it is for the patient. Sometimes the goals are very clear. The depressed patient needs relief from symptoms and the suicidal patient needs to be kept safe. When a patient presents with depression, we know to say, "Mr B, it seems to me that you are having a major depression. What we need to do is to make you feel better. With medication, your sleep and appetite should be back to normal, and you should regain the energy and concentration to go back to work." But we can also set clear goals for problems such as interpersonal difficulties and self-esteem issues. In doing so, we can think about the following:

The urgency of the complaint: Does something have to be done right now? This is true when patients are in danger of hurting themselves or others. You can set layered goals, prioritizing urgent goals while also discussing goals that you will get to later.

The nature of the setting: You and your patient will have to set goals that make sense for the setting in which the treatment is occurring. For example, if you're a trainee who can only treat the patient for a year, you will have to set goals that are different from those that you'd set if the treatment were completely open-ended. The same is true if patients know that they are going to move away after some period of time.

What does the patient think is wrong? When setting goals, you have to work with what patients bring to the table. Even if you have an idea of what the goals should be, the best way to join with patients is to *listen* to what they want to work on *right now*. Start there. Help the patient set realistic goals for that treatment setting. This is not copping out or scratching the surface – it's helping patients and establishing a therapeutic alliance.

Let's look at a few examples to think about how to collaboratively set realistic goals for the beginning of psychodynamic psychotherapy:

> *Ms C is a 34-year-old single, heterosexual woman who presents with the chief complaint that she's been "feeling bad" about herself. She explains that she's upset that all her friends are already married and having children. She says that she keeps getting involved with men who initially seem interested in her but who "turn out" not to be interested in commitment. This pattern has made her confused and frustrated. She has no symptoms of a mood or anxiety disorder. She says that her parents divorced when she was 7 and that her father has now been married and divorced three times. When you ask whether she thinks that her parents' marital history could be related to some of her difficulties, she seems interested in this possibility and begins to talk about further memories.*

Ms C does not have an immediate, urgent problem. There isn't something to fix right now; rather, she wants help with long-term problems. You hypothesize that her difficulty is related to an unconscious process and she seems interested in this idea. She has the resources to engage in an open-ended treatment. She seems psychologically minded and motivated to learn about herself. You recommend psychodynamic psychotherapy, twice a week, with the goals of

- improving her sense of self and self-esteem
- improving her relationships with men

and you say:

> *Struggling with your feelings about being single has made you think about how your relationships with people from your childhood – for example, your mother and father – might be affecting your current life. That's the silver lining of this tough period – you've started thinking about things and it*

has motivated you to come here to talk about them. I think there may be thoughts and feelings of which you're not aware – that are unconscious – that are affecting the choices you've been making about relationships. My sense is that the best goal for us is to try to understand why you've been having relationships that haven't felt satisfying – and that the best way to do this would be in a psychodynamic psychotherapy. Learning about this will help the way you feel about yourself, too. Does that sound like what you're aiming at?

These goals are broad and open-ended. They will not be accomplished overnight. In order to achieve goals like this, your patient has to be able to tolerate delayed gratification. Note that the therapist offered the patient the chance to discuss her feelings about the goals and to add her input.

When patients have more problematic patterns of function, goals may have to be shorter term and more concrete. It also may be necessary for therapists to be very active in the discussion of goals with these patients. It's important to remember that goal setting may be very therapeutic for patients because it offers structure to the psychotherapy, instills hope, and can be personally organizing. Even if someone is having trouble defining goals, you can make this process collaborative by asking questions such as "What would you like to accomplish here?" and offering suggestions about possible specific and realistic objectives. Of course, always ask for feedback, for example, "Does that sound right to you?" While the *general* goals in a more supportive psychodynamic treatment are to reduce symptoms, change behavior, and improve functioning, the *specific* goals for any individual can vary widely depending on the particular patient's array of strengths, vulnerabilities, and needs. Here are two examples of goal setting in a treatment that uses a predominantly supporting stance:

Mr D is a 47-year-old man with bipolar disorder. He has just been readmitted to the inpatient service for depression that occurred after he decided to stop his medication. When you first meet him, he is anxious and depressed, and eager to get better quickly so that he can be discharged. After taking a history, you have this conversation with him:

Mr D	*I just want to feel better, doc. I'm jumping out of my skin. I feel terrible.*
Therapist	*I can only imagine how bad you feel – the first thing we have to do is to get you back on a good dose of medication so that you can feel better.*
Mr D	*That's my goal – I just want to get home as fast as possible so I can get back to work.*
Therapist	*We're definitely in agreement about that. But I wonder if it would also be helpful to figure out what led you to stop taking the medication to begin with?*
Mr D	*I don't know – I just get it into my head to stop and I do and then I get into this mess.*
Therapist	*So that sounds like something we should work on, too – figuring out what it is about taking medication that makes you want to stop, and thinking about what you might be able to do to keep yourself from stopping in the future.*

In this example, there are several short-term goals:

- symptom relief
- understanding why the patient wants to discontinue medication
- improving impulse control when he wants to discontinue medication

Let's also think about the goals for Ms E:

> *Ms E is a 40-year-old woman whose generally good function has temporarily regressed in the setting of depression following a bitter divorce.*

Here's a goal-setting conversation that she had with her therapist:

Ms E	*I feel like I used to be a normal person – now I'm just decked by this divorce. What's happened to me? Will I ever feel better?*
Therapist	*Of course you will – we're just going to have to work during this period to help you to remember all the things you're capable of doing.*
Ms E	*But you know, the thing that terrifies me most is that I picked him to begin with. After all this, will I just pick another jerk?*
Therapist	*That's a great thing for us to work on – it sounds like you're really ready to figure out why you've tended to choose men who aren't really available. Does that sound right?*

Here, there are two goals:

- helping to buoy self-esteem urgently
- working collaboratively to learn about her maladaptive choice of partners

All psychodynamic psychotherapies – whether predominantly uncovering or supporting, time-limited or open-ended – have goals that you can set and discuss with your patients. Remember that goals change as therapy goes on, so you will have to have new goal-setting conversations as the treatment progresses. Note that these goal-setting conversations are not formal – they are part of the natural dialogue of the therapy. Nevertheless, they can and should be explicit.

Once you've done that, the next step is **setting the frame**, which we'll turn to in the next chapter.

Suggested activities

Activity 1: Informed consent

Here is one therapist's effort to give informed consent to her patient. Can you name the elements that are included? What is left out?

> *Ms A, let me try to sum up what you've told me so far. It sounds like you've had real difficulties with work recently, which could be related to the fact that you're not really interested in your field. It also sounds like there are other things in your life that you continue despite the fact that you're not 100% interested in them, like your relationships with some of your friends. These problems suggest that psychodynamic psychotherapy might be helpful. This kind of treatment allows us to learn more about you – even about things that might be out of your awareness – so that you can make choices that feel more fulfilling. I'd suggest that we begin twice a week – we can talk about a schedule that's convenient for you. My fee is $150 per session. How does that sound?*

Comment

The therapist does a fine job of **stating the problem**. She begins to **describe the recommended treatment**, although she does not explain why she recommends the frequency of two times per week. She also gives information about the **cost**. She does not, however, include the **likely course with and without treatment**, **side effects**, **other therapeutic options**, **likely duration**, and **confidentiality issues**. These additions might sound like this:

I'm recommending that we meet more than once a week because really understanding what's below the surface takes some time, and if we meet once a week it's likely to just give us time to hear what's been happening that week. There are other types of psychotherapy available, and we could talk more about these, but my sense is that the kind of longstanding patterns you're describing are best dealt with in psychodynamic psychotherapy. Depending on our goals, this therapy can take a while – sometimes months to years – in order to really help you to understand yourself as fully as possible. What you've been describing to me is that this pattern of sticking with things that are unsatisfying goes on in every aspect of your life, so my guess is that until you understand its cause it will continue. A few other things that you should be aware of – we'll always meet here, we'll have a regular schedule, and of course the treatment is completely confidential. Let's spend some more time talking about these things to make sure that you understand them and to address any questions you might have.

Activity 2: Collaborative goal setting

For each of the following patients, write two goals and a few sentences about how you would present this to the patient.

Patient #1

A 54-year-old man presents for psychotherapy saying that he and his wife are fighting bitterly. As you talk to him, it becomes clear that he has major depression for which he is not receiving any treatment.

- What are the goals?
- How do you present them?

Patient #2

A 25-year-old woman presents saying she feels lonely and depressed after breaking up with her boyfriend. Over the course of the evaluation, you learn that she regularly blacks out after drinking with friends on weekends. She has a long history of difficult relationships, although she is a very successful student.

- What are the goals?
- How do you present them?

Patient #3

A 50-year-old man presents saying that ever since driving his son to college in another state he's been feeling old. He has aches and pains, but his doctor says that he is in perfect health. His father died young – at 56 – and he knows that this has something to do with the way he's feeling. He is happy with his wife, but has started to think about a woman who works with him. He's not sure if he needs therapy but just isn't feeling like himself. He has no symptoms of depression and denies substance abuse.

- What are the goals?
- How do you present them?

Comment

Patient #1

- **Goal #1**: decrease patient's symptoms of depression
- **Goal #2**: help patient understand what is causing difficulties in his relationship with his wife

Since the patient is in the middle of an acute depression, it's not clear whether the trouble that he's having with his wife is persistent or related to his mood disorder. Therefore, your first goal is to help him with his depressive symptoms, while beginning to engage him in a discussion of his relationship. You might say:

It seems clear that you and your wife are having some real difficulties in your marriage and that you've been pretty depressed recently. Sometimes, when you're that depressed, it's really challenging to even begin to deal with what's going on in a relationship, so I think that our first order of business is to help you feel better.

Patient #2

- **Goal #1**: decrease patient's binge drinking
- **Goal #2**: help patient to understand her pattern of unsatisfactory relationships with men

This patient has both short-term and long-term goals. The breakup with her boyfriend prompted her to come to psychotherapy – if she is able to self-reflect, she could use the treatment to begin to examine her unsatisfactory pattern of relationships. However, an important short-term goal is to help her to understand that her binge drinking on weekends is a form of alcoholism for which she needs help. You might say:

I think that taking a look at your relationships will be very helpful. The first step is to notice a pattern, which you've done – this will help us learn more about the kinds of choices you make when you begin relationships, and will help you understand why the relationships you've had have been less than satisfying. I'm also glad that you told me about blacking out on weekends – it sounds like that's been a real problem and that getting your drinking under control will help you in all aspects of your life. I'd suggest that we make that a goal as well.

Patient #3

- **Goal #1** – decrease patient's transient symptoms of somatization and obsessing about other women
- **Goal #2** – help patient to make the transition into a new phase of life

As with Patient #2, this patient has both short- and long-term goals. The short-term goals involve symptom relief, but you can see that his symptoms are related to deeper problems. You suspect that taking his son to college feels like a symbol of the beginning of old age and, given his father's early death, may even feel like the prelude to the end of life. Helping him make this transition and explore his fantasies about growing old will be very helpful. You might say:

> A child going to college is definitely a big milestone. You must be very proud of him. But I think that, whether you're aware of it or not, taking him to college means something else to you, too – something like, "well, now I'm old." I wonder if this is why you're suddenly so worried about your health and are looking around for diversions. Given this, I think that we've got a few goals – we need to help you feel better about your health and understand what's getting you preoccupied with your co-worker – but I suspect that these are connected with another goal, which is helping you figure out where you are in your life and making you more able to see how much of life you still have ahead of you.

Chapter 7: References

1. Rutherford, B.R., Aizaga, K., and Sneed, J. (2007) A survey of psychiatry residents' informed consent practices. *Journal of Clinical Psychiatry*, **68**, 558–565.
2. Frank, J.D. (1982) Therapeutic components shared by all psychotherapies. *Psychotherapy Research and Behavior Change: Master Lecture Series*, Vol. **1** (eds J. H. Harvey and M. M. Parks), American Psychological Association, Washington, DC, p. 9–37.
3. Bordin, E.S. (1994) Theory and research on the therapeutic alliance: New directions, in *The Working Alliance: Theory, Research and Practice* (eds A. O. Horvath and L. S. Greenberg), John Wiley & Sons, New York, p. 13–37.

8 Setting the Frame and Establishing Boundaries

Key concepts

Setting the frame is essential to any type of psychotherapy – it establishes boundaries and sets up a safe relationship in which patient and therapist can work.

Setting the frame must be done actively at the beginning of the treatment.

The frame of psychotherapy includes:

- role
- time
- setting
- money
- contact information
- what to do in the event of an emergency
- confidentiality
- issues relating to traineeship

A **boundary** is defined as the edge of appropriate behavior.

A boundary "crossing" is a benign deviation from the frame that may advance the treatment and does not harm the patient.

A boundary "violation" is a deviation from the frame that is clearly harmful or exploitative of the patient.

The best ways to avoid boundary violations are to:

- actively establish the frame with patients
- establish a usual way of conducting treatments that does not vary from patient to patient
- seek out supervision from a supervisor or peer whenever you have doubts about a boundary

---

Setting the frame

Setting the frame is essential to beginning a psychodynamic psychotherapy. It should be done thoughtfully and explicitly at the start of the treatment. This chapter will

---

Psychodynamic Psychotherapy: A Clinical Manual, Second Edition. Deborah L. Cabaniss, Sabrina Cherry, Carolyn J. Douglas and Anna Schwartz.
© 2017 John Wiley & Sons, Ltd. Published 2017 by John Wiley & Sons, Ltd.

outline the elements of the treatment frame and suggest methods for establishing it in different treatment situations.

Why do we need a frame?

Of all the elements of psychodynamic psychotherapy, the frame is among the most caricatured. The "50-minute hour," "our time's up" and the two chairs facing each other show up in everything from cartoons to movie spoofs. This may be because the therapeutic relationship *is* different from other relationships – and for good reason. We want to separate what goes on in therapy from what goes on outside. We know that psychotherapy is difficult – it reveals vulnerabilities, strong affects, and shame – and we know that in order to tolerate this, our patients need to be assured of the safety of the therapeutic setting. We set up certain things *before* the patient arrives, such as maintaining a clean, quiet office, free of distraction, with discrete places to sit. We set up other things *with* the patient – for example, the schedule and the boundaries. Our personal styles affect the way in which we set the frame. For example, some therapists always answer their cell phones while others use an answering service; some allow patients to contact them at home on weekends while others do not. But whatever we choose to do, we try to do it in a standard way for all patients and in a way that our patients know about. Try to imagine the anxiety a patient would have if she never knew whether her therapist was going to show up at the same time. *The therapist should never imagine that the patient knows the frame without being told* – even experienced patients might have had different frames with other therapists.

One way to think about the frame is that the elements of the frame are the "ground rules." If you're playing a game with one or more people, you need to use the same set of rules or you can't play together. Imagine four people on a tennis court, two of whom are using one set of lines and two of whom are using another set – that's a recipe for chaos and fighting. Or two kids playing a board game, one who says that the first roll of the dice is final and another who allows for "do-overs." Stay tuned for many tears!

The elements of the frame

There are many parts of the frame – some are concrete and some are more abstract, but they are all important. They are (adapted from Gutheil and Gabbard (1993) [1]):

- role
- time
- setting
- money
- contact information
- what to do in the event of an emergency
- confidentiality
- issues related to traineeship

Role

As Gutheil and Gabbard note, defining and communicating the **roles** of therapist and patient is an important part of the treatment frame [1]. A role is a part or function that we play in a particular situation. We play roles in every aspect of our lives. Sometimes we're daughters and sons, sometimes we're weekend guests, and sometimes we're patients. All of these situations go better when roles are defined and all participants accept the definitions. The same is true for psychotherapy. You might think that the roles played by therapist and patient in psychotherapy are obvious, but that's not necessarily true. First of all, different psychotherapists play different kinds of roles. Resident psychiatrists might have to draw blood from patients with whom they conduct psychotherapy sessions. Behavioral therapists might drive with patients to an airport to treat flying phobia. Cognitive therapists might give directions about homework. All of these therapists have slightly different roles.

The concept of role has many different parts. There's **function** – that is, what we do. You can think about the many functions that psychodynamic therapists have, some of which we've already discussed. Making assessments, listening, and trying to empathize and understand in a non-judgmental way are all functions related to the psychodynamic therapist's role. In some therapies, the therapist's role might also include other functions, such as prescribing medication, assessing medication side effects, and speaking to other healthcare professionals or school personnel. These overlap with the therapist's **responsibilities**. A responsibility is literally a duty – something that one person can count on another person doing. Some of the therapist's responsibilities are so obvious that they might seem ridiculous to mention, but they are among the most important. They include showing up when and where you say you will, giving adequate notice of vacations, staying awake during sessions, paying attention, remembering things patients tell you, and adhering to the frame of treatment without crossing boundaries. The fact that you will do these things means an enormous amount to patients – particularly those who never had people in their lives who took these kinds of responsibilities to heart.

Keep in mind that you have to do these things in an average, expectable way – circumstances may sometimes make you late, tired, or forgetful. That's fine and human – it happens to all therapists. The idea here is that if you take these responsibilities and functions seriously, when you deviate from them in benign ways you can use the experience to learn about yourself and your patient.

> *A therapist who has always been on time comes 5 minutes late to a session.*
>
> Patient #1   *I can't believe you're late! Now I'll only get 40 minutes instead of 45.*
>
> Therapist   *Why do you assume that?*
>
> Patient #1   *That's the way it is in this world – everybody's always trying to cheat you.*

Since the therapist has already set the frame and is generally on time, he can use this benign deviation to learn about this patient's rigidity and inability to sustain an image of the therapist as trustworthy.

Patient #2 doesn't mention the lateness until the therapist asks about it.

Therapist   *You didn't mention that I got to the session 5 minutes late.*

Patient #2   *Oh that – that's fine – you're always on time – and I'm sure that it's because you had an emergency on the inpatient unit.*

Here the therapist learns that the patient can hold on to good feelings about the therapist, but also suggests that this might be a person who tends to put his/her own needs last.

If the therapist's role includes listening, understanding, and being reliable, the patient's role includes attending sessions, arriving on time, paying, speaking, and participating in the psychotherapy. Part of the role of each member of the therapeutic dyad includes acknowledging what is and what is not appropriate behavior. For example, psychodynamic psychotherapy is a talking therapy, *thus physical contact is not part of the role for either party*. It is the role of the patient to say whatever comes to mind, but it is not the role of the therapist to say whatever comes to mind. Patients can tell therapists that they are angry with them, but, regardless of the degree of rage, they can't be cruel, make racially or ethnically derogatory remarks, or sexually harass therapists.

Communicating role

Part of setting the frame involves communicating roles and role expectations. Research indicates that this kind of **advance role preparation** (one of the common factors shared across psychotherapies) has positive effects on therapeutic alliance and treatment outcome [2]. Here is an example of how you might communicate roles in an early session of an uncovering treatment:

> *The basic idea here is to say whatever comes to mind, without holding back or editing, as much as possible. Things you might pay particular attention to are thoughts and feelings about the therapy, and dreams – but talk about whatever comes to mind. I'll listen and chime in with questions and comments. Since we're trying to get to material that's out of awareness, and to do that we rely on your ability to follow your train of thought, I might be quiet even when you're quiet in order to let you just get to the next thought.*

With patients who need more support, the *content* of what you say about roles might be somewhat different. For example, patients might need you to suggest a general structure for sessions and/or would feel more disorganized if you suggested they pay attention to their dreams, fantasies, or transference feelings – but it is still important to provide some explanation about roles. It might sound like this:

> *You should feel free to talk about whatever's on your mind – how you've been doing since our last meeting, any difficulties that may have cropped up with the medication, or problems you're having at home. I'll listen, ask questions, make comments, and try to keep us on track so we'll be sure to leave time for other issues you'd like to talk about.*

Sometimes, patients have questions about role that come up in the treatment. For example, patients frequently ask us personal questions. When this happens, we can explain our role with comments like this:

> *Patient*   *How come I have to tell you all of these things about myself and I never get to find out about you?*

> *Therapist*   *You're right – this kind of conversation is different from conversations you have with people outside this room, like with friends and co-workers. It may seem strange but there's a reason for that – this conversation is about you and about helping us to understand more about you. Is there something that we've been talking about that made you particularly interested to know about me just then?*

Acknowledging that the therapeutic roles are different from normal social roles helps patients become familiar with the therapeutic situation.

Common factor – role preparation

Time

Time is one of the most important aspects of the frame. When we set up a psychotherapeutic situation, we set aside a specific, consistent period of time during which our attention is focused exclusively on the patient. When you think about that, it's amazing – who else sits and listens to another person for 45 minutes straight? Nevertheless, patients may have underlying wishes for unconditional or unlimited caretaking by the therapist, which can make the formality of the "set time" or time limit seem restrictive. Your conviction (or your developing conviction) that time limits and predetermined, consistent schedules are protective of the patient will help you convey the importance of the "time" aspect of the frame. What if one day a therapist decided that the session was boring and cut it short? What if the therapist decided to take the day off and didn't tell the patient? What if the patient decided not to come and didn't tell the therapist? What message would be sent to the patient if the therapist decided to extend the session for another hour? Going back to the analogy of the game, time limits are part of the rules – not because therapists are arbitrary and withholding, but rather because we want to protect our patients. Aspects of the time frame that we need to convey include the times of the individual sessions, the schedule of sessions (when they will be held), and some idea of the duration of the therapy. For time-limited treatments, the therapist can convey the duration at the outset ("we'll be meeting for 24 sessions"); for more open-ended treatments this is harder, but not impossible ("psychodynamic psychotherapy usually lasts for more than a year"). See Chapter 11 for further discussion of the frequency and duration of sessions.

When setting a schedule, try to be flexible, but know your limitations. Only offering one or two possible hours per week might be too restrictive, but on the other hand, you should know what your "hours" are even if you're a trainee. You might say that you work 9 AM–7 PM or 8 AM–6 PM, but then you shouldn't offer anything after or before those hours. You set your schedule for reasons that relate to your own life, and if you deviate from that schedule to suit a particular patient, you will undoubtedly become resentful. You also know when you work best: if you're not a morning person, don't agree to a 7 AM session just because your patient is being demanding. Furthermore, you may have limitations that relate to other work responsibilities.

If you have questions about setting schedules, discuss this with a peer or a supervisor. Too often, trainees get "bullied" into meeting with patients at hours that are unreasonable – you can consider this to be a deviation from the frame if you know your limitations. Similarly, the schedule should be fairly reasonable for the patient. Demanding that the patient come to sessions during classes or work time is usually not viable. If your schedule and your patient's schedule really don't seem to have any points of intersection, you may need to make a referral to another therapist.

Beginning on time and ending on time are also part of the frame that you should discuss with your patient. When you say "We'll begin at 11 AM and end at 11:45 AM," you mean it – when the patient comes at 11:15 AM because the train was late, you should still end at 11:45 AM. This conveys the importance of the frame. If patients protest, you can say that you're sorry about the train but that's the time you have for the session. Again, you'll learn about your patients this way. Higher-functioning patients will understand even if they're disappointed; more demanding patients will think that you should adjust your schedule around their lives. This does not mean that you need to be rigid, though – patients who are weeping copiously at the end of a session should get a few extra minutes to compose themselves. On the other hand, you can help to choreograph the session so that patients are ready to go by the end of the allotted time.

Setting

Where the therapy occurs is another critical part of the frame. You don't meet in the park, in a coffee shop, or at a bar – you meet in a place that's particularly designed for psychotherapy. This might be a clinic room or a private practice office, but it's your psychotherapy "space." That conveys that the therapy is a professional arrangement, not a social interaction. Again, this is vital for the protection and safety of the psychotherapy, the patient, and the therapist. Even on the most beautiful day of the year, it is not appropriate to say: "Why don't we have our session out on the front patio?" The patient can expect the setting to be reasonably comfortable and private. Most therapists who have their own offices like to decorate them in a way that feels comfortable, with furniture, lighting, and pictures that reflect their own taste, but a "comfortable" setting generally means that the patient is not bombarded with personal information about the therapist. Thus, pictures of friends and family and overly personal memorabilia are generally overstimulating. For example, while it's appropriate and essential to hang up one's professional license, and it would be fine to display professional certificates or even commendations, displaying one's bowling trophies or scuba certification would not be appropriate.

Money

Ah, money. Psychodynamic lore has it that many people find it more comfortable to talk about sex than to talk about money! People are often ashamed about how little or how much money they have, would like their therapist to treat them for free, and guard their money carefully – these are but a few of the reasons that make it difficult for patients to talk about the fee. Nevertheless, it is another essential element of the frame [3–6]. Once again, a reality of the psychotherapeutic situation is that it is usually a fee-for-service professional arrangement. At some time in your career you will probably have a patient say to you: "If you really cared about me, I wouldn't have to pay for this" – but the fact is, nothing could be further from the truth. It is because we care about our patients and about treating them in the most professional way possible that we insist on payment. Plus, it pays our bills – being a psychotherapist is a profession.

Some fees are set and some need to be set with patients. When there is a sliding scale, the therapist should find out how much money patients make and how much they can budget for psychotherapy per week. Yes, this means asking patients how much money they make and whether they have other income streams (trust funds, parents who can help pay for treatment, insurance, etc.). Some patients have no idea – this is a good time to encourage them to find out and to make a budget so that they can negotiate the fee. When we discuss this in an open and straightforward way, it is actually very helpful for our patients. Sometimes, the discussion of the fee ends with the fact that patients cannot afford to be seen by that therapist – in this situation, the therapist can help them find an affordable therapeutic situation. This is a good outcome. As with the schedule, psychotherapists usually do best when they are somewhat flexible while knowing their limits. And, as with the schedule, therapists who deviate from those limits will find themselves quite angry with their patients in short order.

Once the fee is set, the therapist should communicate to the patient about when and how payment should be made. Some therapists are paid by third-party payers, while others operate on a self-pay basis. This should be clear at the outset:

> I'll give you a bill on the first of the month and I'll ask you to give me a check by the middle of the month. The bill will have everything you need to submit to insurance.

Once the frame is communicated, you can deal with deviations in the therapy. Non-payment of bills should not be allowed – the situation should always be dealt with as soon as possible. It might mean any number of things – the patient might be angry with the therapist, have antisocial traits, or have gotten into an unaffordable psychotherapeutic situation – but each of these should be explored and dealt with to preserve the frame.

Contact information

There are three major reasons why patients might need to contact the therapist outside of session time: emergencies, the need to cancel or reschedule a session, and to request medication refills (when the therapist is also prescribing medication). The therapist should tell the patient this very straightforwardly:

> *Although the therapy will take place here during our scheduled session times, in the event of an emergency, or if you need to let me know that you have to cancel or change a session time, you can reach me in the following way . . .*

This conveys both how to reach you and the appropriate reasons for trying to reach you. Thus, the patient should not call just to "touch base" with you unless that is specifically part of the frame. More fragile patients may call frequently between sessions, particularly early in treatment. This may be because their capacity for self-soothing is so limited that any emotional upset feels like a four-alarm fire, or because their ability to maintain a sense of connection with you between sessions is tenuous. Under certain circumstances, it may be appropriate to provide additional support by making yourself more available between sessions or offering the patient extra time. At the same time, your ultimate goal is to help people develop the capacity to contain their feelings and hold on until they can talk it over with you in person. These are not easy decisions for the therapist, so when in doubt, don't hesitate to seek advice from a peer or supervisor.

This is the age of email, texting, and cell phones, all of which require thoughtfulness if used for therapist/patient contact. Email has confidentiality limitations, and texting and cell-phone calls suggest the kind of constant contact generally reserved for friends and family. People also make the erroneous assumption that their therapist reads their emails and texts as soon as they send them, potentially setting up problems when there's an emergency. Once again, the professional frame calls for limits. If you decide to use email or texting with patients, we recommend being clear that this method of communication is only for scheduling. Otherwise, it's too easy to use digital technology to write about thoughts and feelings that should be communicated face to face. In addition, when using digital communication, make sure that you adhere to the mandates established by privacy regulations and employ additional safeguards and precautions to ensure confidentiality.

In terms of phone contact, you should have a phone number for your practice that is separate from your personal phone number, and you should record an outgoing voice mailbox message that says who you are and what to do in the event of an emergency. Here is an example:

> *You have reached the voice mailbox of Dr John Doe. Please leave your name, the date and time of this call, and your telephone number – even if you think I have it – and I will get back to you as soon as possible. If this is an emergency, please hang up and call 911 or proceed to your nearest emergency room and have the doctors there contact me.*

Individual psychotherapists who know the scope of their practice may ultimately feel that they do not have to include the last sentence of this message; however, it is generally useful for trainees working in an institutional setting. You can discuss this issue with your peers and supervisors.

What to do in an emergency

Discussing what to do in an emergency is an important part of setting the frame – particularly with patients who are at high risk for self-injurious behavior. You can only function as a therapist if you and your patients agree at the outset on what they should do when there's an emergency. The best plan is likely to be that patients either call 911 or, if they are able, take themselves to the nearest emergency room. They can call you from there. Do not try to handle emergencies yourself over the phone.

Confidentiality

Part of the frame is that you provide the patient with confidential treatment. This may be somewhat modified if you are in supervision (see next section), but those modifications are only for training purposes. If you need to speak to someone else about the patient (such as a family member, or another health professional), you need to obtain consent from the patient. You should tell your patient that confidentiality is part of the frame and you must hold to your end of the bargain. You will hear some very interesting things in your psychotherapy office – stories that would mesmerize many a dinner party guest – but resist the temptation! The saying is that there are six degrees of separation, but it sometimes feels as if there are two. Presume that the person you tell could be your patient's long-lost sister – it's definitely a frame violation. Your patients can talk about the treatment with whomever they wish, but you cannot. That said, you might need to talk about the case with your supervisor and occasionally with peers. Peer supervision can be a vital part of your professional life, particularly after training. As a peer supervisor, take your role seriously and professionally, and remember that proper names are usually not necessary. When writing up cases for publication, Gabbard's dictum of "disguise or consent" is the way to go [7]. The same goes for professional presentations.

Supervision and issues relating to traineeship

If you're a trainee, the patient should be aware of your trainee status. The fact that you will discuss their case with a supervisor is part of the frame. There's no reason to hide this. If you were a patient and your therapist was a trainee, you would probably be glad there was a supervisor. That does mean, however, that the case will be regularly discussed with another person. As a trainee, you also may be asked to videotape the treatment. This becomes another part of the frame, which you should discuss and for which you should obtain consent.

Trainees often worry that these frame issues will upset the patient; however, most patients are relieved to discuss them up front and are more upset when they are surprised by them midstream. Here is an example of how to discuss these issues with a patient:

> As you know, all treatment in our resident clinic is free. All the therapists in the clinic are psychology interns – that is, we have finished graduate school and are becoming clinical psychologists. As part of our training, we discuss our work treating patients with senior supervisors. You and I will meet with

a supervisor some time in the coming weeks. This is a helpful consultation for the treatment that also helps me to learn about interviewing and psychotherapy.

As discussed in the chapter on informed consent, do not be afraid of your trainee status. It's what you are and you should let the patient know. Your transparency about this will help build the therapeutic relationship.

Here is an example of a frame-setting conversation:

Therapist	So now that we know we'll be working together, let's talk about how and when we're going to meet. As we discussed, it seems to me that meeting twice a week makes sense for the goals we've outlined, and I've got time available either on Wednesday morning at 9 or 10 or on Thursday afternoon at 2 or 3.
Patient	The earlier times would work well for me.
Therapist	Great – our sessions will be 45 minutes and they'll be here in this office. If you need to talk to me between sessions, you can always call my office line – I generally don't pick up when I'm seeing patients, but I'll get back to you as soon as I can. On weekends, I usually check my messages in the morning and in the afternoon. The clinic fee is $90 per session, and once we set up a schedule, we will charge you for sessions even if you miss them.
Patient	Why is that?
Therapist	Well, I'm going to keep this time open for you so that you always know you can be here for a session. It's like you're renting it. If you choose not to come to a session, that's your choice – it's not for me to say that your reason for not coming is or is not a good one. If you know in advance that you're going to miss a session, I will try to fill your time – and if I do, you won't be charged.
Patient	OK, I get it. Do I pay you each time?
Therapist	Yes – you can pay the clinic receptionist before you come in each week.
Patient	Are you going to talk in the sessions? My friend goes to a therapist who never talks.
Therapist	Of course – we'll both talk. But this time is really yours, to talk about whatever feels important to you. I'll listen, I'll ask questions, and I'll talk in order to help you to talk more and to try to understand what you're thinking and feeling.

Note that the therapist who is taking a predominantly uncovering stance may want to add something like:

Since our goal is to get to thoughts and feelings that are out of your awareness, the best way we know how to do this is to say whatever comes to mind. You should try to do that to the best of your ability – paying special attention to your feelings, dreams, and things that relate to the treatment.

In such a conversation, the therapist addresses many aspects of the frame: time, meeting place, and money.

Changing the frame

Neither life nor therapy is static, and thus we sometimes have to change the frame. This could be on a one-time basis, for example when we have to see patients before their next scheduled session because of a decompensation or crisis (such as worsening depression or mania, suicidal ideation, or a traumatic situation), or when we have to change the schedule for some length of time (such as increasing the number of sessions per week for a few months during a crisis period). When this happens, let the patient know how and why you are suggesting a frame change. For example:

> *It's been working well to meet once a week, but given how depressed you've been I think that it makes sense for us to meet twice a week for the next few weeks. We'll particularly work on ways to get you back on your feet and back to work. Let's check back in about this in about a month to see when it makes sense to go back to our regular schedule.*

If you find yourself changing the frame frequently with a particular patient, it might mean that you have the wrong frame. For example, a patient you see once a week who has difficulty containing affect and who frequently requests extra sessions may be signaling to you that it would make more sense to meet twice a week.

How do you know when to change rather than hold to the frame? Use your judgment about whether it is an emergency, and, if you are unsure, consult a supervisor or trusted peer. If you offer an extra session and find that the situation wasn't an emergency, discuss this with the patient. Remember that the frame is there to help you and your patient create a treatment situation that works for both of you, not to be a rigid firewall when the patient needs something else.

Patients often have questions about the elements of the frame, so it makes sense to think ahead of time about how you will address them. If you understand the rationale behind the frame, you'll have an easier time explaining it to others.

Boundaries, boundary crossings, and boundary violations

As you can see, all treatments have frames, and all good treatments start out with a careful frame-setting conversation. Once the frame is set, deviations from it are clear. A **boundary** is defined as the edge of appropriate behavior [8]; thus deviations from the frame cross boundaries. Some boundary crossings are benign, while others are not. A **benign boundary crossing** is defined by Gutheil and Gabbard as a boundary transgression, "where the ultimate effect of the deviation from the usual verbal behavior may be to advance the therapy in a constructive way that does not harm the patient" [8]. They cite examples such as touching patients in order to help them up after a fall on the way out of the office, or hugging the patient who reaches out for an embrace after getting news of the death of a child. A study of the behavior of psychoanalysts following the events of September 11, 2001 found that the majority of analysts surveyed engaged in some type of benign boundary crossing such as self-disclosure and advice giving to help patients deal with the traumatic nature of the event [9].

Sometimes we consciously engage in benign boundary crossings (keeping patients a few extra minutes while they compose themselves, rescheduling in a way that's a little inconvenient for us because the patient is in some distress) and sometimes we realize this later (for example, in supervision) – either way, it's good to discuss this with the patient. For example, after realizing that you forgot to tell a patient you were going on vacation until two days before you left, you might say, "You're right, I usually tell you with more notice. That was my mistake. What thoughts did you have about that?" You can acknowledge the error, but also allow the patient to express feelings about it.

On the other hand, Gutheil and Gabbard define a **boundary violation** as a transgression "that is clearly harmful to or exploitative of the patient" [8]. Examples of this are socializing with patients, physical contact (other than handshakes) with patients, taking gifts from patients (except small tokens at the holidays or at the end of treatment; see next section) or giving gifts to them, and meeting with patients at odd hours (9:00 PM on Saturday, for example) or in inappropriate settings (coffee shops, restaurants, etc.). Most investigators in this area agree that there is a "slippery slope" between frequent boundary crossings and boundary violations. Thus, while boundary crossings are generally benign, human, and can even be therapeutic, finding that you are making frequent boundary crossings with particular patients warrants reflection – on your own and with a supervisor.

Gifts

Considering the frame and boundaries is a good point to think about gifts. As therapists, we presume that our patients will not give us gifts. Timely payment of the fee is all we expect as compensation for our time and effort. We also try to have patients verbally communicate their feelings to us rather than demonstrating these through gift giving. Every now and then, though, someone will bring a gift. This usually comes up around the winter holidays or at the end of treatment. When patients bring gifts, always open them during the session. This will allow you to do the following:

- Ascertain whether it's an appropriate gift. Inappropriate gifts are things that are very expensive, overtly sexual, or too personal (like a memento that you know was given to the patient by his mother). If you think a gift is inappropriate, sensitively say that while you are touched by the feeling behind the gift, it's not something you can accept. Then explore the patient's feelings about this.
- Talk about appropriate gifts: "Oh, it's that novel you've been talking about so much this year. Thank you. What were your thoughts about getting this for me?"

Like anything else that happens in psychodynamic psychotherapy, understanding the meaning behind gifts helps you learn about patients and their feelings about you and the treatment.

Your initial frame is absolutely essential – for the health of the treatment, and for the safety of therapist and patient. If you begin "setting the frame" as a trainee, this will become a natural part of your practice for the rest of your career.

Suggested activity

Boundary crossing, violation or neither?

1. *A therapist who has expertise in an academic area with which a patient is struggling offers to give the patient 15 minutes extra per session for tutoring.*

2. *A therapist says to his patient, "I think that it might help to bring your husband in next time so that he can learn more about your difficulties with alcohol."*

3. *A therapist says to her patient, "We've got a job in my lab that I think would be perfect for you. Let me give you the name of the human resources person."*

4. *A therapist says to his patient, "I can definitely remember feeling that way when I was about to graduate from high school. It's certainly a scary time."*

5. *A therapist receives a gift of a book from a patient at their last session. He opens it, comments on it, and says thank you.*

6. *A therapist sees that a storm has begun during a session with a patient. At the end of the session, he lends the patient an umbrella.*

7. *A therapist allows a patient to pay the fee two weeks late because the patient has to pay his taxes.*

Comment

1. **Boundary violation**: tutoring is clearly outside of the therapeutic frame. The clue is the "extra" 15 minutes, which is obviously a frame violation.

2. **Neither**: including family members in sessions can be an important part of the therapeutic work and can be essential for psychoeducation.

3. **Boundary violation**: offering to employ the patient may seem friendly, but is a clear boundary violation.

4. **Neither**: although the therapist is disclosing something about herself, it is generic and designed to help the patient learn about an important moment in his life.

5. **Neither**: patients often give small tokens of their gratitude at the end of the treatment.

6. **Boundary crossing**: while it is technically not within the frame to lend something to a patient, helping the patient to stay dry will not threaten the treatment. If lending continues, however, it could lead to boundary violations.

7. **Boundary crossing**: as a one-time allowance, this would be a boundary crossing. Again, if it persisted, it could threaten the treatment.

Chapter 8: References

1. Gutheil, T.G., and Gabbard, G.O. (1993) The concept of boundaries in clinical practice: Theoretical and risk-management dimensions. *American Journal of Psychiatry*, **150** (2), 188–196.
2. DeFife, J.A., and Hilsenroth, M.J. (2011) Starting off on the right foot: Common factor elements in early psychotherapy process. *Journal of Psychotherapy Integration*, **21** (2): 172–191.
3. Schlesinger, H.J. (2003) *The Texture of Treatment: On the Matter of Psychoanalytic Technique*, Analytic Press, Hillsdale, NJ, p. 195–197.
4. MacKinnon, R.A., Michels, R., and Buckley, P.J. (2006) General principles of the interview, in *The Psychiatric Interview in Clinical Practice*, 2nd ed., American Psychiatric Publishing, Washington, DC, p. 62–63.
5. Gabbard, G.O. (2009) Professional boundaries in psychotherapy, in *Textbook of Psychotherapeutic Techniques*, American Psychiatric Publishing, Washington, DC, p. 818.

6. Bender, S., and Messner, E. (2004) Setting the fee and billing, in *Becoming a Therapist*, Guilford Press, New York, p. 109–133.
7. Gabbard, G.O. (2000) Disguise or consent: Problems and recommendations concerning the publication and presentation of clinical material. *International Journal of Psychoanalysis*, **81** (Pt. G) 1071–1086.
8. Gutheil, T.G., and Gabbard, G.O. (1998) Misuses and misunderstandings of boundary theory in clinical and regulatory settings. *American Journal of Psychiatry*, **155**, 409–414.
9. Cabaniss, D.L., Forand, N., Roose, S.P. (2004) Conducting analysis after September 11: Implications for psychoanalytic technique. *Journal of the American Psychoanalytic Association*, **52** (3), 717–734.

9 Developing a Therapeutic Alliance

Key concepts

The therapeutic alliance is the basic trust between patient and therapist that allows them to work together effectively.

It is sometimes called the **working alliance**.

Studies suggest that the state of the therapeutic alliance is one of the best predictors of outcome in psychotherapy.

Therapists actively foster the therapeutic alliance by demonstrating

- interest
- empathy
- understanding
- hopeful, positive expectations about treatment

Therapists have to be particularly active in fostering the alliance when trust is a problem.

What is the therapeutic alliance?

Have you ever tried to change the way you do something? It could be anything – the way you hold your tennis racket, blow into a flute, meditate, you name it. If so, think about that experience. No matter how motivated you were to change, and no matter how much you knew that it would help your serve, musicality, or sense of inner peace, it's difficult and scary to change even the smallest thing. In order to change, you have to give up your old way of doing something before you try the new way. So for a while you're in free fall – you no longer have your old habit and you don't yet have a new one. Now, take the anxiety of trying to change that one thing and multiply it by about a million and you may be close to the terror involved in trying to change something as complex and entrenched as characteristic ways of adapting to stress and relating to other people. Who would do such a thing? Well, that's just what we ask our psycho-dynamic psychotherapy patients to do. Just as you had to trust your coaches and

---

Psychodynamic Psychotherapy: A Clinical Manual, Second Edition. Deborah L. Cabaniss, Sabrina Cherry, Carolyn J. Douglas and Anna Schwartz.
© 2017 John Wiley & Sons, Ltd. Published 2017 by John Wiley & Sons, Ltd.

teachers, your patients need to believe that you will help them through this potentially harrowing adventure. That basic trust is at the heart of what is called the **therapeutic alliance** [1,2].

Establishing a therapeutic alliance

Establishing the therapeutic alliance might be the most important part of beginning the treatment. Many studies suggest that the therapeutic alliance is the best predictor of outcome [3–13]. So what is the therapeutic alliance? Sometimes called the **working alliance**, the therapeutic alliance is the *trust between patient and therapist that allows them to work together effectively*. Trust is the basic ingredient. The patient believes that the therapist is trustworthy and has the patient's best interest at heart – so even if the patient is temporarily angry with the therapist, the patient understands that they can continue to work together productively.

> **Common factor** – therapeutic alliance

This type of trust takes time to develop – in long-term psychodynamic psychotherapy it can take months – but you can begin to establish a therapeutic alliance during the first meeting. Here are some guidelines:

Demonstrate interest

Think about the last time you were seated next to someone you didn't know at a dinner party. Did she ask you questions about yourself or just talk about herself? People who are genuinely interested in you make you want to talk to them – and make you feel that they care about what you are saying. We demonstrate interest in many ways: by being attentive (not answering the phone, or checking email or texts), by asking relevant questions (not just "name, age, serial number" type questions), by demonstrating that we're listening (following up on things that were said a few minutes ago, remembering details), and by making eye contact. You'd be surprised how far remembering a detail goes in developing the alliance. For example, if a patient says, "I was going to go out with Alice last night. She's a woman I work with," and you've heard about Alice before, you might say, "Oh yes, the colleague from the conference in Atlanta." At the beginning of a treatment, this helps patients to know that you've been listening and that you're interested enough to commit brain cells to storing vital information about them.

Demonstrate empathy

Our patients are usually in some sort of pain. They're depressed, getting divorced, recently unemployed, worried – and we have to let them know we understand this.

Although we often show empathy in our facial expressions, it's also essential to actively reflect back our patients' feelings in words. Just nodding your head isn't enough to make someone feel understood. Here are some examples:

Patient #1

Patient   *And then, right in front of Brian, my mother told me that she was sick of the whole wedding thing and wasn't going to pay for any of it. I was mortified. I thought I was going to go through the floor.*

Therapist   *That sounds awful. What happened then?*

Patient #2

Patient   *When I walked into our room there they were – in our bed – Carol and her trainer. I couldn't believe it!*

Therapist   *Oh my goodness! What did you do?*

Patient #3

Patient   *It's getting so that whenever I see Dee at work, I feel a little sick to my stomach.*

Therapist   *That's been going on for a few weeks. Can you tell me more about the last time it happened?*

The type of empathic statement we choose should mirror the feeling the patient expresses. The man who walked in on his wife having sex surprised even the therapist, warranting a dramatic empathic statement. The patient's feeling about her colleague, on the other hand, called for a quieter but equally understanding remark. Being an empathic therapist is a lot like being an attuned mother – you listen to your patients and reflect their feelings back to them in a slightly modified way. Don't be afraid to show some feeling. The bottom line is that when patients tell you something that calls for a human response, say *something*. Remember that silence is also a communication – and early in the treatment, it can communicate lack of empathy and interest.

Demonstrate understanding

You may ask: "How can I demonstrate understanding when it's the beginning of the treatment? I thought that I was supposed to develop my formulation as I go?" This is true, but you have to be able to understand *something*, even from the get-go. You may not understand *why* someone has long-standing relationship problems or behaves in a self-defeating way, but you may understand *that* they do. Saying something that conveys understanding, even in your very first meeting with the patient, is one of the best ways to get someone to join with you in the therapeutic endeavor.

Here are some examples of "understanding comments" that are appropriate for a first (or early) session. In the first example, the therapist conveys understanding of the current state of affairs, not the etiology of the problem:

> *It sounds like this last break-up has made you feel that there's something going on in you that makes it hard to have a long-term relationship.*

In the next example, the therapist conveys understanding of the persistence of the problem:

> *It seems to me that having this recurrence of depression has made you feel that this is going to be a persistent problem, and that's been hard for you to wrap your mind around.*

Finally, the next therapist demonstrates understanding of the impact the patient's defensive rigidity is having on a relationship:

> *For one reason or another, you've found it difficult to respond to your mother in any way other than withdrawing – and that's really straining your relationship with her.*

Offering a plausible, albeit preliminary, explanation for our patients' symptoms can provide an immediate sense of relief and optimism that we "get" them and can help. Note that these comments share many elements – they are stated as hypotheses, rather than as definitive statements, and they convey understanding of the current state of events, rather than of the etiology of the problem. Learning to formulate comments like this is key to "seeding" the therapeutic alliance.

Demonstrate hopeful, positive expectations about treatment

Think for a moment about how patients feel when they first call us. They are often in emotional pain, and may feel hopeless about the future. Our relationships with them begin with that first phone call, and our responsiveness, even our tone of voice, can affect whether they make it to the first appointment and remain in treatment. Although about 15% of patients feel more hopeful simply after making contact with a therapist, most patients need us to

- actively express confidence that therapy will provide relief;
- provide assurance that we will work with them to make that happen [14].

Instilling positive expectations about treatment is another common factor, and patients who have more positive expectations at the start of psychotherapy have been found to experience a greater degree of therapeutic change [15].

Common factor – positive expectations about treatment

Here are two examples of the kinds of comments therapists can make, even in the first session, to instill hope and generate positive expectations about treatment:

> #1: *I'm so glad you decided to come in today. Even though I've just heard some of the story – and I know that there's more to tell – I'm sure that, working together, we'll be able to help you feel better soon.*

> #2: *You've done a great job describing to me what's been going on over the last few months. It can't have been easy to talk about. It shows me how motivated you are for treatment. I know that that's going to help us in our work together.*

Once you have completed an assessment and are recommending psychodynamic psychotherapy, you can be even more confident:

> *What you've been describing is that you're intensely worried about your performance at work but that you are really doing incredibly well there. So your perception is not in line with what you're able to do. Something is preventing you from seeing things as they are – and it's probably something that's out of your awareness. That's why this is exactly the right kind of treatment for you. It will take some work, but I'm confident we'll be able to finally help you to see yourself more realistically and enjoy life more.*

Trainees may have difficulty instilling positive expectations because they're not yet confident about their ability to effect change; in that case it's helpful to borrow some conviction from a supervisor in order to convey optimism from the start.

Other contributors to a strong alliance

The elements we've discussed are critical at the beginning of treatment, but continue to be important throughout your work with the patient. For example, marking progress with comments like "The way you spoke to your mother last night was new; you weren't able to do that when we started" will give patients positive expectations as they struggle to effect life changes (see Chapter 29 on working through). Collaborative goal setting (Chapter 7), providing psychoeducation about the process of therapy (Chapter 7), and facilitating expression of affect (Chapter 19) have also been demonstrated to contribute to the strength of the alliance [3,4,9,13,16,17].

When trust is a problem

How do we foster the alliance with a patient who has difficulty trusting? Patients who

- are paranoid
- have difficulty believing that others are interested in them
- have difficulty believing that others care about them
- find it deeply humiliating to admit that they need help
- expect to be judged harshly by others

often find it hard to believe the therapist is on their side. With these patients, we have to work more actively, both at the beginning and throughout the treatment, to build alliance and enhance the patient's sense of safety. Showing that we're interested in all of the patient's concerns, doubts, criticisms, and negative feelings about treatment; being non-defensive and non-judgmental; and creating a collaborative atmosphere can help [4,18–20]. For example, let's take the following remark made by a patient in an early psychodynamic psychotherapy session:

> When I was in the waiting area, I noticed that you were talking to that other doctor down the hall. I wondered what you were talking about.

If the patient generally trusts other people, you can show interest in her thoughts by asking:

> Can you tell me more about those thoughts?

On the other hand, if the person generally has trouble trusting others, you might need to pre-emptively address potential paranoia by saying:

> Perhaps you're mentioning that because you wonder whether I share what we talk about with anyone else. Remember that everything that we talk about here is completely confidential. If you ever have concerns about that, we can talk about it some more.

Here's another example: a man who has been in therapy for several months arrives 15 minutes late two weeks in a row, and falls silent early in the next session. The therapist asks the patient "What's on your mind?" and the patient responds with:

> This appointment time is really inconvenient for me. It's hard to leave work early and get here during rush hour.

If the patient generally trusts other people, you might wonder if he has other negative feelings that he is not articulating and say:

> I understand that it's an effort to get here for our appointments, but I also wonder if there's anything else about our work together that you're not feeling satisfied with.

However, if the patient has difficulty with trust, you might stay with the stated complaint and say:

> That sounds tough. Would you like to look at our schedules to see if we can find a time that would be more convenient?

Although the patient may well have other negative feelings, the therapist first demonstrates that she's taking the patient's complaint seriously and working collaboratively to address it.

How do you know if you have a good therapeutic alliance?

One indicator of a good alliance is the patient's ability to work actively and productively in treatment. Another very important sign is low anxiety on the part of the therapist. Conversely, substantial anxiety in the therapist may indicate a tenuous alliance.

For all patients, *actively fostering the alliance is essential for beginning therapy*. Remember that you are making an alliance with the healthy part of the patient – you need to find that part to make the connection.

Suggested activity

Read each vignette and write one or two lines about what you might say next in order to convey understanding and enhance the therapeutic alliance.

Patient # 1

> Ms A is a 62-year-old woman who presents to a clinic complaining that her daughter-in-law (B), with whom she lives, hates her and is making her life miserable. The patient's internist recommended the visit when Ms A presented with increased blood pressure after a particularly bad fight with B. In your evaluation, you find that the patient does not have a mood or anxiety disorder. You also find that the patient has few friends. "They're all out for themselves," she tells you. During the session, you feel that Ms A is simply externalizing her difficulties. Your only attempt to see if she sees any of this as problematic – "Do you think that you might have done anything that has upset your daughter-in-law?" – is shot down in short order. You realize that this woman's problem with her daughter-in-law is just the latest in a long line of interpersonal difficulties. The patient is not particularly happy to be at a psychiatrist's office and says, "So, what do you think you can help me with?" You say . . .

Comment

This is very early in the treatment; in fact, it's the first meeting. The surface material is that this woman is suffering – she feels victimized, angry, and misunderstood. Even if you think that underlying characterologic problems are at play, you want her to know that you understand what *she* thinks are her main problems. You say:

> You have really been suffering. I think the first thing we need to do is understand what exactly has been happening at home because it's troubling you so much it's affecting your physical health. I think that if we know more about that, we might be able to figure out ways to make the situation better.

Patient # 2

> Mr C, a 29-year-old man, presents with symptoms of major depression – hypersomnia, hyperphagia, lack of initiative, difficulty concentrating, and low self-esteem. His work functioning is negatively affected. He also complains that he is isolated and frustrated with his romantic life. You tell him that he has major depression and you recommend initiating medication therapy

with sertraline. After six weeks at 150 mg per day, his symptoms are significantly improved – he is eating and sleeping normally, concentrating better, and his work functioning is back on track. He's aware that his depression is better and is happy about that. Yet his interpersonal difficulties persist. He begins to date a woman, D, whom he has met online. He gets very excited about the relationship, then drops her when it is clear that she has some tastes that are not as "cultured" as his. Although always on time when he was depressed, he begins to arrive a bit late and sometimes asks if you have extra time after the sessions. He says, "I don't know if this is working – I'm still having the same problems with women!" You say . . .

Comment

This is a little later in the treatment, although it's at a point when the goals might be shifting. What is on the surface is that the patient is frustrated, and you want to convey your understanding of this. You say:

I think that you're really feeling frustrated that your problems with women didn't clear up as quickly as your problems with your mood. But this is exactly what happens in therapy. People come for therapy when they're in crisis, their symptoms go away pretty quickly, and then they're able to look more closely at other issues in their lives. So we're right on track. Let's talk more about what happened with D . . .

Patient # 3

Ms E, a 34-year-old woman, has been working with you for six months in twice-weekly psychodynamic psychotherapy. She sought therapy for interpersonal difficulties resulting from her intolerance of other people's incompetence. Though she recognizes this is problematic, she still becomes enraged when she is not properly supported at work. She thinks that you are very smart, and is pleased with the treatment. Through your work, she has realized that her standards for herself and others are often too high, and she is getting along better with her co-workers. One day, in a session, you misremember something about her history, confusing it with information about another patient. "I don't have an Aunt Ilene," she roars. "Are you paying attention? I'm surprised . . . I thought that you were different." You say . . .

Comment

This is well into the treatment. The patient has a good alliance with you. You want to convey understanding about her disappointment in you while helping her see that this is exactly what she experiences with others. You say:

You're very disappointed and angry that I misremembered something about you and it makes you feel as if I never pay attention.

Chapter 9: References

1. Bender, D.S. (2005) Therapeutic alliance, in *The American Psychiatric Publishing Textbook of Personality Disorders* (eds J.M. Oldham, A.E. Skodol, and D.S. Bender), American Psychiatric Publishing, Washington, DC, p. 405–420.

2. Ackerman, S., and Hilsenroth, M. (2003) A review of therapist characteristics and techniques positively impacting the therapeutic alliance. *Clinical Psychology Review*, **23**, 1–33.
3. Bordin, E.S. (1994) Theory and research on the therapeutic alliance: New directions, in *The Working Alliance: Theory, Research and Practice* (eds A. O. Horvath and L. S. Greenberg), John Wiley & Sons, New York, p. 13–37.
4. Safran, J.D., Muran, J.C., and Proskurov, B. (2009) Alliance, negotiation, and rupture resolution, in *Handbook of Evidence Based Psychodynamic Psychotherapy* (eds R.A. Levy and J. S. Ablon), Humana Press, New York, p. 201–225.
5. Horvath, A.O., and Symonds, B.D. (1991) Relation between working alliance and outcome in psychotherapy: A meta-analysis. *Journal of Counseling Psychology*, **38** (2), 139–149.
6. Martin, D., Garske, J., and Davis, M. (2000) Relation of the therapeutic alliance with other outcome and other variables: A meta-analytic review. *Journal of Consulting and Clinical Psychology*, **68**, 438–450.
7. Horvath, A.O., Del Re, A.C., Flukiger, C., and Symonds, D. (2011) Alliance in individual psychotherapy. *Psychotherapy*, **48**, 9–16.
8. Owen, J., and Hilsenroth, M.J. (2011) Interaction between alliance and technique in predicting patient outcome during psychodynamic psychotherapy. *Journal of Nervous and Mental Diseases*, **199** (6), 384–389.
9. Hilsenroth, M.J., and Cromer, T.D. (2007) Clinician interventions related to alliance during the initial interview and psychological assessment. *Psychotherapy: Theory, Research, Practice, Training*, **44** (2), 205–218.
10. Crits-Christoph, P.F., Gibbons, M.B.C., Hamilton, J., Ring-Kurtz, S., and Gallop, R. (2011) The dependability of alliance assessments: The alliance-outcome correlation is larger than you may think. *Journal of Consulting and Clinical Psychology*, **79**, 267–278.
11. Bond, M., Banon, E., and Grenier, M. (1998) Differential effects of interventions on the therapeutic alliance with patients with personality disorder. *Journal of Psychotherapy Practice and Research*, **7**, 301–318.
12. Cailhol, L., Rodgers, R., Burnand, Y., Brunet, A., Damsad, A., and Andreoli, A. (2009) Therapeutic alliance in short-term supportive and psychodynamic psychotherapies. *Psychiatry Research*, **170**, 229–233.
13. Barber, J.P., Muran, J.C., McCarthy, K.S., and Keefe, J.R. (2013) Research on dynamic therapies, in *Bergin and Garfield's Handbook of Psychotherapy and Behavior Change*, 6th ed. (Ed M. J. Lambert), John Wiley & Sons, New York, p. 443–494.
14. Cuijpers, P., Driessen, E., Hollon, S.D., van Oppen, P., Barth, J., and Andersson, G. (2012) The efficacy of non-directive supportive therapy for adult depression: A meta-analysis. *Clinical Psychology Review*, **32**, 280–291.
15. Howard, K.I., Kopta, S.M., Krause, M.S., and Orlinsky, E.E. (1986) The dose-effect relationship in psychotherapy. *American Psycholology*, **41**, 159–164.
16. Frank, J.D. (1982) Therapeutic components shared by all psychotherapies, in *Psychotherapy Research and Behavior Change: Master Lecture Series*, Vol. 1 (eds. J. H. Harvey and M. M. Parks), American Psychological Association, Washington, DC, p. 9–37.
17. DeFife, J.A., and Hilsenroth, M.J. (2011) Starting off on the right foot: Common factor elements in early psychotherapy process. *Journal of Psychotherapy Integration*, **21** (2): 172–191.
18. Winston, A., Rosenthal, R.N., and Pinsker, H. (2012) The therapeutic relationship, in *Introduction to Supportive Psychotherapy – Core Competencies in Psychotherapy*, American Psychiatric Publishing, Washington, DC, p. 107–122.
19. Markowitz, J.C., and Milrod, B.L. (2011) The importance of responding to negative affect in psychotherapies. *American Journal of Psychiatry*, **168** (2), 124–128.
20. Safran, J., and Kraus, J. (2014) Alliance ruptures, impasses and enactments: A relational perspective. *Psychotherapy*, **51** (3), 381–387.

10 Technical Neutrality

Key concepts

Technical neutrality is the therapist's ability to listen and respond to patients without imposing judgment.

Historically, the concept of technical neutrality referred to the therapist's ability to remain equidistant from the patient's id, ego, and super-ego.

Technical neutrality is not always the proper stance for a therapist. When patients

- have the potential to harm themselves or others
- are abusing substances
- are engaged in high-risk sexual behavior
- are denying a medical illness, or
- are violating the frame of the psychotherapy

the therapist needs to take a non-neutral stance.

Therapeutic abstinence is the therapist's ability to conduct the treatment without gratifying his/her own needs.

Neither technical neutrality nor therapeutic abstinence connotes the need to squelch one's own personality or effect a wooden stance as a therapist.

Psychotherapists hear it all. Fantasies of every flavor, tales of petty and not so petty crimes, lust, rage, envy – you name it. It's all part of a day's work. Some things are easy to listen to, some are titillating, some are seductive, some are revolting, and some are dull. Unless we hear something that makes us think that either the patient or someone else is in danger, we just listen, try to understand, and attempt to make appropriate and helpful interventions. That's our job. It's not our job to cast aspersions, punish, admonish, convert, or otherwise judge what our patients tell us. That stance, in which we listen impartially and use what we hear to understand rather than judge, is called **technical neutrality** [1,2].

Technical neutrality

No therapist, no matter how experienced, is ever perfectly neutral. Achieving neutrality, like trying to free associate, is an asymptotic task – we may strive for it, but we never quite get there. Over time, we learn which patients and what types of

---

Psychodynamic Psychotherapy: A Clinical Manual, Second Edition. Deborah L. Cabaniss, Sabrina Cherry, Carolyn J. Douglas and Anna Schwartz.
© 2017 John Wiley & Sons, Ltd. Published 2017 by John Wiley & Sons, Ltd.

material make it hard for us to be neutral. This often has to do with our own values, beliefs, background, and history. For example, a therapist whose family was involved in the Armenian genocide might find it hard to remain neutral when listening to an anti-Semitic patient, while a therapist who had lost a sibling might find it difficult to listen to a mother whose child had just died. Supervision and personal therapy can be very helpful in these situations.

It was Anna Freud (Sigmund's daughter) who first defined technical neutrality as the therapist's stance that is equidistant from the id, ego, and super-ego [3]. Although we may not think about the mind in this way any more, the idea that we should try not to "side" with one part of the patient still has great clinical wisdom. Consider the way three therapists approach Mr A:

> Mr A is a 60-year-old man who has been married for 30 years. His wife, while kind, has never been particularly sexual and Mr A has felt sexually dissatisfied for much of his life. His wife is now suffering from Alzheimer's disease and is being cared for by a live-in female nurse, B, who is about ten years younger than Mr A. Mr A and B have become quite close and have recently started a sexual relationship. While this has been exciting and gratifying for Mr A, he is wracked with anxiety and guilt and seeks out therapy.

> Therapist #1 thinks that Mr A has been unfairly sexually repressed during his adult life and feels happy for him that he has finally found a sexually satisfying partner. He tells Mr A not to feel guilty and to enjoy his new relationship.

> Therapist #2 thinks that Mr A is anxious because he knows that he is doing something wrong. He tells Mr A that he will continue to be anxious as long as he is having an adulterous relationship.

> Therapist #3 thinks that Mr A has a conflict – one part of him wants to gratify long-denied sexual needs, while another part wants to be faithful to his wife. He explains to Mr A that the anxiety he is experiencing is probably the manifestation of this conflict. He suggests that talking about this in therapy will help him to understand the choices he is making and will ultimately decrease his anxiety.

Of the three therapists, only Therapist #3 has a technically neutral stance. Therapist #1 sides with Mr A's sexual wishes, while Therapist #2 sides with his prohibitions. Therapist #3 parks himself squarely in the middle – he sees the conflict, outlines it for the patient, and does not take sides.

Taking sides

There are times, however, when a psychodynamic psychotherapist needs to take sides. Here are some examples of situations in which technical neutrality is not the right stance:

When patients have the potential to harm themselves or others

As mentioned before, when patients place themselves or someone else in danger, technical neutrality is trumped by the need to protect them or the other person. For example, if patients are hurting a child or partner, the therapist needs to

- tell them to stop, and
- help them to do so.

This could involve different kinds of interventions, such as referrals to social service agencies or hospitalization.

Substance abuse

If you hear from patients that they are abusing substances, it behooves you temporarily to abandon your technically neutral stance in order to try to get them into treatment. For example:

> *A 35 year-old lawyer comes to her psychodynamic psychotherapy session with a broken nose. You notice this and ask her what happened. She says that she's not sure. On exploration, she tells you that she blacked out during a party and thinks that she might have fallen on her face. She reveals that she frequently has 8–10 drinks on a weekend night and has blacked out several times before. You help her to understand that binge drinking is a form of alcoholism and you tell her that in order for the treatment to continue, she needs to go to Alcoholics Anonymous (AA).*

This non-neutral intervention could save her life.

High-risk sexual behavior

All patients need to be asked about safe sex practices. If patients reveal to you that they are not practicing safe sex, you need to tell them to do so. Subsequently, you can explore the meanings of their behavior, as well as their feelings about your taking a directive stance. Again, this is not technically neutral, but is potentially life saving.

Denial of illness

If patients avoid medical attention in a way that could jeopardize their health, you need to let them know the dangers in a non-technically neutral way:

> *A 34-year-old woman whose mother died of breast cancer and has never had a mammogram tells you that her breast self-examination revealed a small lump. She says she is sure it is a cyst because it was painful to touch. You try to explore her fear of breast cancer and of what mammography could reveal, but she still says she's sure it's a cyst. You then tell her that she has to go for a mammogram, and that you'd be happy to help her find a referral.*

You tried the exploratory route and failed – time to abandon technical neutrality temporarily.

Violations of the frame

If your patient tries to cross a boundary or to deviate from the frame, it's not the time to be technically neutral. For example, if a patient suggests meeting outside of the session or engaging in physical contact, you need to say, "No, that's not part of what we do in psychotherapy." That's not technically neutral, but it's necessary for maintaining the treatment. Similarly, when a patient doesn't pay, you need to explore the reasons for the non-payment – but if it continues you may need to set a payment deadline in order to preserve the frame of the treatment.

Therapeutic abstinence

In psychodynamic psychotherapy, the patient and the therapist have a one-way relationship. That means that the therapist is there to help the patient and not vice versa. There are many moments in psychotherapy when it would be very easy for the therapist to satisfy personal needs – but then it would no longer be psychotherapy [4–8]. Consider these examples:

> *A therapist in a small town is treating the dean of the local law school. The patient has been substantially helped by the psychotherapy and is very grateful. He hears through the town grapevine that the therapist's son is eager to go to law school. He tells the therapist that he would be happy to do whatever he can to help her son gain acceptance to his program. The therapist knows that her child is bright, but that his law school entrance examination scores were a bit below par. This help could be invaluable to his chances of acceptance. Nevertheless, she thanks the patient for his offer, says "no thank you," and explores this interaction with him. They uncover his discomfort with gratitude and his wish to "level the playing field."*

> *A recently widowed therapist is treating a young artist. The therapist's wife was a prominent scientist and her obituary was in the newspaper – thus, the patient is aware of her recent death. The patient is invited to many art openings and invites the therapist to one of them. The therapist, who has been painfully lonely, longs to join his young, vibrant patient, but knows that this is not part of the treatment. He thanks his patient, declines, and asks the patient to explore the offer. The conversation turns to the patient's feelings about his lonely grandfather.*

> *A third-year psychiatry resident is treating his second patient in psychodynamic psychotherapy. The only time that the two could find to meet was on Thursday at 7:00 PM, after the resident's shift in the Emergency Room (ER). The patient notices the bags under the resident's eyes and brings him a cup of coffee during one session. The resident is so tired that he accepts. The patient brings coffee to the next session as well. The resident realizes that this is gratifying his needs and tells the patient that although it is a nice thought, she does not have to bring him coffee. They explore the interaction, and learn about the patient's generally masochistic relationship with her mother.*

> *A research psychologist with a private practice is treating a very wealthy philanthropist. The researcher is in need of $500,000 in order to start a new and very important research center. The philanthropist gives that kind of money and more to worthy causes all the time. The patient has done well in psychotherapy and is very grateful. After the patient gives $1,000,000 to another research venture, the therapist becomes agitated and upset. In the next session, the therapist almost asks the patient for a donation – but stops herself.*

In each of these examples, the pull to violate therapeutic abstinence is intense, but in order to preserve the treatment the therapists must refrain from gratifying their own needs. One might think that in some cases no harm would be done – for example, in the case of the research psychologist – but the balance of the therapeutic relationship would be forever changed. In order for therapy to work, patients need to feel that they are the only one being helped by the psychotherapy.

That said, there are many complications. For example, if you are a trainee, your patients will know that treating them helps you learn. This is a reality of the situation. Patients pay their therapists, thus the therapy allows the therapist make a living. While gaining an educational benefit and receiving a fee do represent gratification of the therapist's needs, this type of gratification is *part of the frame* – patients choose to come to a clinic staffed by trainees, and psychotherapy is generally rendered on a fee-for-service basis. Apart from this, therapists are gratified by knowing that they are helping people, doing interesting work, and learning about new things from their patients, but these are average expectable gratifications of any mental health or medical professional. Clues that we are experiencing more than "average expectable" gratification include

- getting very excited about seeing a patient
- thinking a great deal about a patient outside of sessions or supervision
- choosing special clothes to wear on the day of a patient's session
- engaging in boundary crossings or violations (see Chapter 8)

Again, supervision and personal therapy are generally very helpful in these situations. Therapists sometimes become ashamed of having strong feelings about patients and try to suppress them – this is a sure way to have them lead to trouble. Rather, discussing such feelings in your own personal therapy and/or in supervision will help you to better understand the patient and yourself.

Neutrality, abstinence, and "woodenness"

"Are you going to talk in this therapy?" the first-time psychotherapy patient asks her therapist. Of course therapists talk, but the patient's question didn't come out of nowhere. Scores of movies, television shows, and cartoons portray therapists as bizarrely wooden creatures with stone faces and pursed lips who say next to nothing. Unfortunately, for many years Sigmund Freud's early ideas about neutrality were misunderstood to mean that therapists should be robotic. On the contrary, as a therapist you can smile, furrow your brow, ask questions, and – yes – even laugh, while remaining technically neutral. Consider this example:

> Patient   *I wasn't spying on you, but I saw you coming in today and I noticed that you had the most beat-up umbrella. I hate to say it, but it looked a little weird.*
>
> Therapist   *(laughs and points to her wet shoes) Yeah – and it didn't do me much good today! Did you have any other thoughts about the fact that I had such a crummy umbrella?*
>
> Patient   *Yeah, I thought, "Your kids must take the good ones in the morning too." So maybe my kids aren't as selfish as I think they are.*

No "emotional coldness" is required. In fact, natural moments like this one help patients to remember that their therapists are first and foremost human beings. Expect that it will take you some time to find your way to a technically neutral but natural stance as a psychodynamic psychotherapist.

Some patients with weaker function are especially vulnerable to feeling anxious, demeaned, or mistrustful if the therapist is too silent, wooden, or opaque – especially at the beginning of treatment and at the beginning of each session. Creating a holding environment for these patients may involve being more personal, active, responsive, and conversational than you might be with other patients. Particularly if your natural style is to be reflective and reserved, you may need to demonstrate your "presence" for these patients with a more animated demeanor, a warmer tone, or more facial expressiveness. Sometimes, it might even help to make a joke, share an opinion, offer anecdotes from your own experience, or reveal a little more about yourself in response to questions.

> *A very inhibited patient with whom you are using a predominantly supporting stance is terrified about giving an important presentation at work. She asks you if you have ever been nervous when speaking in public. She has come a long way from the beginning of treatment when she would barely look at her colleagues, and you want to support her freshly minted bravery. You say, "You bet – it's always hardest to speak in front of your closest colleagues."*

Note, however, that adopting a more supportive stance does not give you free rein to talk about yourself without carefully considering what's best for the patient. As always, use what you know about patients' particular needs, problems, and vulnerabilities to decide whether they would be best helped by having this information about you at this time. When in doubt about how open to be or whether to answer a specific question, you can always hold off until you get more information or seek supervision. Here are some graceful phrases that might help you deal with requests for personal information:

> *What brought that to mind just now?*

> *I could answer that, but what would it mean to you, one way or the other?*

> *What got you thinking about that?*

> *Can you tell me what's behind your question?*

Very often, thinking about what you might like to hear from a therapist if you were in the patient's seat can help you make technically neutral but *human* choices.

Suggested activity

To answer or not to answer?

What do you say when the patient says:

1. *I really like your haircut – can I get the name of your stylist?*
2. *Where did you get your PhD? Is that a good school? Did you do clinical work or just research?*
3. *Why do you have your office in this complex? The parking is terrible.*
4. *Why do you think that's what my dream means? That doesn't make sense to me.*
5. *Can you recommend a good book about how psychotherapy works?*

6. *Do you think that I might need medication?*

7. *Are you divorced? I'm not sure you could really understand me if you aren't.*

Comment

1. **Don't answer**: This kind of question is clearly outside of the frame of therapy. Therapists deserve their privacy and boundaries. This kind of question, though, is often helpful because it suggests that the patient might have feelings about the therapy and the therapist. You might say:

   Thank you. I know that your question was about the haircut itself, but I wonder if your asking might mean that you have some feelings about me or about the way I look?

   This kind of answer is implicitly psychoeducational, since it helps promote self-awareness and interest in feelings about the therapist.

2. **Answer**: This is a valid question and part of the informed consent process. It's reasonable for a patient to want to know where and how the therapist was trained.

3. **Answer**: Particularly if this is at the beginning of treatment, it's reasonable to say something about the location of your office. The fact that the patient has asked may indicate that the patient has feelings about the therapist or the therapy. A comment like "I'm sorry that you're having difficulty with parking – but I wonder if you're having other feelings about beginning the treatment that we should talk about" is likely to deepen your understanding of the patient's feelings.

4. **Answer**: Again, particularly at the beginning of the treatment, it's good to be transparent about the comments you're making – no harm in first explaining your idea and then asking why it doesn't seem to resonate.

5. **Answer**: There's no reason why a patient in psychotherapy shouldn't read about it, so by all means make a recommendation. But don't forget to explore whether this request is covering other concerns. You might say: "There are many books about psychotherapy, and I'd be happy to suggest one. It sounds to me like you have some questions about how this process works that we could talk about. Do you have any specific questions that could start us off?"

6. **Answer**: This is a direct question about the treatment. You should answer in a straightforward way, and then explore what brought up this question at this time.

7. **Don't answer**: As in #1, this information is private and does not have to be revealed by the therapist. Again, though, it indicates that the patient has a worry that the therapist should address:

   It sounds like you have some worries about whether I will be able to understand you and what you're going through. Let's talk more about that.

Chapter 10: References

1. Auchincloss, E.L., and Samberg, E. (1990) *Psychoanalytic Terms and Concepts*. Yale University Press, New Haven, p. 1.
2. Gabbard, G.O. (2004) *Long-Term Psychodynamic Psychotherapy: A Basic Text*, American Psychiatric Publishing, Washington, DC.

3. Freud, A. (1937) *The Ego and the Mechanisms of Defence*, Hogarth Press and the Institute of Psychoanalysis, London.
4. Bordin, E.S. (1994) Theory and research on the therapeutic alliance: New directions, in *The Working Alliance: Theory, Research and Practice* (eds A. O. Horvath and L. S. Greenberg), John Wiley & Sons, New York, p. 13–37.
5. Greenson, R.R. (1967) *The Technique and Practice of Psychoanalysis*, International Universities Press, New York.
6. Greenacre, P. (1954) The role of transference: Practical considerations in relation to psychoanalytic therapy. *Journal of the American Psychoanalytic Association*, **2**, 671–684.
7. Freud, S. (1915) Observations on transference-love (further recommendations on the technique of psycho-analysis III), in *The Standard Edition of the Complete Psychological Works of Sigmund Freud (1911–1913), The Case of Schreber, Papers on Technique and Other Works*, Vol. **XII**, Hogarth Press, London, p. 157–171.
8. Freud, S. (1912) Recommendations to physicians practicing psycho-analysis, in *The Standard Edition of the Complete Psychological Works of Sigmund Freud (1911–1913), The Case of Schreber, Papers on Technique and Other Works*, Vol. **XII**, Hogarth Press, London, p. 109–120.

11 Conducting a Psychotherapy Session

> ## Key concepts
>
> Every session has a beginning, a middle, and an end.
>   Each part of the session has particular goals and techniques.
>   The therapist's job is to gently guide the session to give it form and to develop themes.
>   The session begins when we first encounter the patient, which could be in the waiting area, and ends when the patient leaves the room. Comings and goings are part of the process.
>   We make decisions about length and frequency of sessions based on our assessment and formulation.

Sonatas have an exposition, a development, and a recapitulation. Exercise classes have stretching, the workout, and the cool-down. The same is true for a psychotherapy session. Like a sonata or a class, psychotherapy sessions have a form. Each part of the session is different, with distinct goals and techniques. Thinking about these can help us decide what we do and say in sessions.

Once you have conducted whole psychotherapies you will see that the topography of each session is a microcosm of the psychotherapy as a whole – there is a beginning, a time of deep work, and an ending.

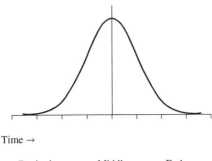

Time →

Beginning----------Middle----------End

Psychodynamic Psychotherapy: A Clinical Manual, Second Edition. Deborah L. Cabaniss, Sabrina Cherry, Carolyn J. Douglas and Anna Schwartz.
© 2017 John Wiley & Sons, Ltd. Published 2017 by John Wiley & Sons, Ltd.

The beginning – opening

People come into therapy sessions from the outside world. They have been dealing with their external lives – work, family, stressors – and when they come into our offices for psychotherapy, something changes. They are now in a place where they are going to think and talk about their internal lives. This is not necessarily an easy transition to make. We need to be respectful of this potential difficulty and help it to happen gently. We can think about it as a gradual opening. Whether the patient comes once, twice, or three times a week, there is the need for a transition at the beginning of the session. This transition doesn't just begin when the patient starts to talk – it starts the moment you open the door or even when the patient is sitting in the waiting area.

Introductions/greeting

Every session has a beginning. This usually involves some sort of greeting. In the very first session, you need to introduce yourself to the patient. For adult patients, it generally makes sense to use formal titles for your patient and for yourself. The relationship begins immediately, from the first interaction, and if you call your patient "Jane" and introduce yourself as "Dr Smith," you're setting up a power differential from the get-go. A handshake is often in order for this first meeting. A smile conveys interest and warmth. No need for extensive chitchat, although it is sometimes good to have something to say as you walk the patient to your office. Remember, this is the beginning of an important relationship, and you're forging the alliance from the very start:

> *Hi, you must be Mrs Jones. I'm Mr Anderson. (handshake) Why don't you come this way – we'll be meeting just down the hall. Did you have any trouble finding the clinic? (as you walk there)*

> *(approaching a busy waiting room) Excuse me, is anyone waiting to see Dr Brown? (patient stands up and approaches) Hi, you must be Mr Wilson, I'm Dr Brown. Nice to meet you. We'll be meeting here in Room B. Did you have to wait long?*

You are a person, as is the patient, so when you meet it's a human interaction. You can be welcoming without being overly familiar as you set up the psychotherapy situation. Note that Dr Brown respected Mr Wilson's privacy by not calling out his name in the clinic waiting room.

In subsequent sessions, you needn't greet the patient in the same way – you can forgo the handshake (although some continue this) and the initial introductions. However, the smile and welcome are always important.

The therapist's opening

Therapy is a little like chess: someone has to make the first move – and it should be you. The silent therapist who comes in, sits down, and says nothing is a caricature. Your job is subtly to shape the session, and this happens from the very beginning. Patients – particularly those who are very upset, disorganized, or pressured – may start the session, and if they do you can let them talk for a little while. However, after a minute or two, it's time to begin the choreography. An effective therapist will control the flow of the session without seeming to, gently nudging the patient like a parent who is guiding a child learning to walk. Openings should be just that – open – and should generally consist of open-ended questions. The beginning of the session is a time for patients to speak freely and your opening should encourage this. Let patients speak in their own way for a little while – perhaps 5 minutes or so. This will help you to hear the patient's speech pattern and thought process. It will also let you see where they begin and what they prioritize:

> *I heard from Dr Z that you were going to call, but he really didn't tell me much about the problem. Let's start from the beginning. What brings you here today?*

> *On the phone, you mentioned that you wanted to have a consultation for psychotherapy – maybe we could start with why you thought that would be a good idea now?*

Later in treatment you won't have to start with the history, but it's still good to say *something* to open the session. What you say will depend on who the patient is, the kind of therapy that you're doing, the current issues and problems, and your own style. If you're doing a predominantly uncovering psychotherapy that stresses free association, you might start with "What's been on your mind?" If you're mostly using supporting interventions, you might say "How has your week been?" or "Tell me how things have been going." Again, you're a person and your patient is a person and sitting down to talk to a person who says nothing is bizarre. You can experiment with using different openings with different patients.

The opening part of the session gives you information about how patients are feeling and what they are thinking about. From this you will begin to pick up themes that you can develop in the middle portion of the session.

The middle – deepening

The middle of the session is a time for deepening issues that emerged in the opening. During this part of the session, you will choose from among the things that you have heard in the opening about which you want to ask more. In terms of the session's topography, this is where the "peak" occurs, as it might in a short story. One important thing to remember is that *when* the "middle" happens might not be at the middle of the time period – it could be after 10 minutes or after 40 minutes. The "peak" does not have to be dramatic, it's just the part of the session in which the most work happens. This could mean many things, but it often occurs when patients connect to fresh affects or realize something new about themselves. Timing it in this way allows for closing during the end part of the session. You do not want patients to leave sessions in a raw state, and you want to give them time to respond to your comments. Thus, the middle of the session is the time to make comments designed to move the patient forward in the therapeutic work:

> *During the opening phase of the session, Mr A spoke about being very angry with his boss for passing him up for a promotion. He also said that he didn't feel like cooking, although this is something he generally finds enjoyable. The therapist wondered to himself whether these things were related, and in*

the middle portion of the session said, "I wonder if one of the reasons you didn't feel like cooking had to do with your feelings about what happened at work." This allowed Mr A to delve into his feelings about work and how they were affecting him.

Ms B began the session by saying that she was feeling anxious but didn't know why. The therapist noted to herself that Ms B had been about five minutes late to the session. During the middle of the session, the therapist asked Ms B, "I wonder if you have any thoughts about coming a little late today." After a brief pause, Ms B was able to begin to think about having been very upset after the last session. They then discussed whether this might have made Ms B ambivalent about coming to the session today.

In both of these examples, the therapist had thoughts early on about what to explore with the patient, but waited until the middle of the session to deepen the material.

The end – closing

Just as the beginning of the session is the transition to internal reflection, the end is the transition back to the outside world. We have to give patients enough time to "close" a bit before returning to their lives. Some of this involves timing – we don't want to introduce new topics or probing questions too near the end because patients will not have enough time for reflection or response. Even if we have things to say, we hold them for another time, rather than introducing them at the very end. Sometimes, we need to be explicit about the closing. For example, if a patient brings up an important topic near the end of the session we can say:

That's a very interesting and important topic, and we should bring that up again next week, when we have more time.

We can also help patients to close by making consolidating comments like:

We've really been able to explore many things about your relationship with your mother today.

This helps frame the session and signals that it's almost time to end. Although the session may just be another 45 minutes in your day, you have to remember that this may be a very important and cherished time in your patient's day or week. This makes the end of the session a time of strong feeling, whether it's communicated and conscious or not. Thus, the gentleness and respectfulness of the opening also hold true for the end. Abruptness is jarring and not necessary – there are many ways to say that it's time to end. For example, "OK – why don't we stop here for today" is much less abrupt than "Time's up" or "We have to stop."

Saying goodbye

Just as we greet patients when they come in, we have to say goodbye when they leave. "See you next week" or "See you next time" are perfectly fine things to say to your patients as they walk out the door. As with the opening, there's no need for extensive chitchat – your closing should be a respectful end for work done together.

Sessions – how long, how often, and how many?

Along with learning how to choreograph a session, we also have to make decisions about session frequency and duration [1,2].

How long should sessions be?

Freud originated the "50-minute hour" – he saw his patients for 50 minutes and then used the remaining 10 minutes for note taking and formulation. Many psychotherapists continue this schedule. The session has to be long enough to allow patients to open up and for themes to develop, but not so long that they become overwhelmed or unfocused. When using primarily uncovering techniques, most therapists feel that they need at least 45 minutes for this to happen. A 45-minute session is also often preferred for more supporting techniques, although patients with limited capacity for managing emotions and attention may do better with shorter sessions. If you decide to use shorter sessions with a patient, be consistent and set this up at the beginning as part of the frame.

Some therapists may decide to make the first assessment session longer, usually 1–1.5 hours, in order to have time to take a full history. If you decide to do this, make sure to explain to your patients that the length of the assessment session is different from the length of your weekly sessions so that they know what to expect.

How often should I meet with patients?

The frequency of sessions in psychodynamic psychotherapy depends on the goals and needs of the patient. Because psychodynamic psychotherapy requires self-reflection, meeting less than once a week makes continuity difficult. There are two indications, however, for even more frequent sessions:

To enhance in-depth uncovering work

When patients are able and motivated to do in-depth uncovering work, and you feel that the goals include major shifts in adaptive functioning, self-esteem management, or relationships with others, psychodynamic psychotherapy is often optimized by having sessions two or even three times per week. Increased frequency of sessions promotes free association, decreases resistance, and enhances discussion of the therapeutic relationship. It also increases the intensity of the work, and thus can boost anxiety and painful affects as well. Note that if you decide to increase the frequency of the sessions and patients worsen, this could mean that they cannot tolerate the heightened level of intensity. Nothing is written in stone – you can always go back to once a week and either remain there or decide to increase again when their functioning improves.

To add greater support during a crisis

Patients with weakened function may need multiple meetings per week to help them cope with the vagaries of everyday life. This could include a brief period of increased suicidal feelings, the weeks after a major loss, or any other crisis situation. Again, whenever you change the frame, discuss both the alteration and the return to the previous frame with the patient.

How long should the treatment be?

Sometimes psychodynamic psychotherapy lasts a few weeks and sometimes it lasts a few years. Discrete goals, such as relief of a single symptom, or sorting out a specific interpersonal situation, may be accomplished in a few weeks or months. The uncovering and supporting techniques described in this manual can be used in a short-term treatment if the goals are well defined. Long-term psychodynamic psychotherapy, which can last months or years, is indicated for the following goals:

- substantial change in domains of function – defined by major changes in characteristic ways of adapting, self-esteem management, and relationships with others
- ongoing need for support of function

As discussed in Chapter 8, the length and frequency are part of the frame and need to be discussed explicitly at the beginning of the treatment.

Suggested activities

Here are some exercises to practice openings and closings of sessions.

Activity 1: Greetings and openings

1. *Mr A is a 55-year-old man who has had paranoid schizophrenia for 30 years. He was admitted to an inpatient unit by the doctor on call last night. At rounds, the admission note is summarized and you learn that he will be your patient. After rounds, you start to read the chart when you notice that he's pacing around the nursing station. A nurse approaches you and says, "You need to meet with Mr A."*

What do you do next? What do you say?

Comment

> *Good morning, Mr A, I'm Dr Z. I'll be your doctor while you're here in the hospital. Do you feel up to speaking for a while now? If so, let's take a few minutes right here near the nurses' station and talk, and then we can talk some more a little bit later.*

No need to be rigid about your intakes – always gauge how appropriate it is to begin talking to the patient at that moment.

2. *Ms B is a 43-year-old woman who was recently hospitalized for a suicide attempt and who was referred to the Day Treatment Program after discharge. She is your Wednesday morning intake. It's time for the session. You go to the waiting area where several people are seated.*

What do you do next? What do you say?

Comment

> *Hi, I'm Mr Y – does anyone have an appointment with me this morning?*

You can protect your patient's privacy in a waiting area by using your own name rather than his or hers.

3. *Mr C is a 62-year-old man who has his first appointment at an outpatient clinic. The patient called to schedule an appointment and told the administrative assistant that it was "for help with depression." All you have is that note. When Mr C comes into your office, he looks older than his stated age and is using crutches.*

What do you do? What do you say?

Comment

> *Good morning, I'm Ms X, one of the therapists here in the clinic. Can I help you with those? Why don't you have a seat? I'm glad you were able to make it in today. I heard from the clinic staff that you wanted to make an appointment but I don't have any other information, so let's start from the beginning. What brings you to see me today?*

Your introduction is designed to help make the patient feel comfortable and able to begin to talk.

4. *Ms D is a 45-year-old woman who has made an appointment with you in your private office. On the phone she said she was having difficulties with her husband that she wanted to discuss. She comes at the appointed time.*

What do you do? What do you say?

Comment

> *Hi, I'm Ms W. Nice to meet you. We just spoke briefly on the phone, but why don't we start now with what's brought you to see me today?*

A friendly, open-ended, clear opening will help your patient begin. Perhaps the problem is with the husband or perhaps that's what she felt most comfortable saying over the phone – this opening gives her the greatest latitude to tell her story.

Activity 2: Closings

1. *You have spent 10 minutes talking to Mr A when you notice that he is starting to fidget in his chair. You have barely scratched the surface of the story of why he came into the hospital. At one point he starts to stand up.*

What do you do next? What do you say?

Comment

> *I'm glad that we had a chance to begin to talk. Why don't we finish up for now and we'll talk more in a little while?*

An agitated patient may not be able to sit through a full assessment session. Attending to the patient's comfort and ability to sustain the interview can be as important as making sure that you get all the information.

2. *You have spent 45 minutes with Ms B. She was extremely tearful and repeatedly said that she was having obsessive thoughts of driving her car into a wall. Although she says that she thinks that she won't do it, you are very nervous and not sure what to do, but time is almost up.*

What do you do next? What do you say?

Comment

Even though you were just discharged, it sounds like things are still pretty rough for you. The time for our session is up, but I think that we still have some things to think about in terms of how best to help you now. Why don't you come with me to speak to Dr Z, my supervisor, a bit more?

You never know what you will learn during an assessment session. Be prepared to extend the evaluation in case of emergency.

3. *You have spent 45 minutes with Mr C, who is recently widowed and is recovering from knee surgery. He has dutifully told you much of his history and says he is depressed and lonely. Despite this, he seems to be getting out, eating and sleeping well, and has recently enjoyed a trip to see his grandchildren. He has no suicidal ideation. You are not sure whether he has a major depression and needs medication. The session is almost over.*

What do you do next? What do you say?

Comment

It's clear to me from what you've told me that you've been depressed in the last few weeks. Before we decide on the best treatment, I think that it makes sense to meet again to see how you're feeling in a few days and to hear more about you. Can we try to find a time early next week?

The evaluation phase can last several sessions – as long as there's no emergency, you should not feel pressured to make a decision about the treatment after one session.

4. *You have spent 45 minutes with Ms D, who has told you that her marriage of 15 years is "on the rocks" and that she has been having an affair. The session is almost over and you know that you only have 10 minutes before your next session. There is no emergency, although Ms D has much more history to tell.*

What do you do next? What do you say?

Comment

You know, we're almost out of time today. I'm glad that we were able to begin talking about the difficulties you're having, but it's clear that you have much more to tell me. That's the way this usually works – it generally takes a few sessions to get the whole story. Let's figure out when we can meet again to continue talking.

Again, conveying understanding while also communicating that this is the beginning of a longer process is an important function of the closing.

Chapter 11: References

1. Gabbard, G.O. (2004) *Psychodynamic Psychiatry in Clinical Practice*, 4th ed., American Psychiatric Publishing, Washington, DC, p. 98–99.
2. Luborsky, L. (1984) *Principles of Psychoanalytic Psychotherapy: A Manual for Supportive-Expressive Treatment*, Basic Books, New York, p. 64–67.

12 Our Patients' Feelings about Us and Our Feelings about Our Patients

Key concepts

In psychodynamic psychotherapy we are interested in knowing about and understanding

- our patients' feelings about us, and
- our feelings about our patients

These feelings are ubiquitous and important to the treatment.

As we begin a psychodynamic psychotherapy, it is important to recognize both sets of feelings so that we can use them in our work with our patients.

The process of recognizing and managing the feelings we have about our patients is called self-reflection.

The heart of psychodynamic psychotherapy is the relationship between patient and therapist. Whether the technical mode is primarily uncovering or supporting, the relationship is key. It makes sense, then, that the feelings that patient and therapist have about each other are integral to the treatment, and that starting to recognize them is an essential part of beginning a psychodynamic psychotherapy.

Our patients' feelings about us

The fact that patients may have strong and complex feelings toward their therapists is not unique to the psychotherapeutic encounter. Relationships with doctors, bosses, teachers, and even spouses are all examples of situations in which expectations, wishes, and fears are heightened. In psychodynamic psychotherapy, our patients' feelings about us, their therapists, give us important clues about their emotional lives. Our aims are to

- recognize these feelings, and
- encourage our patients to take interest in them

Psychodynamic Psychotherapy: A Clinical Manual, Second Edition. Deborah L. Cabaniss, Sabrina Cherry, Carolyn J. Douglas and Anna Schwartz.
© 2017 John Wiley & Sons, Ltd. Published 2017 by John Wiley & Sons, Ltd.

Our patients have feelings about us even before we meet

It's never too early to listen for a patient's emotional response to us; you can even hear it in the initial phone call. Does the patient sound excited, nervous, condescending, or eager to please? Patients may talk about their initial impression in the first session.

> *Mr A was referred for an evaluation by his internist. Within the first five minutes of the interview, he tells the therapist, "I have to say, you're not at all like what I expected. From what Dr Z said about you, and because of your last name, I expected you to be old, stern, and European. I was a bit nervous coming here today."*

Encourage your patients to talk about these feelings

Encouraging patients to take interest in and talk about their feelings toward us is an important part of beginning treatment. Patients who have never been in psychotherapy before may not know that these feelings are of interest to us, or that they are useful to the treatment. Psychoeducation is key. Here's an example:

Patient	*I wasn't sure I wanted to come to this second appointment.*
Therapist	*I'm glad that you mentioned that – I wonder if it had anything to do with your experience here last time or about any feelings you had about me?*
Patient	*I feel funny saying this, but I thought that you probably have much sicker patients to deal with and that you would be bored with my silly problems. You have that big diploma on the wall – I thought that you should be doing more important things.*
Therapist	*No one person's problems are more important than the next. But it's great that you told me about your feelings. As we continue, try as much as possible to talk about thoughts or feelings you have about me or your experience of therapy. Those feelings will not only help us in our work together, they'll help us learn about you.*

It is important to state this explicitly, since many patients need a certain amount of permission to talk about their feelings toward you in the sessions. As you continue, you can ask questions such as:

> *What were your feelings about our last session?*

> *What has your experience been of this conversation?*

> *You were very upset last time – what were your feelings about what I said?*

This will encourage your patients to talk about these feelings in an ongoing way.

Strong early reactions to us can tell us about patients

How patients react to us emotionally at the beginning of treatment can help us learn about how they react to stress and to others. Consider the following examples:

> *Ms B is a young woman who is hospitalized on an inpatient unit. When she first meets the resident assigned to treat her, she says, "How old are you anyway, like 23? Dr Y is much more experienced*

than you are. I'm not sure I'm going to be able to work with you. And by the way, no offense, but that's a really ugly shirt."

Ms C, a middle-aged woman who is at the end of her initial consultation with a new therapist, says, "I can tell you're different than the other therapists I've had. No one else understands how awful my husband is. You really picked up on that, like it's intuitive. I already feel such a connection, it's fantastic!"

Mr D is a man in his 30s who has come for treatment of mild depression and panic attacks. At his second appointment he says, "I felt better after meeting with you the other day. It was reassuring to hear that you think I have symptoms of panic, and that medication will help. I also thought that what you said about why this may be happening to me now made a lot of sense."

Ms B is overly aggressive, devaluing, and insulting to the therapist. We could expect that she relies on splitting-based defenses to help her cope with stressful situations. When she feels insecure, powerless, or envious, she resorts to belittling and attacking – in this case, the therapist.

Ms C is too complimentary of her new therapist. We could suspect that she tends to idealize or devalue people. In order to shore up her self-esteem, she yearns for special feelings of connection with individuals whom she sees as very intelligent, talented, or powerful.

Mr D responds in a generally positive, but not idealized, way to the therapist. We could imagine that he has fairly healthy responses to stress and that his relationships with others are deep and nuanced.

In all of these examples, the patients' early reactions to the therapist give interesting information about their characteristic ways of dealing with stress and relating to others.

Patients convey their feelings about us verbally and non-verbally

The patients in these examples expressed their feelings about the therapists verbally and without prompting. In contrast, many patients' feelings about their therapists are more indirectly expressed. This kind of communication can be non-verbal, for example through affect, demeanor, attitude, or body language. Or it can be expressed via displacement, for example when a patient describes feelings about another person. It is helpful when listening to patients to ask yourself the following questions frequently:

- What is the patient feeling and thinking about me, or about our relationship, at this moment?
- How is he/she expressing this?
- Are the thoughts and feelings in the foreground or the background?

Even the seeming absence of any feelings toward or about the therapist is an emotional response, and something to be noted:

A 19-year-old man comes for psychotherapy with a chief complaint of difficulty in romantic relationships. He doesn't explicitly report his feelings about his female therapist; however, she observes the following behaviors: he blows his nose and strews the used tissues all over the table next to his chair; he frequently pulls out his cell phone to send or receive text messages; he stands up to stretch, turning his back on the therapist; and he interrupts and talks over the therapist.

A 28-year-old woman in therapy for anxiety and low self-esteem has a history of a very close but highly ambivalent relationship with her mother, whom she experiences as extremely critical, intrusive, and controlling. She tends to respond to her therapist's observations as criticisms. She appears eager to please the therapist, but is easily wounded by all but the most overtly supportive statements.

A 40-year-old married woman who has recently begun psychotherapy with a male therapist starts talking about a man at work whom she finds attractive. She spends increasing time in her sessions discussing her flirtation and deepening intimacy with this colleague, as well as her guilt and conflict about "emotionally cheating" on her husband.

The therapist who picks up on verbal and non-verbal communication will learn a great deal about these patients.

Challenges for the beginning therapist: How could I be that important to the patient?

One of the biggest challenges for beginning therapists is becoming comfortable with hearing and acknowledging patients' feelings about them. It can be very difficult to convey an attitude of openness, interest, and acceptance when faced with a patient's aggressive or sexual feelings toward you. But such an attitude is usually the most helpful stance.

> Patient   *I don't think I can work with you, you're just too young. I don't mean to offend you, but I don't see how someone your age can possibly be helpful to someone my age.*
>
> Therapist *I understand that you have some concerns about working with a graduate student who is still in training. I'd like to hear more about them. What about you, more specifically, are you worried that I won't understand?*

In this example, the therapist both validates the "realistic" aspect of the patient's complaint and stays non-judgmental, demonstrating interest and probing for more detail.

As therapists, we may become highly important figures in our patients' lives. It may take some time for beginning therapists to appreciate and become comfortable with this role. Events such as interruptions in treatment for vacations, illness, or other reasons can have tremendous significance. Listen for patients' responses when there is an alteration in the usual therapeutic frame, and don't be afraid to ask questions about it.

> *Because of an emergency on the inpatient unit, a fourth-year psychiatry resident had to cancel a therapy appointment with his patient at the last minute. When he phones the patient to tell him, the patient says, "Oh, that's OK, I'll see you next week." At the next session, his patient doesn't mention it. The resident brings it up about midway through the session:*
>
> Therapist   *You haven't said anything about my canceling our last appointment. That's never happened before, and I wonder how you felt about it.*

Patient	Well, I know that you work in the hospital, and that emergencies happen. That's OK. But I did feel disappointed; I was really looking forward to the session and to telling you about that job interview.
Therapist	You didn't mention that until I asked.
Patient	Yeah, I have a hard time telling people that I'm upset with them, especially when I feel rejected. I'm always afraid they'll get angry with me, especially if it's something like this, where it wasn't really your fault.

Another therapist might not have mentioned the canceled session if the patient hadn't brought it up. He may have felt anxious or guilty himself about having canceled and might not have wanted to face the patient's reaction. However, by introducing the topic and expressing an attitude of curiosity about the patient's response, this therapist invited the patient to reveal feelings of rejection, which may have remained hidden under the guise of a "reasonable" response to the canceled session.

Our feelings about our patients

Just as our patients develop a wide array of feelings toward us, we respond emotionally to our patients. Being able to recognize and manage such feelings is an important component of therapeutic competence. These feelings help us understand what our patients are experiencing, both consciously and unconsciously. We can think of this process of **self-reflection** as the counterpart to empathic listening.

At times our reactions to patients may be dramatic and in the forefront of our attention. At other times they may be subtle and out of our awareness, forming the general backdrop of our interactions with patients. It can be helpful to ask yourself these questions periodically:

- What am I feeling toward this patient now?
- What do I think the patient is feeling about me? How does that make me feel?
- What in the patient's communications (verbal or non-verbal) might I be responding to?
- Does the patient seem to be casting me in a particular "role"?
- What might I bring to this situation (such as attitudes, memories, or biases) that is specific or unique to me?
- Is my response within the range of average, expectable responses that a therapist might have to this patient?
- Do I feel compelled to say or to do something in response to the patient now?

All therapists have all kinds of feelings about their patients

In thinking about our reactions to patients, it is important to remember that, just as we expect our patients to have the full gamut of feelings about us, it is normal for us to have all kinds of feelings about our patients. These can include affection, love, anger, protectiveness, dislike, attraction, disgust, boredom, and excitement. Recognizing and accepting such feelings in oneself are important, as is having the opportunity to talk about them with others, such as colleagues, supervisors, or one's own therapist.

Self-reflection is key

Allowing ourselves to accept and recognize our feelings about our patients will give us some of the most important information we can get about who they are, what they are feeling, and how they experience the world. Sometimes, our emotional response may be very similar to what the patient is feeling:

> You have just admitted a 23-year-old man to the inpatient unit and are conducting your initial interview. He appears to be in an exuberant mood, talking very animatedly, laughing often, and leaping up from his chair at times. He describes his recent work on an important artistic project, which he feels may be a work of genius. He hasn't slept in several days, but feels full of energy. As you listen, you notice yourself feeling energized, despite the late hour. Although you have some trouble following the thread of his story, you find him fascinating. When he laughs, it is contagious and you find yourself smiling.

> A 59-year-old woman is in psychotherapy for mild generalized anxiety and an adjustment disorder. She is somewhat obsessional, and is a self-described "worrier." She is talking about her husband's recent retirement and her anxiety about their finances. "The stock market is tanking," she says, "and the rest of the global economy will follow." She's not sure it was a good idea for her husband to retire, and she's especially worried about her adult daughter, who has three young children and a large mortgage to pay. As you listen, you find yourself feeling a bit anxious and uneasy. At one point, you realize your mind has wandered and you're worrying about your own finances. You think to yourself, "Maybe she's right and we should all feel as nervous as she does."

The first thing therapists need to do when they self-reflect is to note their affect. For example, the first therapist is happy and energized, while the second therapist is anxious. Therapists may see that their affect resonates with the patient's. Then they can proceed to ask themselves the series of questions outlined earlier.

Our emotional responses to patients will often be more complex than a single affect; they may become organized into a set of attitudes, or a role or variety of roles that we feel cast in by a patient. Of course, the role of doctor or therapist is one we expect, and usually take for granted. Yet beyond that, we may feel that our patients respond to us as if we were their parents, siblings, colleagues, friends, lovers, or adversaries. Again, the process of self-reflection can help sort this out:

Patient #1

> A new patient walks into your office for the first time. He greets you in a friendly and casual manner, calling you by your first name, "Hey, Joe, how's it going?" He throws a leg over the side of his chair as he sits down. He proceeds to chat about the trouble he had with the bus on his way to your office.

Here are two potential responses:

> You feel a bit taken aback at first, and unsure of yourself. It feels as though you're meeting someone at a party, and are expected to make small talk. Then you feel yourself relax, and you make a joking comment about mass transit.

Or:

> *You feel a bit taken aback at first, and then you feel irritated. It seems as though you and the patient are in some sort of competition. You think about asking him to put his leg down, and wish that he would refer to you as "Doctor."*

Patient #2

> *A patient you've been treating in psychotherapy often asks for advice and reassurance. She has difficulty making decisions on her own without a great deal of support and input from you or others. She now is asking you, for the tenth time, whether or not you think she should take the new job she's been offered.*

And two responses:

> *You feel affectionate toward, and protective of, this patient. You are tempted to tell her that she should take the job, and to praise her for having landed such a good opportunity.*

Or:

> *You feel a mix of warmth and irritation toward this patient. You are exasperated at being asked, yet again, what you think she should do. You feel tempted to tell her just to make up her mind and stop obsessing!*

In the first example, the therapist may experience him or herself as cast either in the role of friendly peer or in the role of a competitor. In the second, the therapist may feel cast in the role of a loving and approving parent or in the role of a frustrated and impatient parent.

These brief vignettes also illustrate that therapists have unique responses to every patient, determined by their own personality, life experiences, and history with the patient. There is no one "standard" or correct emotional response to a patient.

Preview – transference and countertransference

In psychodynamic psychotherapy, our patients' reactions to us are often referred to as **transference** and our reactions to our patients are often referred to as **counter-transference**. Both are central to many of the techniques that we use in conducting this kind of treatment. You will learn much more about this in Chapters 17, 21, and 22. For now, let's move on to two chapters in which you will see the ways in which self-reflection can help the psychodynamic psychotherapist listen empathically and explore unconscious meanings.

Suggested activity

Read the following vignettes and consider the questions at the end.

1. Mr A

> You are a trainee on the psychiatric inpatient unit, admitting a new patient. The information you have been given from the emergency room resident is that the patient, Mr A, is a 35-year-old man with a history of bipolar disorder who stopped his mood-stabilizing medication a month ago, and now presents with manic symptoms. You knock on the door of the interview room and say, "Hello, Mr A, I'm Dr Z. I will be working with you here on the unit. I'd like to talk to you now about what brought you to the hospital." Mr A is sitting in a chair with his arms crossed, with a faintly contemptuous smile on his face. He looks mildly disheveled. In a scornful tone of voice, he says, "I don't care who you are, and I'm not interested in talking to you. Do us both a favor and go back to wherever you came from, and let me relax. I'm not planning to stay here long."

- How would you describe what Mr A might feel toward Dr Z?
- What are you feeling as you imagine yourself in Dr Z's place?
- What would you say to Mr A?

Comment

Mr A is probably exhibiting symptoms of a manic episode. You don't know exactly what he's feeling, but his response to you suggests that he may be feeling irritable, angry, suspicious, or grandiose. He also might be feeling anxious, frightened, tired, or vulnerable. Whatever his combination of feelings may be, he is directly and indirectly (body language, tone of voice) expressing strong feelings about you. Since you've just met him, these feelings are not based on anything specific or personal about you, but rather on your role and the situation you and he are in. In such a situation, it is important to take your own emotional pulse before proceeding. If you feel frightened or threatened by Mr A, you shouldn't stay alone in a room with him. You might say:

> If you'd like to rest a while before we meet, that's fine. I'll be at the nurses' station – why don't you come by there a little later? We don't have to talk for more than a few minutes today.

Even if you don't feel frightened, chances are that you have some kind of feeling about Mr A. Remember, there is no one "right" emotional response to a patient. The range of emotional reactions to him might include anxiety, irritation, frustration (you were hoping to finish your admission before dinner time), excitement (you've never treated a manic patient before, this will be a challenge), or intimidation or insecurity. If you feel comfortable enough to continue the interview, you might say something like:

> I'm sorry you don't feel like talking now. We will have to meet at some point so I can learn about you and we can make a plan for your time here in the hospital. Could we spend a few minutes doing that now?

2. Ms B

You are treating a 28-year-old woman, Ms B, in twice-weekly psychotherapy. She is a teacher at a local head-start program; you and she have used primarily uncovering techniques to help her understand and solve her difficulties. It is now a year into treatment and she is feeling considerably better. You consider that Ms B has a strong therapeutic alliance with you, and that she genuinely likes and trusts you. You like her very much, and feel that the two of you have done good work together. During a session in which Ms B has talked about trying to meet new friends, she says, "I was at a fun party Saturday night. I met some people who were really great. I'll bet you would have had a good time if you were there. Do you think that if you weren't my therapist and we met at a party we would become friends?"

- What might Ms B feel about you at this moment?
- What are you feeling about Ms B?
- What would you say to Ms B?

Comment

Ms B is talking about her positive feelings toward you. These might include fondness, affection, gratitude, respect, and longing for closeness. They might also include loving or erotic feelings. Moreover she is expressing curiosity about you – what are you like outside of the therapy setting, and what do you feel about her?

As Ms B's therapist, you might have similar feelings of fondness, affection, and a wish to be close to her. In addition, you might have feelings of pride in her and in yourself for the successful work together. Since this treatment has been predominantly an uncovering one, you would want to continue to uncover the thoughts and feelings Ms B has about you now. You might say to her:

You're wondering what I would have felt at that party, and what it would be like to know me outside of this setting. Can you tell me more about these thoughts and feelings?

13 Empathic Listening

Key concepts

Empathy is the capacity to recognize and understand another person's mental and emotional state. Sometimes we say that it is the ability to "put oneself in another person's shoes."

Empathic listening is listening to other people in order to understand how they are experiencing themselves and their world.

Paying attention to our emotional responses to our patients is essential to listening empathically.

In psychodynamic psychotherapy, we oscillate between listening from the patient's perspective and listening from our own perspective.

More than anything else, psychodynamic psychotherapists are listeners. We listen to our patients, and we listen in particular ways. We need to learn not only how to listen, but also how to think about and organize what we hear. We will discuss listening skills more extensively in Chapter 16. However, one of the most important aspects of psychodynamic listening is the capacity to use what we hear in order to understand how patients experience themselves and their world. We call this **empathic listening**.

The ability to understand how another person experiences the world is a powerful ingredient in human emotional connections. Each of us has our own view of reality, but using our imagination and drawing on our experiences can give us an approximate sense of someone else's perspective. This ability is called **empathy**. How do we learn to listen empathically to our patients?

Learning to be an active listener

Asking questions

As empathic listeners, we have to listen *actively* to our patients in order to really try to get a sense of what they're experiencing. Two important principles to guide this type of listening are "don't make assumptions about what the patient means" and "the devil is in the details." Understanding details and nuances makes a big difference. For example, let's say a patient comments that she felt "upset" after an argument with her mother. We might know what *we* mean by upset, but what does *she* mean? The word "upset"

Psychodynamic Psychotherapy: A Clinical Manual, Second Edition. Deborah L. Cabaniss, Sabrina Cherry, Carolyn J. Douglas and Anna Schwartz.
© 2017 John Wiley & Sons, Ltd. Published 2017 by John Wiley & Sons, Ltd.

can have many meanings, such as sad, hurt, frustrated, annoyed, or enraged. Questions such as:

> *You said that you were upset – can you describe what you mean by that?*

or:

> *When you got upset, can you tell me exactly how that felt?*

can help both you and the patient understand her experience more deeply and precisely.

Using reflecting statements

Reflecting statements allow for confirmation or revision of mutual understanding:

Patient	*For my birthday my mother got me a cookbook. But she knows I hate cooking. I was so mad!*
Therapist	*It sounds like you felt that your mother didn't care about what you wanted.*
Patient	*Yes, that's what got me so angry.*

The therapist has heard something and has an idea that she understands her patient's view of the situation, but she uses the reflecting statement to be sure. Reflecting statements often start with words like "It sounds like . . . ," "So what I'm hearing is . . . ," or "It seems that what you're saying is . . . ." Sometimes patients make corrections that help our capacity to listen empathically:

Patient	*I was so happy that my sister said she was coming home for Christmas.*
Therapist	*I guess you'll be glad to see her after all these months.*
Patient	*Maybe, but it really means that I won't have to be with my parents alone.*

Here the reflecting statement helps to clarify the patient's experience so the therapist has a better idea of the way *the patient* sees the situation.

Looking into yourself in order to understand someone else

Aside from making sure that you're as clear as you can possibly be about what your patients are trying to communicate, another way to listen empathically is to use your own reactions to your patients to help understand their experience. You can do this in several different ways:

Putting yourself in your patient's shoes

As you listen to your patients, you may find yourself imagining being in the patient's place. Memories may come to you about similar experiences, situations, or feelings.

You may have the sense that you really "get it," or can relate to what the patient is describing:

> *Ms A is a 25-year-old student who is talking about her anger and resentment at the unreasonable demands one professor is making of her. Her therapist, Dr Z, is a third-year psychology graduate student. As he listens to Ms A, he finds himself remembering a recent experience he had with his thesis adviser, who he felt was being unreasonable and demanding. He realizes that Ms A's anger feels very familiar to him.*

Recognizing the way that your patient's experience resonates with your own can be very helpful. Remember, though, don't assume that you know exactly what the patient means just because you're having this kind of empathic response – test it out with reflecting statements to be sure.

Paying attention to our own feelings

Sometimes we become aware of feelings we have that relate to our patients' experience, even before they are aware of their own feelings. Here's an example:

> *Mr B, a 33-year-old man who is married and has two young children, tells his therapist that in the last week he and his family moved out of their "starter home" into a much larger house in a better neighborhood. Mr B gives many details about the move and talks rationally about how this is a sign of progress. While he talks, his therapist notices that she is having a distinctly sad feeling. When Mr B pauses, the therapist says, "I know that you're excited about this move, but I wonder if you have any other feelings about it." Mr B looks around, and then says that although his wife was very keen to move, he actually loved their previous house and feels wistful about moving. He says that the move also puts more pressure on him financially, which makes him anxious.*

Here, the therapist's attention to her own feelings helped her to listen empathically, even though the patient hadn't directly communicated his experience.

Challenges to empathic listening

When the therapist has strong feelings about what the patient is saying

There can be many challenges to maintaining empathy while listening. For example, if patients talk about something that makes us uncomfortable, it may be more difficult to attend to their point of view. This could be something that fills us with disgust, fear, or sadness. Imagine how challenging it is for a therapist who has experienced racial discrimination to listen to a patient discuss derogatory feelings about a particular ethnic group. Or for a female therapist whose heart was just broken by a man she was dating to listen to a male patient talk about his wish to seduce as many women as possible. Since we ask our patients to talk about whatever is on their minds, some of what they tell us may be hard to listen to. If we notice that our capacity to listen empathically is particularly challenged with a given patient, supervision from a peer or mentor can be extremely helpful.

When the patient describes something with which it is difficult to empathize

Sometimes, the patient may describe something that you feel you can't empathize with because it's just too different from your experience. This might make you feel detached, anxious, bored, or critical. In this situation, being curious about your response can be very helpful. Ask yourself:

- How am I listening to this material?
- Am I listening from the patient's viewpoint?
- Is what I'm hearing and reacting to triggering something specific in me, or does it feel more like something this person is doing to elicit this response?
- What do I imagine that others (colleagues, supervisors) in my position might feel in response to what this patient is describing at this moment?

Maybe this patient's experiences, conflicts, and defenses are fundamentally different than your own. Or it could be that what the patient is describing is inherently difficult to relate to, such as a psychotic experience or evidence of antisocial personality traits. Again, asking the patient for clarifying details and summarizing your understanding can help:

Patient	*I was so mad at my boss when I left work I just had to blow off some steam. I walked home, even though it was late. I saw a stone lying on the sidewalk, so I picked it up and hurled it at the nearest parked car. The window smashed. It felt good.*
Therapist	*It felt good in what way? Can you tell me more about what you were thinking and feeling?*
Patient	*It felt good to do something really physical, to throw that rock. But as soon as the window smashed, I kind of snapped out of it. I didn't feel angry any more, just scared and really sorry. I can't believe I broke that car window!*
Therapist	*So throwing the rock felt like a release of tension, but then you realized you'd done something destructive.*
Patient	*Yeah, I guess so.*

Or:

Therapist	*It felt good in what way? Can you tell me more about what you were thinking and feeling?*
Patient	*I just felt in control. The sound the glass made as it smashed was great. I wasn't at all sorry I did it. If I'd had another rock I would have thrown that too.*
Therapist	*So it felt good to you to do something destructive. You didn't feel any remorse for damaging someone's car.*
Patient	*No remorse. Their insurance will take care of it.*

In these cases, asking questions helped the therapist to understand this potentially hard-to-relate-to experience.

When the patient has strong feelings about the therapist

It can be particularly difficult to stay attuned to our patient's point of view when they are voicing strong feelings about us, such as desire or anger. When this happens, we may be tempted to try to defuse the affect by explaining or defending ourselves rather than staying with the patient's experience:

> *In a recent psychotherapy session, Mr C discussed his ambivalence about an elective medical procedure that he was scheduled to have the next day. In recent weeks, he had talked about feeling that the therapist was not truly supportive of his decision to have this procedure, despite the fact that she had spent many sessions trying to help him to make a decision about it. At the end of the session, as he left the office, he said sarcastically, "You could wish me luck, you know!" In the session after the procedure, he was furious at the therapist for not having wished him good luck, and told her that she was cold and unempathic.*

In a situation like this, a therapist might think, "He is really overreacting! How can he think I'm cold and unempathic when I spent the whole session seriously listening to him and discussing his feelings! OK, so I could have said good luck, but just because I didn't doesn't mean I'm not supportive!" The challenge here is to put aside one's own emotional response in order to stay with the patient's experience. As we will discuss at length later in this book, this does *not* mean that you should ignore your response, since it is likely to help you to understand your patient and his characteristic ways of relating to others. Understanding your patient's experience requires you to register your feelings while staying attuned to his perspective. You might, for example, say to him, "I can see that my not having said good luck to you made you feel that I didn't understand what you needed or wanted." Here's another example:

> *Ms D has a tendency to come 5–10 minutes late for her sessions. One day, she arrives 10 minutes late, and the therapist keeps her waiting for several minutes in the waiting room while he finishes a phone call. As she enters the office she seems annoyed. She starts to talk about feeling irritated at her mother and at her boss. When the therapist comments on her angry affect, she is silent. She then says she is angry with him for keeping her waiting, and that she felt it wasn't fair for him to retaliate for her lateness by being late himself.*

In this example, the patient also accuses the therapist of a lack of empathy, though initially she expresses this non-verbally and indirectly. The therapist may feel a pull to defend himself, thinking, "This patient is almost always late. Why can't she cut me a break for keeping her waiting a few minutes?" Again, the challenge is to put oneself in the patient's shoes and to try to experience things from the patient's vantage point. One response might be:

> *I know that you often feel bad about being late and missing part of your session, so it must have been very frustrating to arrive and have me keep you waiting. Let's look more at your feelings about this.*

When the therapist identifies with another person in the patient's life

A further potential barrier to empathic listening happens when we listen from the imagined perspective of another character in the patient's story. This is often a person with whom the patient has a relationship, such as a family member, friend, or colleague. Sometimes we also listen from the perspective of an outside observer or narrator. You might ask, "Well, isn't that what we're supposed to do as therapists – to look objectively at what the patient tells us in order to try to uncover hidden meanings, affects, and defenses?" The answer is yes and no. Ultimately, we try to help our patients see what they themselves may not see by maintaining curiosity about what they say and what they don't say. However, it's usually most helpful and productive when we don't jump to our own conclusions too quickly. The first step is to try to see and feel things the way the patient does, and to communicate that understanding to the patient:

> Ms E is a woman in her 30s who came to therapy complaining of depression and difficulties in interpersonal relationships. She lives alone and has a few social acquaintances, but no close friends. While trying to launch a career as a singer she has worked at a series of secretarial jobs, all of which ended either when she was fired or when she quit. Ms E complains of feeling persistently lonely and poorly treated by others. She generally describes people as rude, selfish, insensitive, or cruel. She feels she has had terrible luck to encounter such unpleasant people repeatedly, and wonders why she is always the victim. In an early session, Ms E describes an argument she had with a co-worker she had arranged to meet for brunch on a weekend:

> "I had asked S if she wanted to get together on Sunday. She said she could meet for brunch at 11, but I told her I like to sleep in on weekends. She made some excuse about being busy all afternoon, some play she already had tickets for. She probably didn't want to get together with me, but she's too passive-aggressive to say so. So I thought I'd call her bluff, and told her, OK, let's go for brunch. I guess she felt she couldn't back out then, so she agreed. We were supposed to meet at noon at this place near the theater she was going to, which was really inconvenient for me. I woke up late – probably my alarm didn't go off the way it was supposed to. And then the bus never came – even though I was waiting for it for over 30 minutes! I called her and told her I was running late. When I finally got to the restaurant at 12:30, she said, 'Sorry, I already ordered, I don't want to be late to meet my friends at the theater.' Can you believe that? I was so mad, I barely talked to her for the rest of the meal."

Here's how two different therapists responded:

> Therapist #1: Well, I hear that you're quite angry with S. But could it be that you're jumping to conclusions too quickly about her? Maybe she really did want to spend time with you, even though she had already made plans. And how did you feel about being so late? Wouldn't you have been angry if you had been the one waiting?

> Therapist #2: So it really felt to you that S wasn't being sincere in agreeing to spend time with you. And it also sounds like you felt you had gone out of your way to agree to meet her at a time and place that weren't convenient for you. You were frustrated about missing your bus, and then angry to find that she had gone ahead and ordered food without you.

Therapist #1 listened to Ms E's material from the point of view of S, or from that of an "objective" outside observer. The questions he asks are aimed at trying to get Ms E to step *outside* her own experience, rather than to convey an understanding that is *inside* her experience. On the contrary, Therapist #2 describes what he believes to be Ms E's point of view, without critiquing it. Once the therapeutic alliance is strong, and Ms E has some capacity to see things from other people's perspectives, she may be able to hear a gentle confrontation about her behavior. However, the way Ms E describes the situation, we have good reason to doubt her *current* capacity for self-reflection, or for seeing the situation from S's perspective. Particularly if Ms E is in an early phase of treatment, she may hear Therapist #1's comment as unhelpful at best, and as highly critical and unempathic at worst. By helping her to feel understood, Therapist #2's intervention can strengthen the alliance.

Oscillating between our perspective and the patient's perspective

Ultimately, as psychodynamic psychotherapists, we oscillate between viewing things from the patient's point of view and viewing things from our point of view. We may also spend time viewing things from someone else's point of view, such as a person with whom the patient has a relationship [1,2]. All of these perspectives are important to our ability to help the patient. However, if we find ourselves spending too much time in one perspective or another, this could signal that we are having difficulty listening empathically. Here are some things you can ask yourself to help you to know when it's time to shift perspectives:

Am I having a very strong feeling?

This can mean that you are lodged too tightly in one perspective:

> When Ms F talked about her anger at her daughter, the therapist became enraged. This helped the therapist realize that she was identifying with Ms F's daughter (related to her own relationship with her mother) and that she needed to shift perspectives.

Am I feeling disconnected from my patient?

This is another good signal that empathic listening is faltering. Boredom, forgetting things patients say, and getting distracted during sessions are clues that this might be happening.

Learning to shift perspectives in order to listen empathically is a little like learning to shift focus between something that is close up and something that is far away. With practice, it will become automatic, allowing you always to stay close to your patient's experience.

Suggested activity

Give an example of "active listening" – either a question or a reflective statement – for each of the following situations. What is your own emotional response to each?

1. Mr A is an elderly widowed man whom you are seeing for an initial outpatient evaluation. He says:

> Ever since my wife died last year, the meaning has gone out of life for me. Things won't ever be the same. I often wonder, what's the point?

2. Mr B is a 28-year-old man who first came to see you a month ago, complaining of anxiety and mild depression. He just revealed that he is using cocaine multiple times a week, and frequently calling in late or sick to work. In the initial consultation he had denied current drug or alcohol use. He says:

> *I guess I should have told you about my using cocaine, but people tend to be so judgmental. My parents think someone's an alcoholic if they have a glass of wine with dinner. I can get it under control if I want to.*

3. Ms C is a 40-year-old woman who has come for psychotherapy because of conflicts about returning to work after the birth of her second child. In an early session, she says:

> *I feel so torn about this decision. I worked so hard my whole life to get where I am professionally. I never thought I'd want to give up my career, but I also can't stand the thought of being away from the kids so much. It seems so much easier for my husband, he doesn't struggle with this. What do you think I should do?*

4. Ms D is a 35-year-old woman with a diagnosis of schizophrenia. She has come to the clinic for a routine medication management visit. She says:

> *I stopped taking the pills. They told me to take them, but the other ones said no, don't take them. They're not the same color they used to be, and you can't eat things that are that color, they could be poison.*

5. Mr E is a 50-year-old man who was recently diagnosed with coronary artery disease. He comes for a consultation complaining about anxiety and insomnia. He says:

> *It's natural that I'm nervous, I guess. My dad dropped dead of a heart attack when he was 55, and now I've got the same disease. I just need to get used to this new low-fat diet they've put me on and really start exercising. I figured I'd cover all my bases and come see someone about stress management, because stress probably isn't good for my heart.*

Comment

1. Mr A is talking about profound feelings of loss and hopelessness. The therapist should respond empathically to these feelings and also inquire about suicidal thoughts. For example:

> *Losing your wife has been devastating for you. It sounds like you feel pretty hopeless. Tell me more about what you meant by "what's the point?" Do you ever have thoughts about your own death, or about suicide?*

2. Mr B appears to minimize his troubles with cocaine and also his withholding of important information from the therapist. As an initial tactic, reflecting your understanding of Mr B's feelings in a non-judgmental way will probably be most productive (although, as discussed in Chapter 10, if the cocaine use continues the therapist may need to adopt a different stance later). For example:

> *It sounds like you were worried that I would react critically if you told me about your cocaine use. How do you feel talking about it now?*

3. Ms C is struggling with a difficult conflict, and is inviting the therapist to weigh in with an opinion. It's likely that the therapist will *have* an opinion and may feel tempted to answer

Ms C's question. An empathic response would reflect the patient's conflicting feelings and her struggle to come to her own decision. For example:

> *I can see that you feel very torn about what to do, and that it would feel painful either way – to go back to work and miss your children or to stay at home and give up your career. I can't know what the right decision is for you, but I can help you sort through your feelings and choices.*

4. Ms D speaks in a confusing way and, given her diagnosis, the therapist should be suspicious of psychosis or auditory hallucinations. The therapist's first job is to try to clarify what the patient is thinking and feeling. For example:

> *It sounds like you're feeling nervous or scared about your medicine and that's why you stopped it. Could you tell me more specifically who told you what about the pills?*

5. Mr E is clearly anxious about his diagnosis and prognosis. He may be seeking reassurance from the therapist, both about his anxiety and about the fact that he came for therapy. Reflecting this back to him and supporting his decision to seek treatment can be reassuring. For example:

> *I can see why getting this diagnosis would be very stressful for you, or for anyone in your situation. It's great that you're doing so much to help yourself cope with this, including coming to see me.*

Chapter 13: References

1. Fosshage, J.L. (1997) Listening/experiencing perspectives and the quest for a facilitating responsiveness. *Progress in Self Psychology*, **13**, 33–55.
2. Schwaber, E.A. (1992) Countertransference: The analyst's retreat from the patient's vantage point. *Progress in Self-Psychology*, **1**, 43–61.

14 Looking for Meaning

> **Key concepts**
>
> Thinking psychodynamically involves looking for unconscious meaning in what our patients say and do.
>
> The inherent characteristics of our patients' words and behaviors, as well as our reactions to them, are guides to unconscious meaning.
>
> Whether or not we discuss potential unconscious meanings with our patients depends on whether we think this will help them.

Mr A, a 50-year-old man who is very depressed and has never seen a mental health professional, has his first visit with a therapist. During this visit, the therapist asks about Mr A's father and mother. With difficulty, Mr A tells the therapist the story of his father's alcoholism and abusive behavior. At the end of the session, they make an appointment for the next Monday. On the day of the next session, Mr A calls the therapist to tell him that he cannot come in because he is sick. They reschedule for Friday. Mr A arrives 20 minutes late to the rescheduled session, explaining that the train was late.

Why did Mr A miss his second appointment? Why was Mr A late to the rescheduled session? Perhaps Mr A was sick and the train was late. But perhaps Mr A was ambivalent about returning to the therapist after what sounded like an upsetting session. Could this ambivalence have manifested as missing and lateness? While we can never know, we believe *that all words and behaviors have multiple meanings, some of which are unconscious.* Maybe Mr A's ambivalence led him to stall at home just long enough that any difficulty with mass transit would lead to lateness – then both explanations would be correct.

Looking for meaning is essential for thinking like a psychodynamic psychotherapist

Our patients say and do all sorts of things that can have multiple meanings. Difficult thoughts and feelings that are unconscious are often expressed in actions. Aggressive

Psychodynamic Psychotherapy: A Clinical Manual, Second Edition. Deborah L. Cabaniss, Sabrina Cherry, Carolyn J. Douglas and Anna Schwartz.
© 2017 John Wiley & Sons, Ltd. Published 2017 by John Wiley & Sons, Ltd.

and sexual wishes, which can be particularly difficult to acknowledge, are often revealed in behavior. Here are some examples:

- **Missing sessions and lateness:** Although there are always many reasons why patients miss sessions and are late, patients who do so regularly might be communicating something, such as anxiety about sessions, ambivalence about therapy, or a wish to sabotage the treatment.

- **Leaving personal items in the office:** Anyone can forget things, but if patients leave things in your office it could mean something, such as the wish to be remembered or the wish to give you a gift.

- **Eating or drinking in the session:** Patients who routinely eat or drink in sessions could be unconsciously communicating something, such as the wish to make therapy social, or the wish to be your friend.

- **Calling you by your first name:** If you address your patient as "Mr" or "Ms" and introduce yourself the same way, it's noteworthy if your patient calls you by your first name. This could be a manifestation of the patient's wish to deny your role as the therapist or to "cut you down to size."

- **Bringing you gifts:** In therapy, even a cup of coffee is a gift. Patients who bring you gifts could be trying to make sure that you won't be critical of them, or might feel that without the gifts you would lose interest.

- **Clothing choices:** Our patients' clothing choices can tell us things, too. A patient who wears provocative, revealing clothing could be unconsciously communicating erotic feelings, or an ordinarily well-groomed person who comes in looking disheveled could be communicating a wish for care.

This is by no means an exhaustive list – any behavior can have unconscious meanings. Similarly, the possible meanings suggested are just that: possibilities. A type of behavior – for example, lateness – does not always mean the same thing. On the contrary, the meanings of each behavior are unique to that patient.

Beginning to listen for meaning

How do you begin to think about unconscious meaning? Here are three important questions you can ask yourself to help you think about unconscious meanings.

- **What are the inherent characteristics of what the patient is saying or doing?** Is something that your patient says or does inherently aggressive? Entitled? Loving? Even if a behavior seems innocuous, is there something about it that could be construed another way? Let's say a patient slams the door loudly behind her every time she comes into the office. Slamming a door is an inherently aggressive act. Could there be some way in which aggression toward you is part of what she is trying to communicate? Looking at the behavior itself can sometimes give you some clues regarding its unconscious meaning.

- **How do you feel about the words or behavior?** It is also important to register how you feel about the behavior. When Ms B misses a session you feel very little, but when Mr C misses a session you feel neglected. What might that tell you about the unconscious meaning behind Mr C's absenteeism? Your own feelings can often be the best clues to unconscious meaning.

- **Is what the patient is saying or doing incongruous?** If something patients say or do is incongruous with their conscious experience, you can surmise that it may have unconscious meaning. For example, if a patient says that he "loves" psychotherapy but either misses a lot of sessions or doesn't pay on time, you can hypothesize that the lateness and non-payment might be imbued with unconscious meaning.

Should we talk about unconscious meanings with patients?

Just because we suspect that a given behavior might have an unconscious meaning does not necessarily require us to discuss this with patients. We often wait until we have observed the behavior many times before we bring it to the patient's attention. With more fragile patients, our hunches about unconscious meaning may guide our supporting interventions, but we may rarely, if ever, discuss this overtly with them. Here are two contrasting examples:

> Ms D, a 42-year-old married mother of three who is a third-grade teacher, has been in a twice-weekly psychodynamic psychotherapy with a female therapist for two years. In this treatment, Ms D's discussions about her relationship with the therapist have helped her to better understand her relationships with women in general. Initially, Ms D idealized the therapist and felt that she could never attain her level of success. However, as Ms D gained confidence she began to explore the possibility that she, too, could feel that good about herself. One day, Ms D came into her session and told the therapist that she was very sorry but she had spilled coffee on the therapist's new waiting-room rug. The therapist suspected that despite her idealization, Ms D might harbor envious, aggressive feelings toward the therapist and that this accidental spill might be related to them. She asked Ms D if she had any thoughts about having spilled the coffee. Ms D said that although she felt bad, she was secretly glad that the therapist now had a stain on her rug just like the stain on her own living-room rug. As they continued to discuss this, Ms D was able to begin to explore her envious feelings toward the therapist and her feelings about spoiling the therapist's beautiful office.

> Mr E is a 53-year-old physical therapist who has frequent difficulty with aggression that has gotten him into trouble with co-workers. He sought treatment for depression and has been in a once-weekly psychotherapy with a male therapist for six months. In therapy, he has been working productively on alternate ways of handling himself when he gets angry at work. He has made some comments about the therapist's office and "all the money he must have," but has been unable to discuss this further. One day, Mr E came into his session and told the therapist that he was very sorry that he had spilled coffee on the therapist's new waiting-room rug. The therapist noted to himself that this behavior could have aggressive meaning relating to the patient's envy of the therapist but, thinking that the patient could not use this material productively at this time, chose to reassure the patient about the spill and to continue to ask him about how things had gone at work that week. Two weeks later, the patient remarked on the therapist's "cool" response to the spill and said it was in stark contrast to the angry outbursts his father would have had about a similar episode.

In each vignette, the therapist noted the behavior and hypothesized about possible underlying meanings. However, in the first case the therapist felt that the patient could benefit from the exploration of potential unconscious meanings, while in the second the therapist felt that this would not be productive. It is interesting to note, however, that the choice not to uncover underlying meanings does not preclude the eventual exploration of unconscious material – in fact, it often facilitates it down the road.

In the technique section of this manual, we will further discuss how to listen for these behaviors and meanings and then how to use them either to help your patients to make these unconscious meanings conscious, or to help support weakened functioning.

Suggested activity

Think about the possible unconscious meanings of Ms A's words and behaviors:

Ms A is a 50-year-old woman who presents for psychotherapy because she is having difficulty with her family. She explains that after her father's death three years ago on Thanksgiving, her mother "pulled away" from her and seems to spend time only with her two sisters and their families. She is upset and hurt, but denies feeling angry. She says that her husband is "relieved" because he "never liked my family anyway." Her two children are now out of the house and she feels "isolated." She called for an appointment a month ago and canceled, then called again on November 15 but "wasn't sure why." She arrives 15 minutes late, apologizes profusely, then becomes withdrawn as the session nears an end. She makes another appointment that she cancels but reschedules. Before her next session, she calls and leaves a message in which she is in tears. At her next session, she says that she is fine and that the message was just a "blip." She says that she's not sure she needs therapy and makes a negative comment about having to wait in a waiting area with other patients.

Comment

It seems likely that Ms A's canceling and lateness have unconscious meanings. She may be ambivalent about beginning therapy or about talking about these painful family circumstances. She may be ashamed of her show of emotion on the telephone. She may be worried about becoming dependent on a therapist, since she feels that she cannot depend on her mother or her husband. She may also be revealing some ways in which she unconsciously pushes people away, despite her conscious feeling that other people (namely, her mother and her husband) are the ones rejecting her. Finally, calling again in November may indicate that she is having an anniversary reaction to her father's death without being aware of it, and that she has an unconscious wish for more support during this time.

15 Medication and Therapy

Key concepts

In our work as psychodynamic psychotherapists, we shift among different models of etiology and therapeutic action in assessing and treating our patients. One example of this is our need to think about whether medication or psychotherapy will best address a patient's problems and symptoms at any point in time.

Prescribing and taking medication have psychological meaning for both patient and therapist.

When a patient in psychodynamic psychotherapy is also taking psychotropic medication, sometimes the therapist will be the prescriber and sometimes there will be a separate pharmacologist. Each of these situations has different clinical implications.

The patients who come to us for treatment generally do not arrive asking specifically for medication versus psychotherapy. They come complaining of problems, symptoms, and difficulties in their lives. They may already be taking medication or may have taken medication in the past. Some patients have strong opinions about medication, while others may not have given it much thought.

As psychodynamic psychotherapists, our listening is empathic and non-judgmental. It involves asking open-ended questions, looking for unconscious meaning, and helping patients to feel safe. However, we have to simultaneously listen as mental health professionals, which involves listening for medical and psychiatric symptoms and syndromes, side effects, and therapeutic effects. We also have to be able to shift gears in order to be more active when needed, to take the lead, to ask specific questions, and to give recommendations or advice about medication [1].

Using psychodynamic and phenomenological models simultaneously

The DSM takes a descriptive or **phenomenological** approach to psychiatric disorders, without reference to etiology. As psychodynamic psychotherapists, we have to learn to use both psychodynamic and phenomenological models of etiology and treatment simultaneously. Here's an example of how a psychodynamic psychotherapist might do this:

> *Ms A, a 65-year-old widow with a history of recurrent depression, is in weekly psychotherapy for long-standing difficulties with self-esteem, as well as conflicts about intimacy in a new romantic relationship. She has been on several different antidepressants in the past. Six weeks ago, she and her*

Psychodynamic Psychotherapy: A Clinical Manual, Second Edition. Deborah L. Cabaniss, Sabrina Cherry, Carolyn J. Douglas and Anna Schwartz.
© 2017 John Wiley & Sons, Ltd. Published 2017 by John Wiley & Sons, Ltd.

therapist decided to add a selective serotonin reuptake inhibitor (SSRI) antidepressant to the bupropion she was taking, as she had complained of feeling mildly depressed and persistently anxious for over a month. In the first session after a three-week interruption in therapy due to vacations (hers and the therapist's), she described feeling emotionally "flat" and lacking energy and motivation. She remarked that it was the second anniversary of her husband's death two weeks ago, and that she had spent much of her vacation with her children and grandchildren, as well as with her new partner. She said that she did not feel "fully present" for much of the vacation, and was less able to enjoy her time with family. She had a bit more trouble sleeping than usual. However, she felt less anxious than before starting the SSRI.

As we think about Ms A's story, we can approach it from different perspectives. *Thinking psychodynamically*, the salient features are:

- the anniversary of her husband's death;
- the time spent with her children, grandchildren, and her new partner; and
- the recent interruption in therapy.

Thinking phenomenologically, we hear symptoms including:

- mild anhedonia or affective blunting;
- decreased energy and motivation; and
- insomnia.

What is the etiology of these symptoms? Here are questions to help sort that out:

- Did the anniversary of her husband's death reactivate feelings of grief? Is this grief now complicated by conflict over being with a new romantic partner? Could her symptoms be related to trying to integrate her new partner into her relationships with her children and grandchildren?
- Is this a recurrence of a major depression, despite the fact that she is taking antidepressant medication?
- Has the addition of a new medication caused new side effects, such as insomnia, affective blunting, and decreased energy?

Choosing an approach

While it is interesting to think about these possibilities, we have to be agnostic about the fact that we can't really *know* what is *causing* Ms A's problems at this time. The challenge for the clinician is to decide which approach, or combination of approaches, will best serve the patient *at any one time*.

Here are some questions to ask yourself when you are making this kind of decision (adapted from Cabaniss [1]):

- How do I view the clinical picture psychodynamically?
- How do I view the clinical picture phenomenologically?

- Is my current way of looking at the current clinical situation leading me to use therapeutic interventions that are effective?
- If my interventions are less than effective, is there another way of looking at the current picture that might lead to more effective interventions?
- Does the patient present a constellation of symptoms that may be effectively treated with medication?
- Can the patient's symptoms be more fully understood and more effectively treated using a psychodynamic model?
- Which therapeutic interventions (psychodynamic or pharmacological) have been effective in the past, and for which symptoms?
- Is there currently a shift in my thinking about which model – psychodynamic or phenomenological – should guide my therapeutic interventions right now?
- If there is a shift, could it be influenced by something happening in the relationship between the patient and me (such as an interruption in the treatment or change in the frame), or a strong feeling that the patient is having about me or that I am having about the patient?

In the case of Ms A, the therapist might start by asking her some open-ended questions about recent events, including her feelings about the anniversary of her husband's death and the break in the therapy. As the patient talks, the therapist will listen empathically, staying alert to specifics such as symptoms, severity, and timing. The therapist may shift from the mode of empathic listening to one of more active questioning to get more information. Here are some questions designed to get details:

You've been talking about feeling emotionally "flat." When did you become aware of this feeling?

How frequent are these feelings? Do you have them all the time?

How troubling are they?

Are these feelings that you've had in the past during a depression?

Are you having any other symptoms?

Becoming comfortable with uncertainty

In some clinical situations, therapists may feel fairly confident about which model provides the best framework for assessing and treating their patients' problem. In others, the challenge is to become comfortable with uncertainty, and to be able to discuss this with patients. For example, a therapist might say to Ms A:

It seems that you've been experiencing a number of symptoms of depression in the last few weeks. Some of these are similar to the symptoms you've had in the past when you've been depressed. You've had some psychological stresses recently that could be contributing to this – the anniversary of your husband's death, spending time together with your partner and your family, and not seeing me during this time. But another possibility is that the new medication is causing some side effects that mimic your depressive symptoms. Let's make a plan to see if we can sort this out and help you feel better.

Even if you choose to work with one model at one point in the treatment, you should be able to shift flexibly to another model at another point.

The meanings of medication

Prescribing and taking psychiatric medication have psychological meaning for both patient and therapist [2,3]. Depending on their characteristic functioning, patients may react differently to their therapists' recommendation for medication. Here are some common reactions:

- **"It's a biological problem:"** The recommendation for medication may mean to a patient that there is something "biological" at play. This can feel like a relief or a validation. Patients may interpret this to mean that their symptoms are not their "fault" but are a result of something beyond their control. Common ideas are that the problem is caused by a "chemical imbalance" or that "it's not me, it's my brain" that is causing the problem.

- **Medication can feel like a blow to the ego:** Some patients experience the recommendation for medication as a blow to their self-esteem. It may feel as if they are being told that there is something defective about them, and this can be a source of embarrassment or shame.

- **Medication as gift:** The therapist's recommendation of medication can be experienced as a gift or as a "special" form of being taken care of.

- **Medication as mind control:** The therapist's suggestion of medication can be experienced as intrusive or controlling, as if the therapist is, via medicine, invading or controlling the patient's mind and body.

- **"I guess I failed therapy:"** Some psychotherapy patients may feel as if their therapists are giving up on them if they recommend medication. It may also seem like an acknowledgment that therapy doesn't work for them, or that the therapist can't help them

Similarly, for therapists, the decision to discuss or recommend medication to patients can have a variety of meanings:

- **"I failed as a therapist:"** A decision to suggest medication may feel like a failure to therapists because they weren't able to "cure" the patient with therapy alone.

- **Medication as relief:** Alternately, therapists may feel relieved, or powerful, to have the ability to offer patients relief from symptoms or suffering.

- **Medication as enactment of feelings about the patient:** The decision to recommend medication may reflect a shift in how therapists feel about their patient, the treatment, or their own abilities or skills.

- **Medication as gratification of needs:** Prescribing medication may feel to therapists that they are "gratifying" their patients by giving them something special.
- **Medication as shift to a medical model:** Shifting gears from a psychodynamic to a phenomenological model with a patient may make the therapist feel "more medical," and thus alter the relationship with the patient in subtle or not-so-subtle ways.

These lists are not exhaustive; the particular set of meanings about medication will be complex and unique to each therapist/patient pair. The goal is to be able to shift back and forth between medical "fact finding" and advice giving, and psychodynamic exploration of the patient's and therapist's thinking and feelings. Consider this example:

> Ms B is a 35-year-old woman who came for psychotherapy during her divorce from her first husband. She initially complained of significant anxiety symptoms and trouble sleeping, but declined the therapist's suggestion that she consider anxiolytic medication. Over the first month of therapy, the focus was on Ms B's history of difficulty with intimacy, and mistrust of situations in which she felt overly dependent on others. Yet she seemed to struggle with severe anxiety, verging on panic, when she felt isolated and overwhelmed by managing the stress of a full-time job, parenting two young children, and going through a divorce. Her therapist began to point out the conflict Ms B felt about relying on others versus doing it "all by herself," and the anxiety she felt in both situations. Though Ms B reported feeling somewhat less anxious soon after beginning therapy, she continued to complain intermittently about symptoms. During one session, she described feeling exhausted, having been unable to sleep the night before because of worry:

> Therapist   I'm sorry that you had such a rough night. We've been talking a lot about how hard it is for you to rely on others or ask for help. When I suggested that we consider medication back in one of our first sessions, you said that you didn't want to take anything. Let's reconsider that now, in the context of this struggle about feeling dependent. Can you tell me more about what it would mean if you were to take medication for anxiety?

> Patient   I don't want to have to rely on a pill to feel better. I should be able to manage this on my own, or with your help. It's not like I have a mental illness which requires me to take something. It's understandable that I feel stressed, given what I'm going through.

> Therapist   So if you were to take medication, it might mean that you've failed in some important way – failed to take care of yourself, failed to handle the stress in your life. It also might mean that I've failed to help you in the way you'd like to be helped, through talk therapy. Or it might mean that there's something more seriously wrong with you, a mental illness.

> Patient   Yes, I guess that's how I feel. When you put it that way, it also seems kind of extreme, that I wouldn't consider something that would help me feel better in the short term. But isn't there a danger that I might get addicted to the medicine?

> Therapist   Well, "addiction" is a word that's used in a number of ways. You don't have a history of problems with substance abuse, and the medicine I have in mind is not likely to lead to physical dependence. But tell me what you mean by the word "addicted."

Patient	*I guess I'm afraid that if I do feel better on the medicine, I'll never want to stop taking it. Or if I do stop it, what if I go right back to feeling miserable? I don't want to feel so reliant on something.*
Therapist	*That sounds a lot like what you've said about relying on other people.*

In this example, the therapist's focus is on uncovering the meaning behind Ms B's attitude toward medication. However, she also answers Ms B's question about addiction directly and provides some information about the medicine, before returning to further exploration.

Combined versus split treatment

When a patient in psychodynamic psychotherapy is also on psychotropic medication, sometimes the therapist will be the prescriber (**combined treatment**) and sometimes there will be a separate psychopharmacologist (**split treatment**). A separate psycho-pharmacologist may be involved either

- because the therapist is not a psychiatrist; or
- because the therapist has determined that it would be preferable for a separate pharmacologist to prescribe the medication. This may occur when a specialist is needed, or when the logistics of the medication management take up a significant proportion of time in the therapy.

Each configuration has its own set of clinical issues.

Combined treatment

The challenge of combined treatment is for the therapist/pharmacologist to balance discussion of both therapeutic modalities during sessions. Patient and therapist sometimes collude to avoid discussion of the medication, as if it were a less important part of the treatment. On the contrary, much can be learned from the patient's reaction to the medication.

> *Mr C is a 56-year-old man who presents after a divorce. He is being treated by Dr X, a 40-year-old female therapist who is also a psychiatrist. At presentation Mr C had clear symptoms of major depression, and Dr X prescribed an antidepressant. The symptoms cleared within six weeks, and Dr X no longer asked about the medication. Within a few months, Mr C began to date, although he showed no interest in having a physical relationship. Dr X asked Mr C about this, particularly as it might relate to anger at his ex-wife. When Mr X mentioned having gone to a urologist to investigate new-onset erectile dysfunction, Dr X realized that she had neglected to ask follow-up questions about Mr C's sexual function in terms of potential side effects. She wondered whether she and the patient were avoiding discussing this because of a growing erotic transference (see Chapter 21).*

Prescribing medication can also have an impact on the way a therapist conducts sessions. For example, the therapist/pharmacologist may need to be more directive, give advice, or make recommendations. Here are some examples:

1. *Although you feel that your depressed mood is understandable given the circumstances of your life right now, the symptoms you're experiencing have been going on for several weeks and are causing you quite a lot of distress. There's a good chance that medication could help you to feel better fairly quickly.*

2. *Now that we've agreed that medication is likely to help, and you want to give it a try, let me explain the different medication options and the pros and cons of each.*

3. *I've given you a lot of information just now. Do you have questions?*

Prescribing medication may also require the therapist to direct the patient's attention to specific details, such as symptoms, side effects, therapeutic effects, dosage adjustments, and prescription refills. Points at which this is particularly important include:

- when you first introduce the topic of medication
- when you write the first prescription
- the first session after you give a prescription
- when you or the patient first note a therapeutic benefit
- whenever you change a dose, refill a prescription, or change the medication regimen.

The therapist may choose to start a session with questions about symptoms or medication, or may wait to see if the patient brings this up. Sometimes, as in the following example, the therapist/pharmacologist may relegate discussion of medication to the margins of the session:

Therapist   *Our time is up for today. By the way, do you need a refill of your antidepressant?*

This precludes ample discussion of any practical or psychodynamic issues related to the medication, and may signal to the patient that the therapist is not particularly interested in this. Instead, the therapist/pharmacologist should be continually aware of the issue of medication and the impact it could have on treatment, even when it is not a focus of the session.

Split treatment

Split treatment has its own challenges. In split treatment, patients talk about their symptoms to two people. This requires the therapist and psychopharmacologist to collaborate closely in order to share information. Sometimes, patients only talk about certain issues with one or the other professional. This demands close communication to maximize care. Again, you can always learn something from the way the patient reacts to this situation:

Ms D is a 25-year-old woman who is in therapy with Dr W, a 35-year-old female psychologist. She also sees a 55-year-old male psychopharmacologist, who prescribes the medication. She begins to have symptoms of depression, which she only discusses with the psychopharmacologist. He calls Dr W and tells her about this. In their next session, Dr W mentions this to the patient. They ultimately learn that Ms D's competitive feelings led her to hide her perceived "weakness" from Dr W. Discussion of this opens a new avenue of exploration.

Whether or not you will be both therapist and psychopharmacologist, it is important to learn to use both phenomenologic/pharmacologic and psychodynamic models in order to provide optimal, individualized treatments to each of your patients.

Suggested activity

Give a phenomenologic and a psychodynamic description of the following patient:

Mr A, a 37-year-old businessman, calls you asking for an appointment as soon as possible. He was seen in a local emergency room earlier in the week, where he presented with intense anxiety, palpitations, and chest discomfort. He was found not to have had a myocardial infarction and was given a diagnosis of panic attacks. Mr A describes feeling increasingly anxious and depressed over the past month, culminating in several intense panic attacks in the previous two weeks. He has also had insomnia, trouble concentrating at work, and negative ruminations about his work, but no suicidal ideation, hopelessness, or anhedonia. His psychiatric history is significant for two previous episodes of mild depression and anxiety, the last in his mid-20s, which occurred in the setting of starting a new job.

About six weeks ago, Mr A was promoted at work, with a significant pay raise and also increased responsibility. He says that although he enjoys some aspects of his work, including the financial security, he is deeply ambivalent about continuing in his career. He says, "When I was younger I never saw myself becoming a businessman," thinking instead that he would "do something more creative." His father, who founded and ran his own successful small business, developed coronary artery disease in his late 30s and died suddenly of a heart attack in his early 50s when Mr A was a college student.

Comment

Thinking **phenomenologically**, Mr A is a 37-year-old man who has had two weeks of escalating symptoms of anxiety, including full-blown panic attacks, and depression (including insomnia, difficulty concentrating, and negative ruminations). He has a past history of depression and anxiety, and a family history of coronary artery disease.

Thinking **psychodynamically**, Mr A's current symptoms began in the context of a job promotion. The increased responsibility that attended this change may have contributed to his heightened anxiety, but Mr A also has significant ambivalence about his career. The more success and financial stability he gains in this current job, the more difficult it might be for him to think about ultimately working in a more creative field. Additionally, we might wonder about his identification with his father, who was successful in business, and who developed heart disease when he was around Mr A's age.

Combining these approaches to thinking about Mr A will help to develop a comprehensive treatment plan.

Chapter 15: References

1. Cabaniss, D.L. (1998) Shifting gears: The challenge to teach students to think psycho-dynamically and psychopharmalogically at the same time. *Psychoanalytic Inquiry*, **18**, 639–656.
2. Busch, F.N., and Auchincloss, E.L. (1995) The psychology of prescribing and taking medication, in *Psychodynamic Concepts in General Psychiatry* (eds. H.J. Schwartz, E. Bleiberg, and S.H. Weissman), American Psychiatric Press, Arlington, p. 401–416.
3. Busch, F.N., and Sandberg, L.S. (2007) The meaning of medication, in *Psychotherapy and Medication: The Challenge of Integration*, Analytic Press, New York, p. 41–61.

PART FOUR: Listen/Reflect/ Intervene

Key concepts

The basic technique of psychodynamic psychotherapy can be divided into three steps:

- listening
- reflecting
- intervening

Although we don't usually think about it, talking to another person involves a three-step process. We listen to what the other person has to say, process what we've heard, and respond. Ideally, in social relationships people listen and respond to each other in a fairly balanced way. However,the therapeutic relationship, unlike most social relationships, is lopsided. The set-up in psychodynamic psychotherapy is that the focus is exclusively on the patient's problems. Thus, therapists must train themselves to listen and respond in a new way.

In this manual, we will teach you the basic techniques of psychodynamic psychotherapy using three basic steps:

- listening
- reflecting
- intervening

Psychodynamic Psychotherapy: A Clinical Manual, Second Edition. Deborah L. Cabaniss, Sabrina Cherry, Carolyn J. Douglas and Anna Schwartz.
© 2017 John Wiley & Sons, Ltd. Published 2017 by John Wiley & Sons, Ltd.

Listening is the step in which we bring in data, reflecting is the step in which we process that data and decide when and how to intervene, and intervening is the step in which we verbally interact with patients to uncover unconscious material or support weakened function. We will first review each of these steps, and then apply them to the major elements that we listen for in psychodynamic psychotherapy.

16 Learning to Listen

Key concepts

We listen differently depending on what we're listening to.
We can conceptualize three modes of listening:

- ambient listening
- filtered listening
- focused listening

As psychodynamic psychotherapists, we learn to move fluidly among these modes of listening while we listen to patients.
There are particular things we learn to listen for in psychodynamic psychotherapy.
Listening to a patient means listening to sounds *and* silences.
While we listen to words, we also listen for the tone, pitch, volume, and timbre of a person's voice and ways in which these change. These can help us understand the patient's affect and unconscious material.

Listening is the first step of the three-step technique of psychodynamic psychotherapy

Although we have listened to things throughout our lives, as psychodynamic psychotherapists we listen to our patients in particular ways. First we will address *how* we listen, and then we will think about *what* we specifically listen to and for.

How do we listen?

Listening is not a homogeneous activity. We listen differently depending on what we're listening to. Think about the ways you listen to these various sounds:

- the woods
- a symphony orchestra
- street noises
- people talking in a cafeteria

Psychodynamic Psychotherapy: A Clinical Manual, Second Edition. Deborah L. Cabaniss, Sabrina Cherry, Carolyn J. Douglas and Anna Schwartz.
© 2017 John Wiley & Sons, Ltd. Published 2017 by John Wiley & Sons, Ltd.

- a poetry reading
- someone speaking in a foreign language
- your friend talking to you on the phone
- an instructional video on how to set up your computer

As an example, click on the "listening exercise" found at www.wiley.com/go/cabaniss/psychotherapy.

After you've listened to it once, listen to it again, listening only for the background noise. Sounds different, doesn't it?

Now listen again, listening only for the birdcalls. What happened to your listening this time? Did you find that you ignored many of the other sounds as you waited to hear the birds?

Types of listening

What you've been doing is listening differently. You need to listen in many ways when you listen to patients in psychodynamic psychotherapy. Here is how you might conceptualize the modes of listening you have been doing:

1. **Ambient listening:** Ambient listening is what you do when you're not listening for anything in particular. It's allowing sound to wash over you – like listening to all the sounds in a forest, to surf crashing on the beach, or to street noises. Imagine walking into a cocktail party – lots of people are talking and at first all you hear is the din. When you think about it, it's hard to listen without focusing on anything in particular. In fact, we have to train ourselves to listen in this way when we listen to patients, because we have to remain open to everything they say. If we're too interested or focused on one thing or another, we can miss something else that is important. This is particularly hard to do as trainees, when we're trying so hard to learn about things like transference that trying *not* to listen for them is very difficult. Ambient listening is important at many different times in a session, but it is almost always crucial at the beginning, when you never know what the important themes are going to be.

2. **Filtered listening:** Continuing with our party analogy, once you're in the party room you begin to filter out the background noise as you start to pick out particular voices. Maybe you hear someone you know, or maybe you hear part of a conversation that interests you. Something similar happens when we listen to patients. As patients speak, we begin to hear certain things that stand out from the background material, for example repeated themes or strong affects. Although our attention is not yet focused on any one particular element, we begin to screen out some ambient material as we start to hone in on what seems most important.

3. **Focused listening:** Our listening is focused when we fix our attention on something in particular and screen out most of the background noise. At the cocktail party, you've heard a voice you know and you now turn your attention to that person to have a conversation. Although the room is still loud, you begin to listen only to the

person with whom you are talking. This is focused listening – listening to one thing in particular and blocking out most of the background noise. We use focused listening with patients when we pick up an important theme or affect and begin to concentrate on it to the exclusion of other material.

Although ambient listening is particularly important at the beginning of sessions, it is essential throughout a session to be able to move fluidly from one mode of listening to another. Even when focusing on a prominent theme or affect, we have to enable ourselves to disengage from the focus to listen ambiently again. In visual terms, this task is akin to the movie director on her chair, moving in and out of the close-up. This is an analogy that will take us through many aspects of the technique of psychodynamic psychotherapy, as we take in the big picture and then focus in and out on particulars.

What we listen for

Silence

When we think about listening, we generally think about listening for sounds. However, if we're listening closely, we also listen for the lack of sounds – for *silence*. We listen for when sound stops and starts, for the rhythm of the stops and starts, and for how this changes – on a moment-to-moment basis, on a session-to-session basis, and across the broad trajectory of a whole treatment. If you really listen to silence, you begin to realize that it sounds different at different times. Silence can sound peaceful, furtive, or tense – and once you begin to listen to silence you can begin to hear the differences.

Beyond words

We listen for words, of course, but we also listen for the **pace, volume, pitch, and timbre** (particular color or sound quality) of the person's voice, and for how these change. These aspects of the patient's communication can often tell us as much or more about the meaning of the patient's words as do the words themselves. They are often good clues to patients' affects, defenses, and resistances – and missing them deprives us of valuable information about their conscious and unconscious experience. Non-verbal communication is important too, such as facial expressions, eye contact, or the way someone shifts in a chair.

Patterns

We determine which themes and affects are dominant by listening for **patterns and repetitive elements**. If we hear the same thing several times in a session, or in a series of sessions, we hypothesize that it's important. Similarly, we listen for **incongruities** and **slips** – words, sounds, and affects that jar our listening. Think about listening to a melody: we have certain expectations about what the next note might be and if it's very different from what we expect, it sounds jarring. The same is true of incongruities and breaks in patterns. For example, a patient might talk about something that sounds like it was frightening and then say it was fun, or a patient might be talking about one person and then it suddenly sounds like they're talking about another. We want to tune in to these shifts and incongruities.

Slips are formally called **parapraxes** – they occur when someone means to say one thing and instead says something else [1]:

> *Last night I was talking on the phone to my mother – oops! I mean my wife.*

These can be good clues that something is going on in the unconscious, so they're important to listen for.

Negation and double negatives

Listening for the way in which patients say "no" can be very informative. One patient might say "I don't think I'll go to the party," while another says "There's absolutely no way I would take myself to that party – forget it." The affective power behind the second assertion comes through loud and clear. Similarly, listen for the elusive "double negative." Consider these statements:

> *I'm going to go to law school.*

> *I'm not not going to go to law school.*

They both say the same thing – but why does the second person use two negatives to indicate the affirmative? The paradoxical use of the double negative often conveys meaning.

Passive voice

People frequently use the passive voice when they are unconsciously distancing themselves from their own choices and actions. Listen to the difference between these two statements:

> *On Friday night, decisions were made about the way our relationship will move forward.*

> *I broke up with Suzy on Friday night.*

Believe it or not, these two sentences could be about the same thing. Listening to patients' use of the passive voice helps us understand their sense of personal agency.

Nodal points

We can think of the unconscious as being a giant nodal network with points that are connected. Some points have more connections than others. Think of an airline map: hubs have many lines emanating from them, while less well-connected places might be at the end of a single line. When we listen to patients, we listen to everything, but as we begin to filter and focus we listen for unconscious hubs that we call **nodal points** [2]. It makes sense to aim for these well-connected points, as they can lead us down new paths into unconscious territory. It is also likely that these points will be near the surface of consciousness, since we are hearing many references to them. The technique for listening to nodal points involves listening for

- repeated words
- repeated symbols
- points of clarity

Important content to listen for

Here are some of the things we particularly listen for in psychodynamic psychotherapy. They will be discussed in depth in Part Five of this manual:

- affects
- free association/resistance
- transference
- defenses
- unconscious fantasies and conflicts
- dreams

We all listen in different ways

Some of us have been trained to be listeners in other parts of our lives, for example when learning music, languages, or bird calls. Some people are very adept at picking up accents, while others have perfect pitch; some are more aware of ambient noise, while others focus on specific sounds. Part of learning to listen to patients means learning to understand our listening styles. You can begin to think about how you listen and what you tend to listen for. This will help you understand yourself as a listener of patients and think about listening skills you might need to hone.

Once we've listened carefully to our patients, we have to decide how to use what we've heard to help them in the best way. This process is called **reflecting** and is the topic of the next chapter.

Suggested activity

Read the following monologue. What do you hear as you listen ambiently?

I was really excited to come today. I've been looking forward to starting therapy. It's been on my calendar – I even circled it. I know that sounds silly, like it was my birthday or something. And I read a book about starting therapy. I've never been in therapy before. What do I do? I wanted to know what to do – you see people in the movies talking about really important things – I guess I could talk about my mother but I feel like I have silly things to talk about – like being irritated at my wife a lot – I mean, I love her but she drives me crazy. But that's not a very big thing – people have really bad problems. Maybe my problems aren't important enough – I don't mean important, but severe – something like that. But they're upsetting me . . . how much time do we have today? Anyway, what was I saying? Speaking of my family, they always thought that therapy was a waste of time. I don't think so, but I don't really know. I hope that it will help. Do you think it will?

Now read the monologue again. What do you begin to focus on?

Comment

1. **Ambient listening:** The patient talks continuously without pausing. He seems very anxious. There are lots of questions and there is a shift in topic near the end.

2. **Filtered/focused listening:** The patient oscillates between questions for the therapist and thoughts about his family. He seems to make a connection between his wife and his mother. He appears insecure and eager to be a good patient. He is worried that the therapist will find him silly and his problems insignificant. Some of his words sound young – like "silly," which he repeats. The focus on his birthday also has a child-like ring. He sounds conflicted about many things, including feelings about his wife, his family, and whether the treatment will help.

Chapter 16: References

1. Auchincloss, E.L., and Samberg, E. (1990) *Psychoanalytic Terms and Concepts*, Yale University Press, New Haven, p. 188.
2. Freud, S. (1900) The interpretation of dreams, in *The Standard Edition of the Complete Psychological Works of Sigmund Freud, The Interpretation of Dreams (First Part), Vol. IV*, Hogarth Press, London, p. ix–627.

17 Learning to Reflect

Key concepts

Once we listen to the patient's sounds and silences, we process this data in order to understand its meanings. We call this multi-layered process **reflecting**.

Reflecting helps us to:

- understand the meaning of what we have heard
- decide how to focus our listening
- determine what our **therapeutic strategy** will be (how and when to intervene)

Whether we uncover or support, we want to comment on material that is closest to consciousness and that our patients will best be able to listen to and use productively at that moment.

To understand what is closest to the patient's conscious mind, we use what we call the "three choosing principles":

1. surface to depth
2. follow the affect
3. attend to the countertransference

To understand the patient's current ability to listen to/use what we have to say, and to choose whether to uncover or support, we use what we call the "three readiness principles":

1. assess the state of the therapeutic alliance
2. assess the phase of the treatment
3. assess the patient's current functioning

To organize what the patient is saying into themes, we use the "three organizing sources":

1. our working psychodynamic formulation
2. our knowledge of theory and technique
3. our own personal and clinical experience

Reflecting may be conscious and deliberate when we are learning to conduct psychotherapy, but it rapidly becomes a spontaneous skill.

Psychodynamic Psychotherapy: A Clinical Manual, Second Edition. Deborah L. Cabaniss, Sabrina Cherry, Carolyn J. Douglas and Anna Schwartz.
© 2017 John Wiley & Sons, Ltd. Published 2017 by John Wiley & Sons, Ltd.

Reflecting

When we listen to patients, data streams into our mind. The next step is to process this data in order to:

- understand its meaning
- focus our listening
- determine our **therapeutic strategy** (how and when to intervene)

We call this process "reflecting." Reflecting is the second step in the three-step technique of psychodynamic psychotherapy.

Let's think about the word **reflect**. When used as a noun (reflection) it sounds passive (like a reflection in a mirror), but when used as a verb (reflect, reflecting) it's full of activity. It comes from the Latin *reflectere*, which is a compound of *re*, which means *back*, and *flectere*, which means *to bend*; so to reflect means to bend or to throw back, for example light, heat, or sound.

So data comes in and we do something active with it. What we do with it depends on our therapeutic goals. In psychodynamic psychotherapy, we're always trying to think about what's in the unconscious, so we always reflect on how what we hear can help us understand what's beneath the surface. Then we can think about how we can use what we've heard either to uncover unconscious material or to support function.

Now, let's go back to our therapeutic aims. Because our overarching psychodynamic principle is that unconscious elements affect conscious thoughts, feelings, and behavior, our principal technical aim has to be to get to unconscious material. This can consist of affects, thoughts, defenses, fantasies, and representations of self and others – all of which are unconscious. The material we hear – words, silences, tone – is all we have to guide us toward the material below the surface. These are the clues that we have in lieu of an actual map. If we think of each time we listen, reflect, and intervene as a unit, then the goal of each unit can be thought of as moving us a little closer to the uncharted territory of the unconscious.

Exactly how the reflecting process occurs will be different for each person. It's impossible to make it into a linear, cookbook-style process. However, we can think about principles that help guide the way we reflect. In essence, while we're listening to *everything*, we're picking the material that is most likely to move us forward *at that point*. It's about how we make choices – how we focus our listening and ultimately our interventions, on the most salient, meaningful, useful, and usable material. Our interventions will be linked to these elements.

The choices we make when we reflect result in our **therapeutic strategy**. This is our rationale for what we choose to focus on, and how we decide to intervene. We base these choices primarily on two basic sets of principles that we call the "three choosing principles" and the "three readiness principles," and secondarily on the "three organizing sources."

The three choosing principles

The three choosing principles are:

1. surface to depth
2. follow the affect
3. attend to the countertransference

We use the three choosing principles to decide where to intervene and which material will be most productive to address.

Surface to depth

The unconscious is not homogeneous. Some thoughts and affects are more deeply buried than others [1]. The hypothesis is that the more anxiety provoking the thought or affect, the more deeply buried it has to be in order to reduce the likelihood of its coming into awareness. You can think of the unconscious as a stratified paleontological site, with bones fossilized in different geologic layers. If you're interested in the bones at the bottom, you can't go in with a bulldozer to get them; rather, paleontologists painstakingly brush dust off fossils with toothbrushes, gradually revealing layer after layer. In this way, all the bones are uncovered with minimal damage. They will ultimately get to the bottom, but it will take time.

The same is true for the psychodynamic psychotherapist. If you comment about something that is deeply out of awareness, it is likely that the person will reject the comment or, worse, erect more defenses to keep it unconscious. Sometimes, we understand something about someone's mind that is deeply buried. While this can be interesting and can help us with our case formulation, it may be very hard – or even counterproductive – to address this until it is closer to consciousness. This flies in the face of many stereotypes of psychotherapy in which the therapist listens, discovers something deeply buried from the patient's childhood, tells the patient, and the patient says "a-ha!" and is cured. In reality, we want to find the thought or affect that is just below the surface – the one that only needs a gentle tap to shift into consciousness [2]. So when we're sifting through what patients say, we want to get some idea of how their thoughts and affects range from surface to depth.

Reflecting is like riding up and down on a forklift, choosing at which depth to land:

> *A 45-year-old unmarried woman has been in psychotherapy for six months. Generally shy and isolated, she has only recently been able say that she values therapy and feels close to the therapist. When she arrives at her second session after her therapist has moved into a larger office, she carries a small bag. "I brought you a house-warming gift," she says, lifting out a boutique box of Kleenex. "I noticed that you didn't have any last time."*

Bringing the therapist tissues and noting that they were missing in the previous session could be a way of criticizing the therapist. Perhaps the therapist's move to the new, bigger office made the patient feel neglected, or caused her to feel that the therapist was thinking about other things. However, the tissues were presented as a gift by a woman who has only recently begun to express her positive feelings toward the therapist. Thus, the positive feelings are closer to the surface than the negative feelings. According to the principle of surface to depth, the therapist would do well to focus on the positive feelings *now* while remembering the deeper, negative feelings and listening for them in the future.

Follow the affect

Remember the game "hot and cold" that you played as a child? Someone hid something and another person looked for it while the rest of the group shouted "hot!" or "cold!" as clues for the seeker. In the game of psychodynamic psychotherapy, locating affect is the best way to tell if we're close to important unconscious material. If the patient's associations range from topic to topic but only one is tinged with real affect, it's likely that this is closest to something important. In our process of reflecting, it is essential to recognize such clues:

> *A 21-year-old man arrives at his first session and tells you that he has been thinking about coming to treatment for three months and can't believe that the day is finally here. He says he was looking forward to it all weekend and thus was very upset that he was almost late because he couldn't find his wallet when he was leaving the house. He spent the weekend reading books about therapy so he could make sure he said the right kinds of things and focused on the most salient issues. Halfway through this monologue, he looks up and asks, "Am I doing all right?"*

This patient is anxious! Although he is also excited, he is nervous that he will not perform well as a patient, or that he will disappoint the therapist. As we reflect on what he has said, we would choose to comment on this anxiety since it is the affect that is closest to the surface.

Attend to the countertransference

The term **countertransference** refers to the feelings that we as therapists have about our patients (see Chapters 12 and 22). The material that we receive from the patient has to be filtered through our own reactions to the patient and to the material. Like following the patient's affect, attending to our countertransference is an invaluable tool for processing what we hear in sessions. If we have a particularly strong reaction to something a patient says, we have to pay attention to it – although it could be something idiosyncratic related to our own internal experience, it could just as likely tell us something about the patient:

> *In one session, a patient who has been in psychodynamic psychotherapy for four years mentions wanting to end therapy. She reports a dream in which she was in a modernist train station leaving for a new city – while trying to get on the train, she stumbles and falls, but is able to get up and move forward on her own. As the therapist hears this dream, she realizes that she is feeling both proud and sad; on processing this, she thinks that she might be feeling the way a parent does when they sense that their child is ready to "go it alone." This helps her reflect that the patient might in fact be ready to end therapy.*

If you listen for what's on the surface, follow the affect, and attend to what you're feeling in the session, you're most likely to pick up the most important themes.

The three readiness principles

Once we have a sense of what is on the surface and what the patient is most affectively connected to, we have to assess what the patient will be able to hear and work with. To do this we use what we call the "three readiness principles":

1. assess the state of the therapeutic alliance
2. assess the phase of treatment
3. assess the state of the patient's current functioning

Assess the state of the therapeutic alliance

As we discussed in Chapter 9, the therapeutic alliance is a measure of the trust between patients and therapists. This builds as therapists demonstrate over time that they understand their patients, have their best interests at heart, and can help them. A therapist might be able to say something that is quite painful to the patient once the alliance is strong, which the patient wouldn't have been able to tolerate at the beginning of the treatment. Time alone doesn't strengthen the alliance – that takes effort on the part of the therapist and trust on the part of the patient. A paranoid patient may never be able to have a strong alliance, while a patient with a history of trusting people may develop a strong alliance early on. The state of the alliance can wax and wane, depending on what's happening in the treatment:

> Ms A is in her second year of psychodynamic psychotherapy and has felt very helped by her therapist, Mr Z. At one point, Mr Z forgets to tell Ms A that he is going on vacation until the week before he is scheduled to leave. Ms A becomes convinced that this means that he does not care about her and for a few weeks she is unable to process comments that she was able to use readily just a few months before.

Assess the phase of the treatment

There are three basic phases of treatment: the beginning, the middle, and the end. As patient and therapist work together over time, certain types of comments generally become easier for the patient to use:

> During the early months of Ms B's treatment, she insisted on writing Dr Y a check the moment she got the bill. When Dr Y asked Ms B about this, she was annoyed and said that she didn't see anything wrong with paying bills on time. During the middle phase of treatment, Dr Y commented on this again, and at this point Ms Y was able to explore her fear of being in a position of "owing" anyone anything and to deepen her understanding of their relationship.

Assess the state of the patient's current functioning

As discussed in Chapter 4, it is important to be continually aware of the patient's current functioning in key areas such as self-perception, relationships with others, and ability to adapt. Even though you assess this at the beginning of the treatment, it can change at any point, for example when the patient is under stress, medically ill, or regressed for some other reason. A patient who is generally able to use certain types of interventions might be unable to use them during periods of stress:

> During their work together, Dr X frequently used humor to help Ms C notice when she was avoiding certain topics. For example, he would say things like ". . . see, there you go again!" in a way that helped Ms C notice her avoidance in a non-threatening way. However, when Ms C's husband developed cancer, she snapped at Dr X when he used humor to point out the way she arranged to have business meetings during all of her husband's radiation treatments.

Using the readiness principles will help you to learn when your patients are ready to listen to and use things that you have to say to them.

Three organizing sources

Three sources of information help us to organize and focus what we hear from the patient into themes we can listen for, follow, and address:

1. our working psychodynamic formulation
2. our knowledge of theory and technique
3. our own personal and clinical experience

Our working psychodynamic formulation

As outlined in Chapter 5, we construct the psychodynamic formulation by DESCRIB-ING the problems and person, REVIEWING the patient's developmental history, and LINKING what we have described with what we have reviewed to create a hypothesis about the etiology of the patient's difficulties and what we can do to help.

When we create a psychodynamic formulation, we identify themes that dominate the patient's inner life. For one person it might be difficulties with self-esteem, while for another it might be problems with attachment and relationships. When we reflect, we think about how what we hear relates to those dominant themes. For example, if a man whose mother left his family and who has a lifelong pattern of mistrusting people tells us that his boss is ready to "throw his 20 years of work out the window," we reflect that this story may relate to his theme of abandonment, and we develop a therapeutic strategy to connect this latest episode to his past experiences.

Our knowledge of our patients' personal history also helps us to reflect on what they say. This includes information about the patient's life prior to therapy as well as the therapist's experience with the patient. For example, if a single, female patient says that she is interested in a married man, we reflect on this differently if we know

- she has done this before
- she has never done this before, or
- her parents were divorced because her father had an extramarital affair.

Our knowledge of how patients responded in the past, either in or out of therapy, will affect the way we process what they tell us and how we decide to intervene.

Our knowledge of theory and theory of technique

It almost goes without saying that our knowledge of theory and theory of technique affects the way we process our patients' material. For example, if we notice that a patient tends to use defenses based on splitting when describing his officemates, we will be especially attuned to splitting in the therapeutic relationship. Although this is inevitable, we have to be wary of thinking about theory excessively while with patients, since it can hinder our capacity for ambient listening and fluid processing.

Our own clinical experience

Although the reactions of each patient are unique, as we begin to see patients we start to recognize patterns that can help us process information. For example, if we have had several patients who idealized us early on and then suddenly fled treatment, we listen and process a patient's early idealizing comments with this in mind. Similarly, once we have ended a few treatments, we begin to anticipate certain reactions and will be more attuned to them when we process the material of a patient in that phase. Note that initially you may lean on your supervisors or knowledge that you've gleaned from books for clinical experience.

You can also judiciously use information from your own experience *outside* of the therapy room to help you understand what patients tell you. For example, if you had extensive experiences with teenagers as a camp counselor, this will inform the way in which you listen to your adolescent patients.

We use the data from the organizing sources cautiously because our best clues are the immediate data – the patient's affect, our countertransference, patterns (nodal points), and breaks in patterns (slips, incongruities).

Developing a therapeutic strategy

We can think of the reflecting process according to the following schematic:

PATIENT'S MATERIAL: INCOMING DATA		WHAT WE FILTER THE DATA THROUGH		
Affect		Surface to depth		
Resistance		Follow the affect		
Transference		Countertransference		WHAT
Defenses	→→→		→→→	WE
Unconscious fantasies		Phase of treatment		FOCUS
Dreams		State of therapeutic alliance		ON
		Current function		
		Psychodynamic formulation		
		Knowledge of theory and technique		
		Therapist's clinical experience		

Sometimes we're consciously aware of reflecting and sometimes we're not. But when we review what happened in a session, we should be able to articulate the process we used to come up with our therapeutic strategy, that is:

- how we used the **choosing principles** to decide what to focus on
- how we used the **readiness principles** to decide when to intervene
- how and why we decided whether to uncover or support
- how we used the **organizing sources** in this process

It's a good exercise to take a moment after sessions to outline the principles you used to determine your therapeutic strategy, either in writing or as you explain it to a supervisor.

Once we've reflected, we're ready to **intervene**, which is the topic of Chapter 18.

Suggested activities

Activity 1: Surface to depth

For each of the following vignettes, list four things you hear. Then order them from surface to depth.

1. Ms A is a 55-year-old woman who lives with her elderly mother. Here is some material from a session with her therapist:

   My mother wandered off again yesterday. It took hours to find her – she left when I was sleeping. I was out in the neighborhood in my nightgown – me with my old flabby body. Poor thing. My sister was so angry with me for calling her, but I needed help. I don't get it – here I am, no life of my own, taking care of Mom 24/7 – and I call my sister for help and she's concerned that she won't get to her kid's soccer game on time. It's funny, because she was the favorite when we were little. Mom hardly knows who I am now, but it's what I have to do. How could I not do it? I'm eating so much – I have to figure out a way to stop.

Comment

Listen:	Empathy for her mother, who is getting more symptomatic
	Anger at her sister for not helping more with mother's care
	Anger at her mother for favoring her sister
	Resignation about her situation
	Contempt for the state of her body
Reflect:	
Surface	Anger at sister
	Empathy for mother
	Contempt for her body
	Resignation about her situation
Deep	Anger at mother

2. Ms B is a 39-year-old single lawyer:

I'm so worried about my friend Jane – she had an abortion yesterday. She's miserable. I went over there, brought her soup. Her boyfriend just went to work, but I can be there for her. He's a jerk – men are like that. She's worried that she'll never have a baby. Do you think that that's true? Does having an abortion make it harder for you to have a baby? I was on the internet all night researching that – I didn't see anything like that. I hope that this doesn't make her depressed. When I had that abortion when I was 25, I didn't even think of that. I'm glad that I'm not fixated on babies – I would never have been able to make partner if I'd had a kid. Maybe I should stay at her house tonight, just to make sure that she's comfortable.

Comment

Listen: Concern for her friend
            Professional ambition
            Disappointment that she never had a child
            Wish for a child of her own
Reflect:
  Surface   Concern for her friend
            Professional ambition

  Deep   Disappointment that she never had a child
            Wish for a child of her own

Activity 2: Developing a therapeutic strategy

"Listen" to the first few minutes of this psychotherapy session. Write the major things that you "hear." Then, use the reflecting principles outlined in this chapter to write

- what your therapeutic strategy would be, and
- why

Mr C is a 35-year-old married banker whose chief complaint is difficulty in his relationship. Growing up, he lived with his father after his mother died when he was an infant. He now has a 2-year-old son, Jamal. He says:

Terri and I had a big fight last night. I guess it started when were talking about sending Jamal to nursery school. I don't know what's wrong with her, she's totally resisting sending him to a 2's program. He's so ready – he walks, he talks, he's toilet trained – and he's whip smart. Only yesterday he picked up my phone and was pretending to check messages – just like I do. I know, I know – I think he's smart because he's my kid, but he is, and he's got to get out there and be in the world. He can't always stay home with her. Maybe she doesn't want to go to work – and honestly, that's fine, we have plenty of money, she doesn't need him to be home as an excuse. I always went to day care – I mean, I had to – and it did me a world of good. I can go into any situation and be comfortable – talk to anyone. I'm convinced it's from there. So OK, Jamal has a mom and so we don't need day care, but I don't want him dangling from her apron strings. That won't make him into a man.

Comment

- What I heard:

  Affect – anger at his wife

  Resistance – externalizing the problem ("it's all my wife's issue"), potential difficulty mentalizing

  Major theme – "It's a problem to rely too much on your mother. It makes you a weak man."

- How I reflected: Anger at his wife seems to be on the surface, and is the dominant affect. However, he's having trouble seeing things from her side, and based on my formulation that's probably because it's so painful for him to imagine that his son would have to suffer the way that he did. Yet the feelings of grief related to losing his mother are deep – he's focused more on the way that being independent at a young age was helpful to him. My goals are to have him mentalize more with regard to his wife, and to begin to experience some of his deeper feelings about losing his mother. This will help him with his parenting – his denial of those feelings could lead him to get in the way of the relationship his son has with his wife. So my therapeutic strategy will be primarily uncovering, but will be slow. I will empathize with his feelings, see if he can imagine how his wife might feel, and then slowly begin to uncover his feelings about his own mother, starting with a confrontation about being independent at the age of 2.

Chapter 17: References

1. Freud, S. (1923) The ego and the id, in *The Standard Edition of the Complete Psychological Works of Sigmund Freud (1923-1925), The Ego and the Id and Other Works, Vol. XIX*, Hogarth Press, London, p. 1–66.
2. Fenichel, O. (1941) *Problems of Psychoanalytic Technique*, Psychoanalytic Quarterly Press, New York.

18 Learning to Intervene

Key concepts

An intervention is something we communicate to a patient, either verbally or non-verbally. There are three types of interventions in psychodynamic psychotherapy:

- basic
- supporting
- uncovering

We use basic interventions in all psychodynamic psychotherapies in order to gather history, teach patients to use the treatment, and convey understanding.

We use supporting interventions when our goal is to support a patient's function.

We use uncovering interventions when our goal is to enhance a patient's awareness of unconscious thoughts and feelings.

Both supporting and uncovering interventions are used in all psychodynamic psychotherapies.

Interventions also include non-verbal communication, such as facial expression and tone of voice.

After we intervene, we listen for what the patient says next in order to gauge the effect of our intervention. Decreased anxiety or improved function indicates that a supporting intervention was successful. Further associations and deepening affect indicate that uncovering interventions were successful.

Intervening is the third step in the three-step technique of psychodynamic psychotherapy. An intervention is simply something that we communicate to a patient. In psychodynamic psychotherapy, we have three types of interventions:

- basic
- supporting
- uncovering

Although some psychodynamic psychotherapies will have a preponderance of either supporting or uncovering interventions, *all* psychodynamic psychotherapies use all three types of interventions at some point in the treatment. In addition, no single technique is ever *exclusively* supporting or uncovering. What defines an intervention as supporting or uncovering is the therapist's *primary aim* in using that technique at any

Psychodynamic Psychotherapy: A Clinical Manual, Second Edition. Deborah L. Cabaniss, Sabrina Cherry, Carolyn J. Douglas and Anna Schwartz.
© 2017 John Wiley & Sons, Ltd. Published 2017 by John Wiley & Sons, Ltd.

given moment in the treatment. You can determine your aim by asking yourself whether you are hoping to

- directly improve function and change behavior (supporting aim), or
- enhance the person's understanding of unconscious processes (uncovering aim).

Interventions can be non-verbal

It is important to remember that we also communicate with our patients non-verbally. Smiling, making good eye contact, and speaking in a soothing tone of voice are all interventions. Our tone can be encouraging or containing, and is a critical component of both supporting and uncovering interventions. Remember that this never involves physical contact – facial expressions and tone of voice will suffice.

Determining the success of our interventions

Once we make an intervention, we listen to what the patient says *next* [1]. New memories, further associations, and deepening affect indicate that an uncovering intervention was successful, while decreased anxiety or a direct change in behavior signals the success of a supporting intervention. An increase in defensive behavior of any sort is usually an indication that our intervention was

- too deep
- poorly timed
- incorrect or off the mark

That's good information, too – it helps us recalibrate our reflection so that we can intervene more effectively the next time.

Section 1: Basic Interventions

Key concepts

Basic interventions can be used regardless of your aim. They are used in all psychodynamic psychotherapies. They include:

- directions and psychoeducation
- questions
- information
- empathic remarks
- calls for associations
- reflective statements
- silence

Sometimes, trainees think that the only interventions we make in psychodynamic psychotherapy are interpretations. They think that they shouldn't ask questions or give directions, and they apologize for interventions like this when reporting their work to supervisors. Nothing could be further from the truth. In psychodynamic psychotherapy, **basic interventions**, like questions and information, are essential to the process. They help us take a history, learn details, teach our patients how best to use the treatment, and convey our understanding.

Basic interventions

Directions and psychoeducation

Trainees are usually intuitively aware that more impaired patients who have trouble organizing themselves need their therapists to provide structure, direction, and information. However, psychoeducation is not only for low-functioning patients – helping our healthier patients learn how psychodynamic psychotherapy works is critical at the outset and throughout treatment. We ask them to say whatever comes to mind, teach them to talk about dreams, and tell them that thoughts and feelings about the therapist are particularly important. For example, a patient who relates a dream early in treatment will often try to tell us what she thinks it means – we have to instruct her that a good way to use dreams in this type of treatment is simply to associate to the various elements. Patients frequently think that talking about banal thoughts is a waste of time – we have to tell them that we want to hear everything so that we can learn about how their mind works. Once we've said this a few times, we can then begin to think about the patient's difficulties or reluctance to associate as resistance – but without instruction that's unfair!

Questions

Learning about how another person's mind works and how it came to be the way it is can be quite a project. Sometimes the person gives us lots of information spontaneously, but sometimes there are things that we want to know that the patient doesn't freely offer. Every psychodynamic psychotherapy must begin with a careful evaluation and diagnosis, including a personal, family, social, and sexual history. If patients don't volunteer this information, we have to ask for it. Conducting psychodynamic psychotherapy doesn't mean forgetting that we are well-trained mental health professionals. Asking questions is an essential part of technique throughout the treatment. If patients say something that we don't understand – like jargon from their field, a foreign expression, or a piece of their history that they think we know but we don't – we have to ask. It's not interrupting – patients are glad to know that we are interested and invested in having the whole picture. Finally, it's important to remember that many secrets of the unconscious are hidden in details. When the patient says, "I apologized to my mother but she was still angry," we have to ask, "What did you say?" If you find that you need to ask more questions with a particular patient, you may be learning about that person's defensive style, and this might ultimately be something to interpret.

Asking questions also demonstrates interest. Following what the patient says and asking relevant questions is one of the best ways to communicate that we are paying attention and are interested in what they tell us.

Closed-ended and open-ended questions

We ask two basic kinds of questions – **closed-ended questions** and **open-ended questions**. We ask closed-ended questions when we want a particular answer, such as an amount, time, or number. Closed-ended questions can often be answered with "yes" or "no" and can be helpful if we need to know whether or not something happened. Here are a few examples of closed-ended questions:

When did you first start feeling suicidal?

What did you hope your mother would say to you at your graduation?

How many times did you pass the refrigerator before you started your binge?

In contrast, open-ended questions do not have specific answers. They invite patients to open up and deepen what they're saying. Open-ended questions often begin with "how" rather than "why." For example, "How does that make you feel?" is a very different question from "Why did you feel that way?" Asking "why" presumes that patients could tell you – and if they could tell you, they probably wouldn't need your help. When starting out as a psychodynamic psychotherapist, try asking "what?" or "how?" every time you think of asking "why?" We want to get our patients to *describe* rather than to *interpret*.

Learning to ask open-ended questions is a core skill for psychodynamic psycho-therapists. Many phrases are helpful in shaping open-ended questions, for example:

Can you tell me more about (how you felt, the dream, cutting yourself . . .)?

How did that make you feel?

What was your experience of (the dinner, this session, the consultation . . .)?

You can think of many more. Contrast these open- and closed-ended questions:

Closed-ended   *So the conversation with your boss made you really angry?*

Open-ended   *Can you tell me more about the experience of speaking with your boss?*

Closed-ended   *Why are you crying?*

Open-ended   *Can you tell me more about how you're feeling right now?*

Asking open-ended questions helps our patients to deepen their account of their feelings and inner lives. In the beginning phase of treatment the majority of the therapist's interventions are open-ended questions and comments designed to expand the field of inquiry and discussion rather than solve problems. Simple open-ended questions like "Can you tell me more about *x*?" are mainstays in the therapist's repertoire at all phases of therapy.

Information

During the course of treatment, we impart all sorts of information to patients. We tell them when we have times available, when we're going on vacation, and how much we charge. It is also sometimes appropriate to give other types of information to our patients, such as referrals for friends and relatives. If we think that patients are developing symptoms that require medication, we have to give them information about diagnosis, treatment options, consultations, dosages, and side effects. In addition, we always have to think about what it means to the patient to ask for information from us and also to receive information from us. For example, a patient's frequent requests for referrals could be a wish to have one's whole family cared for by the therapist. Similarly, patients have many feelings when receiving information about medications from a therapist who is also the pharmacologist. This should not preclude us from giving information, but it should be in our mind as something that can help us to understand the patient's defensive style and that we might ultimately need to explore and address.

Empathic remarks

We use empathic remarks when we want patients to know that we're listening or that we think we understand how they feel. These can be very powerful interventions. A woman who is overwhelmed by but ashamed of her hypochondriacal fears might feel very understood by the therapist who observes, "It takes an enormous amount of energy to be so consumed by those thoughts every day," while the executive with fragile self-esteem, who has to pretend to be confident to his family and business associates, might feel relieved when the therapist says, "That must be very hard for you." Patients often remember these comments years after we say them.

When our primary goal is to uncover, we can make empathic remarks while also exploring our patients' feelings about them. For example, a man who seems to need an endless stream of empathic remarks may unconsciously want the therapist to be a warm and caring parent. We would also not be surprised to discover that he needs this level of empathic attunement from other people in his life and that this demand strains all of his relationships. Ultimately, we will want to interpret this to him so that he can understand this wish and the way in which it affects his life.

When our primary goal is to support, it may be less important to have patients become conscious of the effect of our empathic remarks. Remember that whether we are primarily uncovering or supporting, our patients are usually in a great deal of emotional pain and need to know that we understand their experience. Trainees conducting psychodynamic psychotherapy sometimes feel inhibited about making too many empathic remarks, as if they're doing something wrong by intervening in this way.

Calls for associations

Calls for associations are the kinds of comments that frequently appear under therapy cartoons, such as the famous "What comes to mind?" One of the reasons these comments are so often spoofed is that they really make people think – and that can be hard. These interventions are invaluable tools for the psychodynamic psycho-therapist. While people tend to think of "free association" as a technique reserved for patients in more uncovering treatments, calls for associations ("Any thoughts about that?") are simply another way to encourage patients to elaborate on and be more aware of their inner experience. Calls for associations in more supporting treatments can have the goal of enhancing patients' self-awareness and helping them understand how their mind works without necessarily exploring deeper unconscious material.

Reflective statements

As discussed in Chapter 13, reflective statements help with empathic listening by allowing the patient to hear how you understand their experience:

Patient	I'm just so fed up with my boss. I'm ready to quit.
Therapist	So it sounds like you're very angry.
Patient	No, it feels more like frustration.

Hearing reflective statements allows patients to be more specific about their thoughts and feelings, enhancing the therapist's ability to understand their experience.

Silence

In psychodynamic psychotherapy, silence *is* an intervention. We make a conscious choice to be silent in a variety of situations. If patients can tolerate it, our remaining silent helps them continue associating on their own in order to move toward unconscious material. Silence can also help slow a patient down, and can sometimes be soothing after a patient has talked about something very difficult. Silence is a potent intervention that we have to titrate carefully according to the patient's comfort level.

Basic interventions

- Directions and psychoeducation
- Questions
- Information
- Empathic remarks
- Calls for associations
- Reflective statements
- Silence

Section 2: Supporting Interventions

Key concepts

Supporting interventions are designed to support deficient or weakened function.
  We support function in two basic ways:

- by *supplying* what patients cannot provide for themselves at that moment
- by *assisting* patients as they try to use their own, weakened function

---

What is support?

Many people think of "being supportive" in psychotherapy as "just being nice" to the patient. It's certainly true that providing a supportive relationship is centrally important in all psychodynamic psychotherapies. Whatever the overarching goals of the treatment, we always offer patients implicit support in our **holding attitude** of acceptance, compassion, and respect, and in our commitment to working together.

But how do we actually offer this support?

To answer that question, let's begin by thinking about the various meanings of **support**. The word comes from the Latin *supportare*, meaning *convey*, *carry*, or *bring up*. Now let's see how many additional meanings you can pick out in the following statements:

> *Flying buttresses support the walls at the Palace of Westminster.*
>
> *His wife's love supported him throughout the long ordeal.*
>
> *She was willing to accept any job to support her family.*
>
> *Leading doctors supported his testimony.*
>
> *Three hundred gathered at Seneca Falls in support of a woman's right to vote.*
>
> *The star was supported by a talented newcomer.*
>
> *Technical support enabled the hospital's computer system to remain in operation.*

Buttressing, holding up, reinforcing, sustaining, supplying, providing for, endorsing, backing, assisting – these words represent the range of therapeutic effects that we hope to achieve in using supporting techniques in psychodynamic psychotherapy. Patients need support when they either lack or are unable to mobilize adequate inner resources. When this is true, rather than simply commenting on their difficulties, we either give them the function they lack, or help them use their own weakened capacities. We offer support to people who – at least in the moment – are unable to provide it for themselves. Consider two examples. First, Ms A:

> Ms A   *I can't make a decision about which accountant to choose – I'm too stupid to know what to do.*

Therapist A   *You feel as if you can't choose an accountant because you are worn down from the divorce and you have grown to feel that only your husband could make decisions.*

The therapist's comment is an *uncovering intervention* ("You feel *as if* you are stupid because you are worn down by the divorce") – it presumes that the patient *has* the capacity to make the decision and just *feels* as if she doesn't. The strategy is to make this assumption conscious so that she can explore it, understand it, and overcome her inhibition. Now consider the situation with Ms B:

Ms B   *I can't make a decision about which accountant to choose – I'm too stupid to know what to do.*

Therapist B   *But actually yesterday you made a terrific decision about your son's school, so I know that you can do it. Let's think together about some of the pros and cons.*

This is a *supporting intervention* – or more accurately, a combination of several supporting interventions. Here, Therapist B presumes that the patient does *not* have the ability in that moment to make the decision on her own and needs the therapist's help to supply or bolster the missing or weakened function. Let's look more closely at what the therapist said and the aim behind his interventions:

But actually yesterday you made a terrific decision about your son's school, so I know you can do it. Let's think together about some of the pros and cons.

In these two sentences, the therapist uses a combination of praise, encouragement, and problem-solving techniques to help the patient reach a decision. But what exactly is being supported? Hearing the patient's own harsh judgments about herself, the therapist praises ("you made a terrific decision") and encourages ("I know you can do it") in order to buoy her **self-esteem**. He helps her to **test reality** by reminding her of her capacities. He supports her ailing **problem-solving (cognitive) abilities** ("let's think about the pros and cons") and strengthens her ability to work in a **relationship** ("let's think together"). The therapist supports these functions to help the patient in the moment, but does it in a way that she might be able to use on her own in the future.

To summarize: *we use supporting interventions to support acutely or persistently weakened function.*

Supplying and assisting

We support function in two basic ways:

- by **supplying** what patients lack and are unable to provide for themselves
- by **assisting** patients to use their own functions

A famous Chinese proverb provides an apt metaphor for these two ways of supporting:

Give a man a fish and you feed him for a day. Teach a man to fish and you feed him for a lifetime.

When we *supply* support, we directly give patients something we think they cannot supply for themselves at that moment (the "fish"). *Assisting* patients to use their own functions is more of a "teaching to fish" approach. We assist when we think that, with some help, patients can mobilize their own resources. In psychodynamic therapy – as in parenting – we continually balance our patients' need for support with their need for autonomy. We want to supply them with as much support as they require while looking for every opportunity to promote self-reliance.

Supplying interventions

Supplying interventions provide the most direct and immediate way to support weakened function. We use supplying interventions when we think that the person is in most need of emergency assistance. It's the tourniquet – if someone is bleeding, we don't say "Oh, look you're bleeding" or even "Now, let's think about some ways to stop that blood" – we just find whatever we can and tie it tight.

Here are some of the major interventions we use to supply missing or grossly impaired function. Remember that many of these, such as encouraging and soothing, can also have non-verbal components, such as facial expressions and tone of voice. The supplying interventions are grouped in clusters according to similarity of aim, and each is followed by specific examples:

Encouraging cluster

In order to have the energy and will to accomplish things, we have to have the feeling that there is a chance that we could succeed. The interventions in this group are designed to provide encouragement to people who can't muster this for themselves. They include the following:

Encouraging

Give it another try – things are usually easier the second time around.

You've done it before. I'm confident you can do it again.

Inspiring and motivating

When I was struggling with calculus as a pre-med, it really helped to get some tutoring.

You really did well on that last report – I'm looking forward to seeing what you do with the next one.

Offering optimism and hope

Your anxiety should lessen over the next few weeks as the medication takes effect.

Your cancer is advanced, but some patients with your condition have had their lives prolonged by years with treatment.

Praising

You made a good decision when you chose to call the emergency room.

You walked away from the fight, which was just the right thing to do.

It took real courage to admit you needed help.

Reminding patients of their capacities

Last time you felt like cutting yourself, you were able to hold off by writing in your journal and calling your friend. I think you can do it again.

You're feeling like you can't take care of your baby, but look at what a great job you've done with your two older children.

Naming cluster

Being able to name things helps patients understand their feelings and experiences. This can enhance self-awareness and their ability to manage emotions. When people can't put things into words, we may have to do it for them. Here are some interventions that involve naming:

Naming emotions

You say you didn't really care about what he said, but you looked as if you wanted to cry just then. I imagine it felt humiliating.

Putting experiences into words

That sounds overwhelming – although you're not saying it directly, what you're telling me is that you had to take care of all those children by yourself.

Redirecting cluster

Sometimes, the best thing we can do to for ourselves is to turn away from a noxious idea or behavior. Often, however, people cannot do this for themselves. This can impair stimulus regulation and their ability to manage emotions. We have many interventions that can help to supply this function in order to lessen anxiety:

Interpreting up

This supports weakened function by offering patients an alternate and generally more positive explanation for what they are feeling:

You're worried that you're not able to make a decision, but it sounds to me like you're carefully weighing your options.

Redirecting

This helps the therapist consciously alter the direction of the conversation:

I can see that worrying that you're going to be in a car accident is upsetting you, but let's start by thinking about how things have been going in your relationship with your daughter in the last week.

Supportively bypassing

Here, the therapist chooses not to address material that might overwhelm or disorganize the patient:

Patient   *I really think that this therapy is helping me and I also think that the dress you're wearing is beautiful.*

Therapist   *I'm glad that you're feeling so good about the work that we're doing.*

Reinforcing and discouraging

This approach consciously and deliberately reinforces more adaptive behaviors and discourages others. These are key interventions for working with defenses in a supporting mode:

Your instinct about taking a friend with you when you visited you mother worked out well last time – you might think about doing it again.

It sounds like doing the hard sell during that job interview didn't work out so well, but you really had success the time you were prepared with lots of questions.

So when the guys on the loading dock make racial slurs, screaming back just seems to make things worse. You've done better when you've avoided that area of the plant whenever possible.

You've said you always feel calmer after yoga classes. Have you considered going more often?

Soothing cluster

Many people have acute or persistent difficulty soothing themselves. This is related to problems with self-esteem regulation, managing emotions, stimulus regulation, impulse control, and capacity for play. Many soothing interventions, including reducing guilt and reassuring, can be very helpful with overly harsh self-appraisal. Note that soothing can sometimes be accomplished with non-verbal interventions, like facial expressions or a calm tone of voice. There are also many verbal interventions that we can make to supply this essential function:

Soothing

Why don't you relax for a minute before you go on – it sounds like you were very overwhelmed today.

Take your time, you're doing a really good job telling me what happened.

Nurturing

I know that Friday is the anniversary of your father's death. Would you like to try to meet that day? I could see you in the afternoon, if that works for you.

Reassuring

I know you're frightened for your daughter, but from what the doctor said it sounds like she's going to be fine.

You'll be all right.

Reducing guilt

You're taking responsibility for something you had no control over.

You did your best with your kids under difficult circumstances.

Remaining calm

Sometimes the sheer act of not getting excited about something can be extremely therapeutic:

Patient	*I just feel completely panicky, like when I leave here I don't know what I'll do.*
Therapist	*I'm sure that we can figure this out together. Now let's think about your options.*

Empathizing

It sounds like that must have hurt you deeply.

Your experience of my canceling the session was that I was leaving you all alone.

Demonstrating interest and understanding

I'd like to hear more about what it felt like during your first year in this country.

I think I understand how desperate you felt when you lost your home.

Explicitly joining

Don't worry, we'll figure this out together.

You're not alone in this – we'll make sure you get the best treatment.

Protecting cluster

When our patients have impaired judgment and impulse control, they may put themselves or others in danger. When this happens, we may have to actively protect them. Here are some ways in which we can do that:

Protecting

It would probably be a good idea to meet in a public place for the first date. You really don't know much about this man other than what is in his profile.

I hear it's really not safe to run alone in the park after dusk.

If you're not wearing a condom, you're taking your life in your hands.

Setting limits

Can we agree that if your weight falls below 75 pounds it will signal that you need to be hospitalized?

You can't come to sessions drunk.

Advising cluster

Although we'd rather have our patients come up with their own ideas, sometimes they can't. This may be related to problems with judgment, cognitive function, or impulse control. When that happens, we supply this function by judiciously **advising, suggesting, guiding,** and **offering opinions**:

Why don't you try writing down your questions before you see the doctor?

Sometimes it helps to have a friend look over your profile to help you put your best foot forward.

You might try acting differently than you feel for just a minute – you can learn to project self-confidence even when you're feeling very insecure.

It's not always the best strategy to tell your wife all your thoughts – sometimes editing might help you not to hurt her feelings.

Structuring cluster

When our patients can't organize their lives and/or their thoughts, we can help them with this:

Slowing down

I know that what your boss said made you want to quit your job immediately but let's take some time to think about how you're going to deal with this.

Structuring

This can help people manage their time in and out of sessions:

> *People generally feel better about themselves if they get out of bed, shower, and get dressed every morning. We should also think about what else you might do during the day so you don't have so much unstructured time on your hands.*

> *Do you feel we've said as much as we need to say about your problems at work, or should we keep talking about that?*

Organizing

This can be supplied or assisted (see later). When we supply, we can help people to organize many aspects of their lives:

> *Because you're so upset, it's hard to know what to do first, but it sounds like after your father's funeral you're going to need to drive your mother home, make sure your aunt has a place to stay, and arrange for a babysitter for the kids.*

Breaking things into manageable parts

People are often overwhelmed by tasks and projects because they don't know how to break them into manageable parts. We can help them with this by supplying or assisting (see below):

> *Getting organized after you're discharged seems overwhelming to you, but there are really only three things that you're going to have to do today – fill your prescriptions, buy some food to put in the refrigerator, and do some laundry.*

Supplying perspective cluster

People can lose varying degrees of perspective on an acute or persistent basis. This can be related to problems with reality testing and lack of self-awareness. When patients are unable to regain perspective, we can supply it for them in the following ways:

Correcting misperceptions

> *You feel that you have no friends in the office, but it's clear to me that Jane and Jill really went out of their way for you. I don't think that you have to feel that no one is in your corner.*

Reframing

> *So another way to look at being single again is that you now have an opportunity to spend much more time with your children.*

Universalizing

Most people feel a sense of loss when their last child goes to college.

In this economy, lots of people are worried about their retirement funds.

Validating

Of course you're exhausted after moving your family cross-country!

That kind of experience would be frightening for anyone.

From everything you've told me, it does sound like your mother doesn't always have your best interests at heart.

Providing practical support outside of the therapeutic relationship

When our patients require even more support than we can provide, our job is to help them get the help they need. This can include hospitalization, a consultation, or offering to speak to their internist. These interventions can supply needed judgment, stimulus regulation, and impulse control:

> *Right now, I think that the chaos in your household is making it even more difficult for you to recover from your depression. Plus, it's clearly so hard for you to stay away from marijuana when it's constantly available there. Coming into the hospital will give us a chance to address your symptoms, and you'll get a quiet place to recuperate, and think about new ways to cope with your anxiety.*

Supporting interventions – supplying type

Encouraging cluster
   Encouraging
   Inspiring and motivating
   Offering optimism and hope
   Praising
   Reminding patients of
      their capacities

Naming cluster
   Naming emotions
   Putting experiences into words

Redirecting cluster
   Interpreting up
   Redirecting
   Supportively bypassing

Soothing cluster
   Soothing
   Nurturing
   Reassuring
   Reducing guilt
   Remaining calm
   Empathizing
   Demonstrating interest and understanding
   Explicitly joining

Protecting cluster
   Protecting
   Setting limits

Advising cluster
   Advising
   Suggesting
   Guiding
   Offering opinions

Reinforcing and discouraging	*Providing practical support outside of the therapeutic relationship*
Structuring cluster	*Supplying perspective cluster*
Slowing down	Correcting misperceptions
Structuring	Reframing
Organizing	Universalizing
Breaking things down into parts	Validating

Assisting interventions

Assisting interventions help people to use their own weakened or faltering functions. This is essentially "function building." We can break these interventions into groups depending on how we're assisting:

Modeling

This is an implicit way to show someone a new way to do something. We consciously model behaviors and ways of thinking to our patients in the hope that they will copy, amend, and incorporate aspects of them:

> *When Mr A said that he wanted to quit therapy, the therapist didn't get upset; rather, he asked Mr A to think about the pros and cons of leaving treatment. This modeled to Mr A a measured way of thinking about a decision.*

Instructing

We can explicitly teach our patients things that they can do to help themselves, such as relaxation exercises, ways to organize themselves, and problem-solving techniques:

> *Since you've been so anxious, I'm going to teach you some practical relaxation exercises. You can practice them at home and we'll go through them here, too. Ready? Close your eyes gently as I count down from five, and just focus on your breathing. Now try to imagine a soothing scene – you love the seashore, so it might be something like floating on a raft. Try to imagine yourself in the scene. Imagine what you smell, what you feel on your skin, what you see.*

Collaborating

We always work alongside our patients, but when we collaborate we're explicit about working jointly. Think about how people learn – actively doing something while working with a teacher is generally more effective than passively listening to a lecture.

When we collaborate, we're essentially saying to patients, "So, now you need to perform a new function. Let's walk through it together. Then you'll have a model for how to do it yourself." This can be done in myriad ways – by talking, by making lists or charts together, or by assigning practice homework. We can collaborate with our patients to assist with almost any function. Generally, if you put the word "joint" in front of a supporting intervention, it becomes collaborative. The basic intervention sounds something like this:

> *Let's work together to . . . (consider alternatives, problem solve, set goals etc.).*

Here are some important examples:

Joint goal setting

> *Let's think about what you want to work on . . .*

This helps people learn to set goals, focus, and organize their thinking. If patients are having trouble defining their own goals, try to make them partners in this process by asking questions like "What are we trying to accomplish here?" Offering suggestions about possible specific and realistic objectives is also helpful:

Patient	*Now that I'm feeling better, what do you think I should work on?*
Therapist	*That's a great question – maybe you can think about some of the things that you usually talk about here to help you answer that.*
Patient	*Well, I always talk about my anger, that would be good to fix.*
Therapist	*Yes, that does come up a lot – sounds like a good goal – although what do you think about saying that it would be good to learn new ways to deal with your anger, rather than saying that you need to "fix" it?*

Joint inquiry

> *Let's think about this together . . .*

This helps people learn how to examine a problem. It involves slowing down enough to deliberate, and thinking about how to analyze something. It can facilitate functions such as judgment, self-awareness, and impulse control. It can also help to manage emotions if the inquiry is about feelings:

Patient	*Julie broke up with me last night – they all do. Why is that?*
Therapist	*That's an interesting question – let's think about it together. Can you think about things that make your last few relationships similar, and things that make them different? This might help us begin to understand what's going on.*

Jointly exploring alternative ways of thinking or acting

> *Let's think about other ways to look at that/other things you could do . . .*

We use this intervention when we think that our patients' rigid thinking disrupts their ability to think of alternatives. It can help with reality testing, judgment, cognition, relationships with others, and impulse control:

> *I know that you feel that you have no alternative but to stay in this job that you hate, but let's think together about whether there might be other alternatives. What about that job you were offered last year in Washington, DC?*

Joint reality testing

> *Are there other ways to think about . . . ?*

As opposed to correcting misperceptions (which supplies a function), this engages the patient in thinking about whether there might be other ways to perceive a given situation. This can be helpful when trying to assess whether someone is psychotic; it can also be helpful when trying to help someone to assess his/her capacities in a realistic way. You can think of this as a special category of **jointly exploring alternatives**, but it's so important that it deserves to be considered on its own.

> *You've said that you think the boss is always talking about you – but can you think of other reasons that he might have been talking to your co-worker in his office today?*

Jointly thinking through consequences

> *Let's think about what would happen if . . .*

Patients often get in trouble because they can't see ahead to the consequences of their actions. If we see that this is a problem, we can work with them to develop this function. It often involves planning and predicting contingencies together. This can help to improve judgment, impulse control, and executive functions:

> *I know that your anger at your wife makes you want to leave immediately, but where would you go? Let's think through this together.*

Joint problem solving

> *Let's try to figure this out together . . .*

We do this so naturally that we may forget that some patients lack effective ways to solve problems. Collaborative problem solving involves weighing options and considering pros and cons together. This can also help to improve relationships with others, judgment, stimulus regulation, managing emotions, and executive function:

> Patient   *I'm so wound up about which internship I should take, I can't do any of my schoolwork. I just don't know how to decide.*
>
> Therapist   *We can try to figure this out together . . . Why don't you tell me about both of them and then we can think about the pros and cons of each.*

Jointly organizing/structuring

> *Let's think about how you can organize this . . .*

As before, we can either supply organization or assist patients in coming up with their own plans:

> *I think that you're getting stuck on writing this paper because it seems like a big, amorphous roadblock. Why don't we work together to figure out a plan for how to begin? Why don't you start by thinking about what all of the components are, and then we can start to prioritize them together.*

Jointly working on projects

> *Let's work on this together . . .*

This includes projects such as formulating schedules, organizing activities, or developing a budget. These projects can be worked on in sessions, or they can include work done at home that is brought in for review. This type of intervention presumes that the person has limited capacity to do projects like this without some assistance. It can help with almost any function:

> *Sounds like you're having trouble putting together a budget. You need that in order to figure out how much you can spend per month on an apartment. Why don't you make a list of all of your monthly expenses and bring it to your next session? Then we can work together on putting together a budget for you.*

Encouraging mentalization

> *How do you imagine that might make me feel?*

As discussed in Chapter 4, the ability to understand one's own mind and be able to imagine the minds of others is called **mentalization**. Patients who have difficulty mentalizing often presume that others feel exactly as they do. We can support problematic mentalization by asking patients to describe their own feelings and the feelings of others – particularly those of the therapist:

> *When I canceled the session last week, you said that it was because I'm tired of hearing you complain about your mother. Can you think of any other reason why I might have cancelled?*

> *Can you think of any other reason why your wife might have been angry with you last night?*

Supporting interventions – assisting type

Modeling

Instructing

Collaborating

> joint goal setting
>
> joint inquiry
>
> jointly exploring alternative ways of thinking
>
> joint reality testing
>
> jointly thinking through consequences
>
> joint problem solving
>
> jointly organizing/structuring
>
> jointly working on projects
>
> encouraging mentalization

Supplying and assisting – a comparison

Supplying and assisting interventions target many of the same functions – the difference is the way in which they provide support. For example, **correcting misperceptions** is a supplying intervention and **joint reality testing** is an assisting intervention, but they both address the person's faltering capacity to *test reality*. Here is an example of each to demonstrate the difference:

Correcting misperceptions

Patient	*I think you made my session first thing in the morning because you want to get it over with.*
Therapist	*I can see that you're upset about that, but actually, if I remember correctly, you wanted to be seen early because of your old work schedule. If your schedule has changed, we could try to find a time that is better for you.*

Joint reality testing

Patient	*I think that you made my session first thing in the morning because you want to get it over with.*
Therapist	*I can see that you're upset about that, but are you sure that that's true? Do you think that there could be any other reason?*

It's also important to remember that many supplying interventions implicitly assist function because helping one function supports others. For example, *encouraging* someone supplies self-esteem, and this could help them to engage in a relationship, make a decision, or solve a problem.

Section 3: Uncovering Interventions

Key concepts

Uncovering interventions make unconscious material available to the conscious mind. They include:

- confrontation
- clarification
- interpretation

Uncovering interventions

There are two definitions of the word *interpret*:

- to explain the meaning of, make understandable
- to translate

Both of these definitions are relevant to the way we use the word in psychodynamic psychotherapy. When we interpret, we explain the meaning of something that has been unconscious – to do this, we have to translate it from the language of the unconscious (**primary process**) to the language of consciousness (**secondary process**; see Chapter 2). This is quite a task, and is best thought of as a process, rather than as a stand-alone intervention. Many of the basic interventions discussed in the basic interventions section of this chapter must occur before the formal process of interpretation begins. We need to give directions about free association, ask questions about behavior, and call for associations in order to get the information we need to begin to understand unconscious meanings. Once we think that we are dealing with something unconscious, we can begin the interpretative process, which is usually thought of as consisting of three steps:

- confrontation
- clarification
- interpretation [2]

Like the process of going from ambient listening → filtered listening → focused listening, the interpretative process is like the movie director going from the panoramic shot to the close-up. Remember that we should only begin this process if we think that our tripartite measure of readiness (phase of treatment, state of the therapeutic alliance, and current function) indicates that the patient is ready/able to use the unconscious material that we aim to uncover.

Confrontation

In everyday conversation, we generally use the word "confrontation" to describe a situation or interaction that is somewhat aggressive or that involves some force. For example, someone might say, "I confronted my daughter with her bad behavior and then grounded her." In psychodynamic psychotherapy, however, we use the word differently. Here, confrontation is the process by which we interest patients in what is going on in their mind. When we think that we might be nearing something unconscious, our first step is confrontation.

For example, let's say that Mr A is talking about something and suddenly stops. We hypothesize that this might be the result of an unconscious thought or feeling. We don't know what it is, but we are interested and want the patient to be interested too. A confrontation in this situation might be:

> I noticed that you just stopped talking.

We observe a phenomenon and hope the patient will be curious about it, talk about it, and in this way help move us toward the unconscious thought or feeling that stopped the associations. The patient might then say, "I feel blocked – like I have nothing to say." Now we have an idea that the patient stopped talking because his mind shut off at that moment. We can then begin to think about why that might have happened. If patients make slips of the tongue, abruptly change topics, or obviously avoid talking about affect, we use confrontation to bring these phenomena to their awareness. Although we are not using the word confrontation to mean "calling someone out" on their behavior, we are pointing out something to patients that they might not have noticed.

Clarification

Clarification helps bring the unconscious into focus by linking similar phenomena. For example, if we notice that Mr A always seems to stop talking right after coming into the Monday session, we can comment on this – it's no longer merely a confrontation of a single event. When we use clarification, we're not only commenting on the feeling of being blocked (confrontation); instead, we're linking times when the patient felt blocked and suggesting that the fact that this always happens on a Monday might have meaning. A good clarification might be:

> It seems like it is always hardest for you to talk on Monday mornings.

Clarifications are aimed at helping you and your patients elucidate patterns. A good way to encourage them to do this is to ask, "Does that feel familiar to you?" Here's an example:

Patient	I thought that doing extra work for my boss was going to impress him, but I just ended up feeling like he was taking advantage of me. It was so frustrating!
Therapist	It sounds frustrating – does that situation feel familiar to you? Have you ever felt like that before with someone else, maybe even someone in your family?
Patient	Now that you ask, it always happened with my dad. He just wanted us to help around the house – always complained that we never did anything – so I used to wake up early to

do things, like make his breakfast, or empty the dishwasher, and all he did was complain that I didn't do other things. I couldn't win.

Therapist   *So that's a pattern that feels familiar.*

Interpretation

An interpretation is an intervention that explains a conscious feeling or behavior as being caused by something unconscious. Thus, it can always be reduced to what we'll call the **because schematic**:

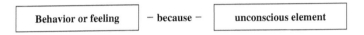

Going back to Mr A, let's say that in his Thursday session, the patient is talking about a dream when he becomes tearful and says:

I can't believe that I have to wait until Monday to come back. That feels like forever. I'm so open now – opening up again feels so painful.

Now we have some data on which to base an interpretation of his blocking behavior. We hypothesize that his wish to avoid a painful feeling is what stops him from talking freely. The interpretation could sound something like:

Maybe that's why you find it so difficult to talk at the beginning of your Monday sessions – you're protecting yourself from the pain of opening up again.

Here it is in the **because schematic**:

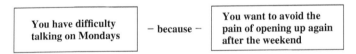

This is more than an observation, it's an attempt to explain the phenomenon by linking it to something unconscious.

Here are some interpretations so that you can hear what they sound like:

Perhaps you frequently pick women like Ann because you're less afraid they will reject you.

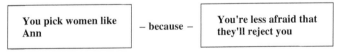

I wonder if your impulsive decision to become pregnant, which has left you feeling so anxious, was your attempt to keep your husband from leaving you.

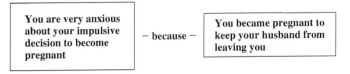

Maybe you're having trouble paying me on time because you feel that if I really cared about you I'd treat you for free.

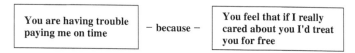

Note that all of these interpretations start with words like "perhaps." This is intentional: *interpretations are speculative by definition – they're hypotheses.* We invite patients to speculate with us, rather than giving them the "word from on high." We're always interested in engaging patients in being curious about their behavior, and the more our interventions convey this to them, the better.

Genetic interpretation

A genetic interpretation is one that not only explains unconscious material, but also links it to the person's early past [3]. The "because schematic" for a genetic interpretation looks like this:

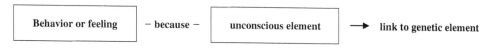

For example, let's say Mr A tells us that his parents were divorced and had joint custody, and that he split his weeks between his mother's and father's homes. Just when he felt comfortable, he had to go to the other place, where it took time for him to "warm up." Given this, we could speculate that the defensive blocking is something he has been doing since childhood. If the patient seems affectively connected to this historical material, we could venture a genetic interpretation that might sound like this:

I think that your trouble talking on Mondays is a way of protecting yourself from painful feelings, just like it was when you had difficulty warming up when you got to one parent's house from the other's.

Here's the schematic:

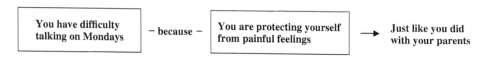

The genetic interpretation adds that last piece – the link to the patient's early history. Genetic interpretations should be used sparingly and carefully, and only when the patient's affect is clearly linked to the early material. Otherwise, genetic interpretations can take the patient away from the heat of the "here and now" situation in the treatment and can foster intellectualization.

Constructing new narratives

In the early days of psychodynamic psychotherapy, therapists talked about **reconstruction**, which meant literally trying to reconstruct what happened in the patient's early history [4]. This used to be a major therapeutic goal of psychoanalysis and psychodynamic psychotherapy. These days, however, most people think that this can never be done – that even with photographs, videos, letters, and stories, we can never really know what happened during a person's childhood. Now we generally think that the best we can do is to try to construct a meaningful narrative of the past that helps patients make sense of their thoughts and feelings about early relationships and experiences [5]. We frequently intervene in a way that helps facilitate the construction of personal narrative, and this often involves uncovering unconscious material. For example, as Mr A talks about the difficulty of being shuttled from house to house each week, we might begin to suspect that he has blocked out a childhood theory that he had to keep moving because his mother wanted more time to see new boyfriends. So we could say to him:

> *It sounds like you now have the idea that the reason that you had to suffer through being shuttled from house to house was because of your mother's wish to have more time to date.*

Here, we're not saying that we *know* this was true, but rather that the patient is developing new ideas about why things happened the way they did. Helping patients construct personal narratives can be enormously helpful to them as they try to make sense of themselves, their lives, and the workings of their minds.

Now that we have reviewed the basic elements of the listen/reflect/intervene model, we can begin to apply it to the major kinds of data that we hear from our patients:

- affect
- resistance
- transference
- countertransference
- unconscious fantasy, conflict, and defenses
- dreams
- working through (Part Seven)
- ending (Part Seven)

Uncovering interventions

- Confrontation
- Clarification
- Interpretation
- Genetic interpretation
- Constructing new narratives

Suggested activities

Activity 1

Consider the following exchange between a therapist and her patient and see if you can:

- list the different supporting interventions the therapist uses
- decide whether the intervention is supplying or assisting
- determine what functions are being supported

> *The patient is a 24-year-old college senior who presented several weeks earlier with "out of the blue" panic attacks. His parents divorced when he was 3 and he was raised by his mother until age 10, when she placed him in foster care because "she couldn't take me anymore. I had temper tantrums. Plus, she needed to be able to go on the road for her singing career." He tells you he "lucked out" with his foster parents who are caring and, recognizing his intelligence, helped get him a college scholarship. The patient's major preoccupation is escalating tension in his relationship with his girlfriend of one year. This has been the latest and most long-lasting in a series of tumultuous relationships. The patient is currently sober, but when these relationships end disastrously – as they invariably do – he spirals into binge drinking and cocaine use. He had to drop out of college on two occasions to "get myself straightened out."*

Patient	*I can't decide what to get my girlfriend for our first anniversary. That's the paper anniversary, right? Aren't you supposed to get presents that match the anniversary?*
Therapist	*I suppose that depends how important that sort of thing is to your girlfriend. Maybe it would help to focus on what she might like.*
Patient	*That's the problem! She's so hard to please.*
Therapist	*Have you asked her what she'd like?*
Patient	*She gets upset if I don't automatically know what she wants, (sarcastically) like I should be able to read her mind by this point.*
Therapist	*(smiles) That sure would make things easier. (more seriously) I guess it's frustrating not knowing for sure what would please her, especially when it seems like it would be so easy for her just to tell you.*
Patient	*Exactly!*
Therapist	*What's the worst thing that could happen if she hates the gift?*
Patient	*Sometimes I feel like I have to do everything right, or she'll break up with me.*
Therapist	*Do you think that's really likely?*
Patient	*Well, no, not really. But she'll be, like, all sulky about it.*
Therapist	*That would be disappointing, but not the end of the world, I guess. If that happens, maybe you could offer to take her out shopping for something she might like better.*
Patient	*(skeptical) I don't know. I guess so.*

> Therapist   (silently noting that patient seems to feel he isn't getting what he needs from her,
>   too) Why don't you tell me a little more about her and maybe we can come up with
>   some ideas together.

Comment

The patient starts with a seemingly innocuous request for **information** to help with his
decision about buying a gift, which the therapist provides. She then asks a series of
questions in an effort to engage him in **joint problem solving**. The therapist notes
(silently) that the patient seems to see himself as a well-meaning, caring boyfriend trying
his best to please a difficult girlfriend who won't give him the answers he needs; she hears
a similar pattern echoed in his childhood experience of abandonment by his mother, and
wonders if the same sort of pattern may already be emerging in therapy. However, she
decides to **supportively bypass** any mention of these patterns, at least for the time being,
because:

- It is early in the treatment.
- The therapeutic alliance is still tenuous.
- The patient describes a history of problematic function, including tenuous impulse
  control, poor tolerance of anxiety, and stormy relationships.

By observing that the "not knowing" makes him "nervous," the therapist is **naming
the emotion** and **validating his feelings** (without suggesting that his anger might
be a way of fending off awareness of his anxiety about losing an important
relationship). She **thinks through consequences** with him and the patient
responds by letting down his guard and volunteering his deeper fears of abandonment. The therapist ends by making a concrete **suggestion** about alternative
behavior that might minimize his anxiety and uses the collaborative intervention
of **working on a joint project**.

Activity 2

How would you describe the therapist's strategy in this vignette?

> The patient has been late for sessions a few weeks in a row due to problems with her childcare
> arrangements. Today, her sitter told her that she will be unable to come on Tuesdays, which
> is the day she has therapy at 4:00 PM. She asks the therapist if she can move her session to
> another day. The therapist offers her the 4:00 PM session time on Mondays. The patient
> begins to cry, stating that she knows she deserves to be punished for having been late and for
> having to make this request. Here is the interchange that follows:
>
> Therapist   It sounds like you are having a very strong reaction to my offer of a Monday
>   session. Can you tell me more about what you are feeling?
>
> Patient   I think you must not want to see me every week since Mondays are often holidays,
>   and it means we will not meet on a regular basis. I think you are tired of my coming
>   late and frustrated by my repeated requests for time changes. This way you will
>   have a break from me whenever there are holidays.

Therapist   *It does sound like you are having a strong reaction to my offer. In fact, I wasn't thinking that when I offered you the Monday time. It is just that Monday is the only day when I have a 4:00 PM session, which is what you have now. I can look for other possibilities, but first, let's also try to understand your reaction. Without knowing why I offered you the Monday session, you assumed that I was angry and acting punitively toward you.*

Comment

The therapist is exploring the patient's reaction to the schedule discussion. By correcting the patient's misperception of why she was offered a Monday session, the therapist is encouraging **mentalization**. This helps the patient imagine that the therapist may have separate reasons for offering this time other than those the patient fears. This is a helpful moment to also consider whether the patient has similar reactions to other people in her life outside of therapy.

Activity 3

How would you label the following interventions?

1. Patient   *Whenever I come in here after I've just gone swimming, I feel really disoriented.*

   Therapist   *You said the same thing last week.*

2. Patient   *So I had a dream last night that I was in jail and didn't know why and there were two black horses in there with me. What do you think that means?*

   Therapist   *Sometimes before we know what a dream means, we can look at different parts of it to see what comes to mind about them. For example, I wonder what comes to mind about black horses?*

3. Patient   *This divorce is going on forever. When I started, I thought we'd be done in a year. I can't even think about what it's doing to the kids.*

   Therapist   *It's taken a lot out of you this year.*

4. Patient   *The office always smells bad after that patient leaves. I prefer Mondays, when he's not here before me. There's no smell then.*

   Therapist   *Maybe you'd prefer to feel like I didn't have any other patients.*

5. Patient   *I was fine when you were on vacation. No problems at all. In fact it was nice to not have to get up so early in the morning to come here. It's funny, though – I couldn't sleep in – I kept waking up at the same time as if I were coming to a session.*

   Therapist   *Although it does sound like you were fine, maybe you had some feelings about not being here.*

6. Patient   *This whole thing with my mother is looming in front of me like a black hole. I don't even know how to get started on it – I just feel like sleeping for a few days.*

   Therapist   *Let's look at it together – why don't we start with the feelings that you had when she forgot your birthday?*

7. Patient	*My son hates me. That's why he never calls. I think that he's been calling and hanging up a lot. My wife thinks that I'm crazy, but I'm sure that that's what's going on.*
Therapist	*Do you think that there's any other way to look at what's been happening?*

Comment

1. **Clarification**: This brings together two phenomena that are related.

2. **Psychoeducation and call for associations**: First the therapist instructs about exploration of a dream, then she directly asks for associations.

3. **Empathic remark**: The therapist is simply empathizing with the patient's difficulties.

4. **Interpretation**: This brings unconscious material to the surface. It could be rewritten as: "You are bothered by the smell on Monday because you would prefer to be able to feel that I don't have any other patients."

5. **Confrontation**: The therapist is calling some potential ambivalence to the patient's attention.

6. **Collaborative intervention**: Breaking things into parts, questions – the therapist helps the patient to look at something that looks impenetrable by suggesting that they work together and then asking specific questions to get started.

7. **Joint reality testing**: The therapist explores the patient's ability to look at his conviction another way.

Activity 4

Are these interpretations?

1. You missed a few sessions the last time I was away, too.

2. You're feeling anxious, but I think that you're actually very angry.

3. Maybe it was your mother's selfishness that made you stay on the west coast for all those years.

4. Do you think that your anxiety about getting married is what is making you delay looking for a wedding dress?

5. What do you make of the fact that you keep changing the subject?

Comment

Remember that all interpretations can be put in the **because schematic**:

1. **Clarification**: This just links like behaviors.

2. **Interpretation**: "You're feeling anxious because it's too uncomfortable to feel angry."

3. **Interpretation**: "You stayed on the west coast because you were escaping your mother's selfishness."

4. **Interpretation**: "You are delaying looking for a wedding dress because you are anxious about getting married."

5. **Confrontation**: This just calls a behavior to the patient's attention.

Chapter 18: References

1. Schlesinger, H.J. (2003) *The Texture of Treatment: On the Matter of Psychoanalytic Technique*, Analytic Press, Hillsdale, NJ.
2. Greenson, R. (1967) *The Technique and Practice of Psychoanalysis*, International University Press, New York. For an alternate conceptualization of confrontation and clarification, see Caligor, E., Kernberg, O.F., and Clarkin J.F. (2007) *Handbook of Dynamic Psychotherapy for Higher Level Personality Pathology*, American Psychiatric Publishing, Washington, DC.
3. Auchincloss, E.L., and Samberg, E. (2012) *Psychoanalytic Terms and Concepts*, Yale University Press, New Haven, p. 121.
4. Auchincloss, E.L., and Samberg E. (2012) *Psychoanalytic Terms and Concepts*, Yale University Press, New Haven, p. 219–221.
5. Schafer, R. (1992) *Retelling a Life: Narration and Dialogue in Psychoanalysis*, Basic Books, New York.

PART FIVE: Conducting a Psychodynamic Psychotherapy: Technique

---

Key concepts

As our patients talk in psychodynamic psychotherapy, we hear many things.
Listening for certain important elements helps us to understand our patients in order to:

- uncover unconscious material
- support weakened function

These important elements include:

- affect
- resistance
- transference
- countertransference

Psychodynamic Psychotherapy: A Clinical Manual, Second Edition. Deborah L. Cabaniss, Sabrina Cherry, Carolyn J. Douglas and Anna Schwartz.
© 2017 John Wiley & Sons, Ltd. Published 2017 by John Wiley & Sons, Ltd.

- unconscious fantasy, conflict, defense
- dreams

All psychodynamic psychotherapies use both uncovering and supporting techniques. Regardless of the predominant mode, the therapist should be prepared to shift flexibly from one to the other depending on the patient's needs.

All patients need some support in order to feel safe and understood in the therapy.

Listening for important elements

In any given psychotherapy session, many themes emerge. As we discussed in Chapter 16, we use ambient listening at the beginning of the session, allowing our attention to be drawn from topic to topic by the patient's flow of associations. However, as we begin to filter and focus, there are certain elements on which we hone in. These include patients' **affect**, ways in which they work against the treatment process (**resistance**), their feelings about us (**transference**), as well as their **fantasies**, **conflicts**, and **dreams**. We also listen carefully to our own feelings about the patient (**countertransference**). These elements are particularly helpful in moving the patient toward unconscious material and in pointing us toward areas of compromised function. Each chapter in this part of the manual will discuss one of these essential elements. When you conduct a psychotherapy session, you should be able to name the dominant affect, resistance, transference, countertransference, unconscious fantasies, conflicts, and defenses in that session. The review activity at the end of this part will allow you to practice this.

Using a mix of techniques

Based on what you have learned in the initial evaluation about the patient's strengths, problems, and needs, you are now able to make decisions about whether the basic overarching approach that will best help your patient is:

- uncovering unconscious material, or
- providing support

Although this will help you understand your predominant therapeutic strategy at the beginning of treatment, the reality is that *psychodynamic therapists typically use a blend of supporting and uncovering techniques in all treatments*. The particular "mix" varies from patient to patient, and sometimes from moment to moment with the same patient. Your choices about this are guided by your understanding of what aspects of the patient's emotional and mental functioning need "support," and how able the patient is to tolerate learning about unconscious material. If you have chosen a predominantly uncovering approach you can still use supporting interventions, and if you have chosen a predominantly supporting approach you can still make uncovering interventions.

All patients need some support

Remember, however, that *all* patients need some support. Healthier patients often need nothing more then the implicit support present in all psychodynamic psychotherapy – the feeling of being heard and understood in a non-judgmental atmosphere. Some patients may need more support at the beginning of treatment to help them feel safe in the therapeutic relationship. Still others may need more support later in the therapy when a crisis occurs. Finally, some patients may require consistent support throughout the treatment.

With this framework, let's move on to listen, reflect, and intervene with the major themes in a psychodynamic psychotherapy session.

19 Affect

> ## Key concepts
>
> Generally, the patient's primary affect leads us to the dominant theme of the session. This is called the **principle of affective dominance.**
>
> Understanding the patient's dominant affect is the best way to choose where to focus and how to intervene.
>
> Affects can be:
>
> - conscious and unconscious
> - conveyed through words and behaviors
>
> Supporting techniques help patients manage their feelings more adaptively.
>
> Uncovering interventions help patients become aware of unconscious affects, improve negative affects, and use affects to understand other unconscious material.
>
> Helping patients to clarify and express feelings has been consistently linked to more positive outcomes in psychodynamic psychotherapy [1].

Why is affect important in psychodynamic psychotherapy?

What are the things we remember most in life? The times we were sad, joyful, frightened; the moments that moved us and were full of feeling. Insight without affect is like a sunset without color. Affect is primary – it fluidly connects us to early, unconscious experiences in a way that mere thoughts cannot. As a psychodynamic psychotherapist, affect is your compass and your weathervane. If you stay close to the patient's affect, even when you're lost you'll have an idea of where to take your next step.

Yet affect can also cause tremendous difficulties for our patients. Many disorders we treat relate to problems with affect, such as anxiety, depression, mania, irritability, and panic. Identifying these affects and how our patients manage them is central to making a diagnosis, assessing function, and selecting treatments. In psychodynamic psychotherapy, we focus on patients' affects not only to make a diagnosis, but also to elucidate aspects of their unconscious experience and to improve their affect management.

Affects can be conscious or unconscious, verbal or non-verbal, expressed openly or defended against. As psychodynamic psychotherapists we have to learn to hear all of these and to use them in the following ways:

Psychodynamic Psychotherapy: A Clinical Manual, Second Edition. Deborah L. Cabaniss, Sabrina Cherry, Carolyn J. Douglas and Anna Schwartz.
© 2017 John Wiley & Sons, Ltd. Published 2017 by John Wiley & Sons, Ltd.

To understand what is most important to patients at any given time

During psychodynamic psychotherapy sessions, patients talk about many things. The best way to determine what is most important to them is to listen for the elements that are most closely connected to affect. For example, let's say a patient spends 20 minutes talking in a near monotone about his work, but then becomes almost tearful during a momentary reference to the going-away party for his research assistant. Follow the affect – it's a sure bet that there's something about this departure that is important to him.

To help patients to better understand their feelings

In order to understand ourselves, we need to understand our affects. Patients can have different kinds of problems related to understanding their feelings, and we can help with all of them:

- **Difficulty experiencing feelings:** Patients who are unaware of their feelings have problems in many aspects of their lives. Not knowing what we feel impacts our ability to make choices, impedes our ability to connect to other people, and decreases our enjoyment of life.

- **Difficulty identifying feelings:** Some patients enter treatment unable to identify and express what they feel. It can be frightening to experience feelings without knowing what they are. In addition, some emotions, such as anger, fear, envy, competition, and shame may be particularly difficult to identify and acknowledge. The capacity to label our affects gives us a sense of control and ultimately a way to reflect on what we feel, to communicate with others, and to understand our reactions.

- **Difficulty linking feelings and experience:** For some patients, feelings may appear to come out of nowhere. As with learning to identify and label one's feelings, making links between affect and experience can also be a tremendous relief and can replace helplessness with a sense of control. Connecting feelings and their precipitants gives patients the capacity to communicate more clearly with others, get what they need from the world, and ultimately develop insight into how they make others feel.

To help patients manage affects

Some patients are flooded or overwhelmed by their feelings. Almost all patients need help with this, but for some this may be a focus of treatment. As the therapist, your ability to tolerate the intensity of the patient's affect, to stay calm, and to help put feelings into words offers a healthy model for managing affects and can serve a powerful "containing" function [1–4]. Helping people learn about the behaviors they employ to manage or defend against affects can also be helpful.

To help patients improve negative affects

Some patients exhibit an abundance of negative feelings, such as a tendency to be angry in close relationships, despairing about the future, or full of shame. As psychodynamic psychotherapists we listen for factors in their early history that may account for these pervasive negative affect states and guide our uncovering work to link their mood and their history. Negative affects in the transference can also be a focus of this work (see Chapter 21).

To help patients express feelings

Talking about feelings can be enormously therapeutic. Having bottled-up feelings is enough to cause mood and anxiety symptoms. There are myriad reasons that people don't talk about their feelings, including being ashamed of them and not having someone with whom they feel safe enough to talk. A lot of what we do as psychodynamic psychotherapists is designed to help patients talk about feelings. It has also been found that helping people express feelings in therapy is positively correlated with outcome – so talking about affects is another **common factor**.

> **Common factor** – being able to talk about feelings

Now let's move on to our techniques for working with affect.

Technique
Listening

If you think of yourself as a hiker looking for a path through the woods, affect signals the trailhead. If you start with the affect, you will generally proceed toward the dominant themes in the session. This is sometimes referred to as the **principle of affective dominance** [2,3]. Thus, as we begin to listen to the patient during a session, our first order of business is to determine the dominant affect. This is not always so easy, since the dominant affect may be unconscious. So how do we do this? Here are some questions to ask yourself while you are listening to patients that can serve as guidelines for identifying the dominant affect:

What is the patient feeling?

When patients directly express feelings that connect to what they are saying, the affect is obvious. For example, a 35-year-old single mother of two comes to her session crying because, once again, she has been thwarted in her effort to obtain a green card. She is sad and frustrated, and she exhibits this using both words and behavior. Remember, though, that there may be deeper, unconscious feelings that patients don't express directly.

Is there an absence of feelings?

Sometimes patients talk about something that seems significant, yet do not express any emotion. For example, if a patient shows no emotion while telling you that his girlfriend just broke up with him, you experience the absence of feelings. This is often a clue that the patient is defending against a painful affect. Depending on the patient and the particular circumstances, you may choose to ask more about it or to respect the patient's defenses and **supportively bypass** the moment. Also, remember that the absence of feelings may be the symptom of a mood disorder, such as depression.

Do the affects match what the patient is describing?

Ask yourself whether the affect that patients express matches the content of what they are saying. As we discussed in Chapter 16, listening for this type of incongruity can help lead us to important material. For example:

> *A 65-year-old retired barber chuckles as he tells you that he has just lost money on the stock market.*

The patient's affect does not match the experience he's describing, suggesting that this is something to explore further.

Does the affect change during the course of a session, and if so, why?

There are many reasons why patients' affects change during sessions. They may be hesitant and anxious at the start of a session and relax as they start talking, be upset by something that you say, have a thought that changes how they feel, or close up as the session comes to an end. For example, a young patient may begin excitedly to tell you about her relationship, and then become more subdued as she remembers that you are about to go on vacation. The patient's ability to express emotions has decreased because of her feelings about the upcoming separation from you.

Does the patient's behavior in the session indicate an affect?

If patients do not directly express their affect in words, they may express it in behavior. Sitting rigidly, fidgeting, talking softly, pounding the chair, giggling, or crying all convey affect in subtle or obvious ways. Ask yourself whether the affect-laden behavior is consistent with the content. Thinking about how patients look in the waiting area and how they come into your office can also be very good clues to their dominant affect. For example, a patient who is sitting with his head in his hands in the waiting area or who comes bounding into the office is clearly communicating affect.

Does the patient's behavior outside of therapy suggest an affect?

The patient's behavior outside of therapy may suggest an affect that is not directly verbalized. For example, a newly married 32-year-old woman says that a conversation with her mother about weekend plans was "no big deal," but then went home and ate an entire box of Oreos. In this case, the patient's behavior outside of the office gives you a good clue to how she is feeling.

What is the quality of the affect? Is the patient's affect excessive or superficial?

Sometimes patients appear to express more emotion than we would expect in a given instance. How much crying is appropriate when one gets a bad grade on a paper? How angry should one be after sitting in traffic? There are no right answers to these questions, but it's important to wonder about the meaning of reactions that seem excessive or superficial. An example of a superficial affect could be a 40-year-old man whose wife has just miscarried for the third time after their fourth trial of *in vitro* fertilization, who calmly states, "I guess we have to go back to the drawing board." In this case you might wonder what he feels about having a baby and why he is so emotionless about this disappointment.

How do patients manage their affects? Do they seem overwhelmed by what they feel?

Some patients become overwhelmed by intense feeling states and may engage in self-defeating behaviors to soothe themselves, avoid, or manage their discomfort. Some manage intense affects with shopping sprees, drinking excessively, sexual acting out, and even suicidal thoughts. Listen for these and other behaviors as clues that patients are not able to manage their affects.

Reflecting

Next, we turn to the choosing and readiness principles to consider how to intervene. Ask yourself whether the dominant affect is near the surface and check in with your countertransference. Think about the phase of treatment, the therapeutic alliance, and the patient's function.

One guiding principle is that affect is almost always a good place to start. Empathizing with an expressed emotion or labeling an inchoate one is almost always a helpful, safe approach that offers relief, provides support, and points the way toward deeper material.

Which affect do I choose?

People are complex, and they do not express isolated emotions. How do we know which affect to focus on? As we begin to reflect, we think about which affect or affects seem to be closest to awareness. Which affect is mentioned most? Which affect explains the patient's behavior? The dominant affect may or may not be the one the patient says is most important. Our job is to discern whether it is conscious or not, using the questions and clues listed in the earlier section on listening.

Choosing the surface affect

Sometimes the best choice is the affect that feels most pressing to the patient. For example, a 30-year-old woman is clearly anxious as she tells you that she and her husband are trying to have a child. She says that she knows she just ovulated, but that it is too early to know whether she has conceived. Despite her anxiety, she says that if she knew that she weren't pregnant, she'd at least be able to drink at the party she's going to that night. In this case, the surface affect is the patient's anxiety regarding her potential pregnancy. Her comment about drinking, however, suggests to you that other, deeper affects might be present – such as ambivalence about becoming a mother and giving up certain pleasures. Given the patient's anxiety, the better part of valor is to stay with the expressed affect and to empathize with the patient's anxiety, saying something like, "That limbo state of not knowing is very difficult. Can you say more about that feeling?" This tack is particularly helpful for new patients, patients who are overwhelmed by anxiety, or patients who have difficulty identifying their feelings on their own [2].

Choosing an unconscious affect or an affect that is being defended against

Sometimes, in contrast, the better choice is the deeper, hidden feeling. With an established patient with whom you have a good alliance, focusing on feelings that are being defended against can be extremely helpful. Your countertransference is often your best guide to identifying hidden feelings. For example, let's say that a patient who has been in treatment with you for many years and with whom you have a good alliance seems cheerful as he tells you that he was just turned down for a job he really wanted. Having heard all the details of the job pursuit and interview process, you realize that you were rooting for him and that you feel deflated as he tells you about the rejection. You reflect that you are experiencing the feeling that he is defending against, and you say:

> *I know how much you wanted this job, yet you seem almost cheerful as you talk about this. Maybe it's too hard to think about being disappointed.*

This helps the patient to learn more about himself and to use his feelings to deal more effectively with this blow.

Intervening

Basic interventions

Psychoeducation, **direction**, **questions**, and **empathy** are essential for helping the patient focus on affects. They are often stepping-stones toward working interpretively or supportively in sessions.

Let's return to the patient who ate the box of Oreos after discussing weekend plans with her mother. You might first intervene with some **psychoeducation** and a **question** to let her know that one way to understand her binge is to think about what she might have been feeling right before the episode. You might phrase this as follows:

> For some people, binging is often a way of coping with uncomfortable feelings. What were you feeling right before you started eating cookies?

Or:

> What were you feeling after the conversation with your mother?

If the patient says that she felt guilty because she had to tell her mother that she was going to her in-laws for Mother's Day, you could **empathize** by saying, "That must have been difficult." Expressing your empathy communicates interest and understanding to your patients and helps them discuss difficult, shame-filled affects.

Supporting interventions

We select supportive interventions when our aim is to:

- lessen (or contain) intolerable affects that threaten the patient or the therapeutic relationship, and/or
- improve the patient's ability to manage and regulate affects.

We all get overwhelmed by our emotions now and then. One aspect of psychological health is the ability to manage these feelings and to continue functioning productively, either by seeking appropriate help and comfort from others, or by finding ways to soothe and calm oneself. However, some people are unable to manage intense affects on their own. Their emotions overwhelm them, impairing their everyday functioning. As has already been mentioned, they often rely on self-destructive activities (such as drinking, using drugs, binging, cutting themselves, and engaging in unsafe sexual activity) to manage strong feelings. Impaired affect regulation can be acute or persistent. Its causes vary from psychiatric disorders (such as mood, personality, and substance abuse disorders) to a variety of stressful life situations (such as trauma and medical conditions). For example, a new college freshman with fundamentally good affect regulation might develop dramatic mood swings from a combination of sleep deprivation, anxiety about being away from home, and the demands of an academically rigorous university.

When patients are overpowered by intense emotions, it is difficult, if not impossible, for them to try to explore what they are feeling [4,5]. A capacity for regulating affect, containing anxiety, and self-soothing is a necessary foundation for self-observation and reflection. Until these capacities have been sufficiently developed, focusing on overwhelming affect is likely to escalate anxiety and further impair functioning [6]. In these situations, we use a variety of supporting interventions to *lessen and contain intolerable affects*, and to *improve the capacity to tolerate and manage affects*.

Lessening or containing affect

Infants are born unequipped to manage emotional distress on their own. They rely on the help of emotionally attuned, supportive caregivers to modulate their overwhelming affects. Caregivers do this by using both verbal and non-verbal responses to convey their empathic understanding and ability to tolerate and endure the baby's distress [7]. Similarly, when our patients are very upset and unable to manage their own affects, we intervene in order to help them lessen and contain affects:

- **Lessening** affect involves using supplying interventions such as **naming emotions**, **nurturing**, **soothing**, **reassuring**, **empathizing**, or **validating** to reduce a patient's overpowering or intense feelings in a direct and immediate way.

- **Containing** affect refers to the ways in which therapists help their patients from being overwhelmed by their feelings [8]. Some of this is communicated non-verbally as a function of the **holding environment** (see Chapter 3) in which therapists tolerate and accept their patients' strong feelings. Containing affect is also accomplished using a variety of supplying interventions. These include **remaining calm** in the face of intense feelings, **putting words** to patients' inchoate and threatening experiences, **demonstrating interest and understanding**, **interpreting up**, and **supportively bypassing** extreme feelings.

Here is an example of using supporting interventions to lessen or contain affect:

Patient	When he left the house, my mind sort of went nuts. I went and got his best suits and cut them up with scissors. (begins to sob uncontrollably) Am I going crazy?
Therapist	No, I don't think you're going crazy. What I hear is that he really hurt you. I guess in the moment cutting up his suits was the only way you could think of to hurt him back – although it sounds like feeling that you were losing control frightened you. (**reassurance**, **empathizing**, **reframing**, **naming emotions**)
Patient	I'm shaking just thinking about it – I wanted to trash his TV, too, but at the last second, I couldn't do it.
Therapist	Given how upset you are, it's great that you're able to talk about it. Maybe you can take a little comfort in knowing you were able to exert some degree of self-control in the middle of feeling so angry? I'm thinking of that time last month when Rick really disappointed you and you felt like binging, but you were able to rein it in and come talk about it here, which was great. (**praise**, **soothing**, **reducing guilt**, **reinforcing**, **reminding patient of her capacities**)
Patient	(Drying her eyes) A lot of good that did me today.
Therapist	It's discouraging to see yourself doing the same old things. But you know Rome wasn't built in a day. It takes time to change the automatic ways we react to things. The next time you're feeling that way, maybe you could try . . . (**validating**, **offering optimism and hope**)
Patient	. . . a good stiff drink? (smirks)
Therapist	(smiles) I guess that works for some people, but for many, alcohol just takes the lid off and makes them more aggressive. There's a good book on anger management I'd like you

to read. It describes a lot of useful tips I think could help you. (**soothing, informing, suggesting**)

Patient   *I feel better just talking about this – calmer. Maybe it gets a little easier each time.*

In this example, the therapist helps to calm the patient down by tolerating her strong affects, listening without judging, and lessening/containing affect using a variety of supplying interventions.

Improving the capacity to manage affect

While it's sometimes necessary for us to lessen and contain our patients' affects, we also want to help them to develop the ability to manage strong affects on their own. Recall from Chapter 18 that **assisting** interventions are aimed at strengthening the patient's existing but faltering functioning. Here, we're assisting weakened affect regulation with the ultimate goal of enabling patients to manage emotional distress independently.

Consider the following examples of supporting interventions that we might use in *assisting* patients to tolerate and manage strong affects:

Patient   *I couldn't sleep. My mind was going a million miles a minute. I felt desperate, like I just had to cut myself to calm down. It felt good when I saw blood. I could finally relax.*

Therapist   *I realize this behavior has been a way of coping for you . . . but my hope is that together we can figure out other, less self-destructive ways to manage your feelings.* (**demonstrating interest and understanding, explicitly joining, joint goal setting**)

Patient   *I try to do that – I can sort of see myself going down the wrong road – but then I'm cutting again.*

Therapist   *That's great that you have some sense of that – and it's true that this can be hard to do on your own. Why don't we try to work on it together? Don't get too discouraged if you can't change the behavior right away. It's hard to break old habits, but it can be done. Have you found anything that ever works to stop that cutting impulse?* (**praise, explicitly joining, encouraging, offering optimism, jointly exploring alternative ways of acting**)

Patient   *A girl from group taught me how to do guided imagery, and I like that – I've done it in the past – sort of tried to drift off to some scene in my mind – but sometimes the impulse is too strong.*

Therapist   *That's a great place to start, and we can practice that in our sessions.* (**praise, jointly working on a project**)

Supporting interventions can also facilitate uncovering work. For example, helping patients manage feelings more adaptively often involves uncovering affective triggers:

You're usually inclined to drink when you're feeling angry or burdened and feel you deserve a reward.

You tend to call old boyfriends when your partner is out of town and you're feeling abandoned and lonely.

These can then become topics for exploration.

Uncovering interventions

We use uncovering interventions when our aim is to:

- help patients become aware of unconscious affects
- use affects to understand other unconscious material, and/or
- understand unconscious factors leading to negative affects

Confrontation

The first step in constructing an interpretive intervention is **confrontation**, which calls the patient's attention to their affect. We confront the dominant affect in order to:

- focus patients on their feelings, and
- stimulate patients to talk about their affects.

For example:

> A 38-year-old recently married lawyer presents for psychotherapy because his wife says he is emotionally distant. He has just told his parents that he cannot be home for Thanksgiving because he and his wife decided that they would spend the holiday with her family this year. He tells you that he told his parents of this decision by phone, which was difficult. After the phone call, he left work early, missing an important client meeting.

When you listen, you are struck by the vagueness of the word "difficult." In your reflection, you wonder if guilty feelings about his parents caused him to skip out on work. Since your aim is to learn more about what is happening in his mind, you decide to confront by calling the missing affect to your patient's attention. You say:

> You said the call was difficult, but I am still not clear about what you felt. It must have been a strong feeling if it led you to skip out on work and miss an important meeting.

The patient responds by telling you that he enjoys the rapport he has developed with his father-in-law, who is also a lawyer, and that he feels that this new relationship could help his career. He also says he feels guilty about having this "new father" because he always wished that his parents were more professional. Thus, your confrontation of the missing affect was successful because it uncovered his guilty feelings and helped him articulate affect.

Clarification

Clarification highlights patterns by linking related examples. We use clarifications to work toward interpretations and to help patients see that something unconscious is operating. This technique helps us get to deeper layers of the patient's experience, and opens up the possibility of making interpretations. To continue with the example of the lawyer, let's imagine that he says that Thanksgiving with his in-laws was "fine." You reflect that, once again, he has chosen a very nondescript word to describe an emotionally charged situation. At this point, you could offer a clarification, saying:

> You know, you used a word like "fine" when you said that the call to your parents was "difficult." My sense is that you often use words like this when you're describing situations that are actually filled with a lot of feeling.

This invites the patient to think about his use of these vague words and what that might mean about his avoidance of affect.

Interpretation

Once you think you understand something about why the patient is avoiding strong feelings, you can venture an interpretation. Perhaps in response to your clarification the patient says:

> Well, using these words is better than screaming all the time like my mother did. I just can't bear that.

Your interpretation could then be:

> So I guess that in order to differentiate yourself from your mother, you choose to distance yourself from your feelings by using these very vague words.

The interpretive process has helped uncover an unconscious motivation for the patient's emotional disconnectedness. As therapy continues, this will repeat many times as he works through the way in which he distances himself from feelings to differentiate himself from his highly emotional family.

Uncovering approaches to persistent negative affects

Uncovering approaches are very helpful for patients whose persistent affects of anger, shame, envy, despair, or other negative feelings seem connected to unconscious factors:

> Ms A, a 26-year-old history graduate student, presents with persistent negative feelings about herself. Having gone to public school, she feels that her private school–trained classmates seem better prepared. She feels perennially inadequate in class and despairs that she will never be able to complete her degree. Her therapy sessions are filled with feelings of envy about her classmates. Supportive interventions that reframe her viewpoint do not help. As winter arrives, she also talks about feeling "too shabby" to be in this graduate program. When asked, she says that the other students actually dress just as she does, in sweatshirts, jeans, and sneakers. Her therapist notes to herself that Ms A looks attractive and youthful, and wonders if her experience relates to her feelings about the therapist's clothes. The session proceeds as follows:

Patient	My classmates don't seem to care about what they are wearing, but I really just feel like a slob. I would love to have some nicer boots and sweaters to wear, but my stipend won't allow it.
Therapist (who is wearing boots and a sweater)	You mention boots and sweaters, which make me think about how I dress. I wonder if you feel you would like to have clothes more like mine? **(confrontation of the transference)**

Patient	Not really. You are a doctor, so of course you dress like that.
Therapist	That's true, but it does seem like you consistently find something to envy. With your classmates it's their schooling. With me it could be my clothes, even though it would make no sense for you to dress like me. It seems you keep feeling envious, even when there is no need – you are managing in your classes and you aren't expected to dress the way I do. **(clarification of transference and interpretation of unconscious affect, envy)**
Patient	It's funny, my mother used to always talk about what others had that she didn't. A nicer car, a better job, or even being young.
Therapist	Well, it could be that you learned from her to respond to difference with envy. **(interpretation of an identification with her mother)**

In this example, an uncovering strategy of confrontation of the transference, clarification, and genetic interpretation helps elucidate the origins of the patient's persistent feelings of envy.

We're now ready to move on to **resistance**, another important aspect of psychodynamic psychotherapy.

Suggested activity

Read the following clinical vignettes and then consider the study questions that follow:

1. Ms A comes in and slumps into the chair. Her hair looks unkempt and she's not wearing any lipstick, which accentuates how tired and worn-out she seems. After a brief silence, she begins:

   I just don't feel like talking about the same old things. It feels like we are not really getting anywhere. I feel stuck in my life. And like I've lost hope for this therapy as a way to change things. I just feel bored at work, not really sure what my goals are. Do I even care about making deals? I just feel like I'm not really sure I am qualified to do this job. I promised myself I would sign up for one of those internet dating sites, but I haven't done that either and don't really want to. My friend has been doing that for six years and doesn't like any of the people she's met. I went on a bird-watching hike in the park, and the only other single person was a nerdy, geeky guy carrying a canvas bag with alternative energy buttons all over it. I'm so done with this. All of the good guys are married by now.

   - What affect is most on the surface? How did you decide?
   - What might you say to this patient at the end of this passage?
   - What interventions would be appropriate if she were a new patient and you weren't sure about her level of functioning?
   - What interventions would be appropriate if you had a strong alliance and she functioned well in most domains?

Comment

The surface affects are hopelessness and despair. This is clearly communicated by her thoughts and behavior. She also seems angry (expressed at the therapist indirectly and at herself by her frustration and self-punishing comments), but because she does not express this directly, we can hypothesize that it is a bit deeper. You might say, "You sound hopeless," or "So many things are frustrating you." In a supportive mode, you might stay with labeling the affects and/or suggesting ways in which she might help herself or reframe things. In an interpretive mode, you might focus on the anger, which is being defended against and is likely to signal areas of unconscious conflict, including her relationship with you.

2. Ms B comes in 15 minutes late, which is unusual for her, and is out of breath.

> *So sorry to be late! You would not believe what happened! It turns out that I have genital warts! It's probably from that football guy I ended up sleeping with during homecoming weekend. I am sure that this will be the end now. No one will ever want to be with me again. This happened to my roommate last year and she hasn't gone on a date since. What am I going to do – it is like having a Scarlet Letter!*

- What affect is most on the surface? How did you decide?
- What might you say to this patient at the end of this passage?
- What interventions would be appropriate if she were a new patient and you weren't sure about her functioning?
- What interventions would be appropriate if you had a strong alliance and she functioned well in most domains?

Comment

The surface affect is panic. Other affects present are shame and feeling sexually damaged. To intervene supportively you might say, "You've just found out and are clearly alarmed, but let's take a moment to think about this. Have you spoken yet to your gynecologist to find out about treatment?" To intervene interpretively after providing empathy about her panic and fear, you could say, "A Scarlet Letter? . . . tell me more about that" in order to deepen the exploration of her shame and feeling of being damaged.

Chapter 19: References

1. Diener, M.J., Hilsenroth, M.J., and Weinberger, J. (2007). Therapist affect focus and patient outcomes in psychodynamic psychotherapy: A meta-analysis. *American Journal of Psychiatry*, **164**, 936–941.
2. Fenichel, O. (1941) *Problems of Psychoanalytic Technique*, Psychoanalytic Quarterly, New York, p. 17–22, 44–49.
3. Caligor, E., Kernberg, O.F., and Clarkin, J.F. (2007) *Handbook of Dynamic Psychotherapy for Higher Level Personality Pathology*, American Psychiatric Publishing, Washington, DC, p. 150–152.
4. Mayes, L.C. (2000) A developmental perspective on the regulation of arousal states. *Seminars in Perinatology*, **24** (4), 267–279.

5. Arnsten, A.F.T. (1998) Catecholamine modulation of prefrontal cortical cognitive function. *Trends in Cognitive Science*, **2** (11), 436–447.
6. Gabbard, G.O., and Horowitz, M.J. (2009) Insight, transference interpretation, and therapeutic change in the dynamic psychotherapy of borderline personality disorder. *American Journal of Psychiatry*, **166** (5), 517–521.
7. Fonagy, P., Steele, M., Steele, H., *et al.* (1995) Attachment, the reflective self, and borderline states: The predictive capacity of the Adult Attachment Interview and pathological emotional development, in *Attachment Theory: Social, Developmental and Clinical Perspectives* (eds. S. Goldberg, R. Muir, and J. Kerr), Analytic Press, Hillsdale, NJ, p. 233–278.
8. Ref to come.

20 Free Association and Resistance

Key concepts

Free association is the patient's attempt to say what comes to mind without editing.

The flow of associations consists of thoughts, feelings, and memories that link together and lead us to material that was previously out of awareness.

Resistance is anything that opposes the work of the treatment and the flow of associations.

Resistance can also be thought of as defense in the context of therapy. It is an expectable part of treatment that helps us to

- understand our patients' characteristic patterns of behavior
- hone in on unconscious material that is particularly difficult for our patients to access

Supporting techniques use our understanding of resistances to help patients make more adaptive choices.

Uncovering techniques aim to understand the unconscious meanings of resistance and to make patients aware of new unconscious material.

How do we get from the conscious to the unconscious mind? We have no map and we don't know where we are going. The one thing that helps us is that our thoughts are linked in a non-random way. We call this **psychic determinism** [1]. We exploit the principle of psychic determinism all the time when we lose our train of thought and follow our associations to get back to what we were thinking. If each thought is connected in a meaningful way to the next, it makes sense that if you keep following thoughts, you'll ultimately get to the unconscious. Thus, if we help patients wander freely from thought to thought, we are likely to travel into unknown territory that is meaningfully connected to conscious experience. For example, a patient says that she feels sad but doesn't know why. She then just starts talking freely in the session, saying:

> *I was feeling this way on the bus coming over. I was sitting next to the window. It's so gray today. I hate gray days like this. They remind me of rainy days at camp. They were so lonely.*

Psychodynamic Psychotherapy: A Clinical Manual, Second Edition. Deborah L. Cabaniss, Sabrina Cherry, Carolyn J. Douglas and Anna Schwartz.
© 2017 John Wiley & Sons, Ltd. Published 2017 by John Wiley & Sons, Ltd.

By freely associating, the patient has stumbled onto an early memory, and we can bet that something about that memory or the feeling invoked by the memory is related to the way she's feeling today.

Free association

This kind of verbal wandering is what we call **free association**. Free association is the patient's effort to say whatever comes to mind without editing [2,3]. It's a very different way of communicating than most people use in social situations. For example, in a non-therapy setting you might choose not to tell your friend that you hate her dress, or you might hide the details of your wedding plans from a colleague who is in the middle of a divorce. We all edit all the time – consciously and unconsciously – in order to protect ourselves and the people with whom we communicate. If you try to talk or think without editing, you'll find that it's nearly impossible. So when we ask our patients to free associate we are asking them to do something that's quite difficult. Nevertheless, we instruct them to do just that because it's the best way we have to move toward the unconscious and to understand how their thoughts and feelings are linked.

Recall from Chapter 8 that helping patients to learn to free associate (or speak freely) is important to do early in treatment. Once the assessment phase is complete, it is important to help patients understand how they can best participate in the treatment. This involves explaining:

- the importance of free association
- how to try to speak as freely as possible

As a review, here are some things that you might say in order to do this:

> As we begin this treatment, try to say whatever comes to mind without editing. It's impossible to not edit at all, but if you notice that you are, see if you can let us know.

> Try to let yourself say whatever comes to mind, with particular attention to how you're feeling, any dreams you may have had, or any thoughts that you have about the treatment.

You can experiment with different versions of this until you find the one that feels right for you.

Do we always want patients to free associate?

Sometimes, clinicians worry that encouraging patients with compromised function to speak freely might overwhelm or frighten them, as if it is inviting them to "take the lid off Pandora's box." The reality is that with the exception of some people with severe personality disturbances or psychosis, very few patients present in a state of such extreme vulnerability that an invitation to speak freely would result in rapid decompensation. In the unlikely event that the therapist's invitation to free associate results in anxiety and disorganization, the therapist can step in with supporting interventions to reduce anxiety:

> *A patient with obsessive-compulsive disorder is talking about what he did over the weekend:*

> Patient   *I had a good weekend with Jane. We saw a movie – oh, I can't believe that I just thought about the movie because it totally sent me into a tailspin. It was really violent and I kept having violent images all weekend. Now I'm afraid that that will start up again.*

> Therapist   *Well, let's get back to the rest of the weekend. Sounds like you had fun – what else did you do?*

Here the therapist **redirects** the patient away from his obsessive thoughts in order to contain affect and prevent him from feeling overwhelmed.

Breaks in free association offer clues to the presence of material that is difficult to bring into awareness

In addition to following the patient's free associations, observing how and when patients are *unable* to free associate is another important way to listen for unconscious material. Breaks in free association signal the presence of difficult material and the defenses that are keeping it out of awareness. For example, let's say a patient comes into session, greets you, and, while talking, notices you are wearing the same shirt she just bought at the store. She then becomes quiet. This break in her verbal communication lets you know that something has made her uncomfortable. When you ask about her thoughts, she says that telling you that she owns the same shirt felt too "familiar." Her discomfort prevented her from associating freely, and we call this a **resistance**.

What is resistance?

Resistance is anything that the patient does that opposes the process of therapy [4,5]. Early psychoanalysts likened free association to the flow of electrons in a circuit; thus, whatever the patient did to impede the "electron flow" was resistance. Anything can function as resistance – silence, hiding thoughts or feelings, being too agreeable, missing sessions, not paying one's bills – anything. Resistances can be conscious or unconscious; they can be expressed verbally or in action.

One way of thinking about resistance is that it is defense manifested in therapy. Here's an example:

> *Mr A has been in therapy for two years and has found it very helpful. He is always on time for his twice-weekly sessions. Recently, Mr A has started to talk about his relationship with his wife in the context of her threats to leave him. His therapist suggested that there might be some things that he was doing that were contributing to the problems in the marriage. In the next few weeks, Mr A was uncharacteristically late to many sessions. Together, he and his therapist came to understand that this lateness related to Mr A's wish to avoid dealing with this topic.*

Mr A is defending against looking at his behavior. When it manifests as lateness to therapy, we call it resistance.

Why do we look for resistance?

One might think that because resistance is the patient's way of opposing the work of the therapy, it is a problem that we should eliminate. This is the way that early analysts thought about resistance. However, the more we learn about resistance, the more we realize that understanding resistance is a very good way to understand our patients and to identify things that are particularly hard for them to think and talk about. For example, patients who don't pay their bills or who come late to sessions are showing us quite clearly that they are ambivalent about their treatment. Resistance is to the therapist what pain is to the doctor – it helps us to know "where it hurts" [6].

Given this, let's look again at the example of the patient who does not tell you she just purchased the shirt that you are wearing. Perhaps she is afraid of feeling closer to you by acknowledging she has the same shirt. Perhaps she worries that you would feel invaded by this comment about your clothing. Whatever her reason, her silence helps us see that this situation has made her uncomfortable. Her resistance thus points the way to unconscious feelings she has about you. Understanding these feelings will undoubtedly help you to understand her better.

Technique

Listening

Listen to the train of associations

In addition to affect, free association and resistance are central to what we listen for during therapy sessions. Having explained to our patients the importance of saying whatever comes to mind, our job is to follow their thoughts on a journey to their unconscious. Some have described this listening stance as "evenly hovering attention" [7]. This type of listening is appropriate whether we are working in a primarily uncovering or a supporting mode.

Listen for breaks in the train of associations

Once you have explained the importance of associating freely, you can then view everything that impedes the process of free association as a potential resistance. Clues that breaks are occurring include silence, hesitation, rapid changes of topic, and losing one's "train of thought." Here's a common example:

> After her Christmas vacation, Ms B talked about everyone she had seen in her family until she got to her sister – she then forgot what she had been talking about and changed the topic.

The break in Ms B's free associations signals to us that feelings about her sister are especially difficult to bring into consciousness.

Listen for other examples of resistance

Resistance can appear in many forms, including skipping over thoughts, having a secret, coming late, forgetting to pay bills, or always starting the session with a dream. Some resistances occur in the form of actions either inside or outside sessions. They function as resistances if they allow patients to express feelings rather than discussing them. **Acting out** refers to behaviors that occur outside of sessions, such as getting off at the wrong subway stop on the way to a session, or starting to date a psychologist at the beginning of the therapy. **Acting in** refers to behaviors that occur within sessions, such as getting up and browsing through the therapist's books or falling asleep. Free association itself can be a resistance if the patient simply talks on and on without engaging with the therapist in a meaningful way. Transference, which we will discuss in Chapter 21, can function as a resistance if patients speak exclusively about the therapist without referring to problems that are occurring in their lives. Good clues to the presence of resistance are the therapist's boredom and stasis in the treatment [8].

Reflecting

Once you have identified a resistance, the next step is to reflect on whether to call it to the patient's attention – and, if so, how and when to do it. If we are primarily trying to uncover unconscious material, helping a patient to notice a resistance can be very fruitful; if we are primarily trying to support, we generally take note of the resistance without highlighting it to the patient. Since resistance is the patient's way of avoiding something painful, shame inducing, or frightening, we have to use careful judgment to avoid seeming to attack or criticize the patient. Remember, when patients are resisting they are just showing us "where it hurts."

Get to know the resistance, respect it, and live alongside it

Once you think that a resistance is operating, your task is to *get to know it* [9]. Understanding a patient's characteristic way of resisting is a good way of getting to know the patient. In addition, you want to know a resistance pretty well before you begin discussing it with the patient. Your goal is not to eliminate the resistance – your goal is to use it as a way of understanding the patient. For example, if patients are late to sessions, your goal is not to get them to come on time, but rather to understand *why* they arrive late. In order to do this, wait until you notice it over a series of sessions and until they bring it up themselves. In addition, give yourself some time to monitor your countertransference. For example, when patients are late it's natural to get annoyed – but that's not usually the best time to comment on the lateness.

Think about why your patient resists

When you notice a resistance, it is helpful to think about why the patient uses it. This can help you empathize with the patient and decide if and when to comment on the resistance. Some possible reasons patients resist include the following:

Fear

Patients are afraid of change, feel threatened by the unknown, and are reluctant to let go of the adaptations they have made in life. The familiar is always a comfort and is generally developed for good reasons. It is hard to relinquish past adaptations, even though they are no longer needed in the present.

For example, let's say you have a patient whose mother was depressed and insecure about her parenting. In therapy, you notice that your patient agrees with everything you say, always pays bills in advance, comes to sessions on time, and speaks only in glowing terms about treatment. When you reflect, you wonder whether her perennially positive, cheery style is a resistance. You imagine that she might be afraid to express negative feelings for fear of angering others. Although this behavior, which may have been adaptive in her relationship with her mother, is no longer adaptive, it may nevertheless be difficult for her to relinquish.

Loss

Resistance to change may also be prompted by the wish to retain the gratifications that are afforded by habitual ways of thinking and behaving:

> *Mr C, a 35-year-old businessman, pursues psychotherapy to understand why he consistently makes poor financial choices that threaten his family's stability. In treatment, Mr C learns to recognize these choices, but persists in making them. You identify this as a resistance and then learn that the patient receives "bail-out" checks from his wealthy parents every time he makes a financial mistake. You realize that he continues (unconsciously) to make bad choices because he is loath to give up the gratification these checks provide. In order to mature, he would have to mourn the loss of this parental support.*

Sometimes these losses are real and at other times they are imagined, but in either case loss is involved.

Occasionally a helpful therapy can precipitate real loss. For example, in an unhappy marriage, exploration of previously avoided feelings can sometimes lead to separation and divorce. In this case, resistance could be a way of avoiding this potential outcome.

Guilt

Resistance can also be a way of avoiding unconscious guilt. For example, patients who use their difficulties to magically atone for fantasized sins may unconsciously feel that they would have to grapple with guilt if they were free of their symptoms:

> *Mr D is a 40-year-old man who presents for therapy because he consistently sabotages himself at work. Taking a history, you learn that he has two disabled siblings who live at home and will never be*

independent. You wonder whether he unconsciously keeps himself from succeeding in order to avoid guilt about surpassing his siblings.

This patient may also resist letting himself benefit from treatment in order to avoid guilt.

Shame

In psychodynamic therapy, patients frequently feel humiliated and ashamed when they become aware of their unconscious fears and fantasies. Avoiding these feelings is another common source of resistance:

> *Mr E is a 28-year-old man who came to treatment after having sexual problems with his fiancée. In the opening months of therapy he revealed having had homosexual fantasies since early adolescence that terrified him because he says that his family was homophobic. In therapy, he resists full disclosure about his sexual fantasies because he fears the shame of discovering that he is gay.*

Therapist error

Resistances can also be a response to therapist error. If we misunderstand our patients, fail to empathize, or show a lack of interest, our patients may consciously or unconsciously resist our help. For example, if a patient is silent during a session to which you were late, you might consider that your tardiness is the reason for the resistance.

Reasons for resistance

- Fear
- Loss
- Guilt
- Shame
- Therapist error

Adapted from Sandler *et al.* [10].

Consider whether patients are ready to look at their resistance

Just because we identify a resistance doesn't mean that the patient can think about it in a way that will deepen the process. In order to make this decision, we consult the choosing and readiness principles. Ask yourself whether the resistance is near the surface, connected to the dominant affect, and related to your countertransference. Think about the phase of treatment, the therapeutic alliance, and the patient's current level of functioning.

Many patients become curious about their own resistances and will let you know when they are ready to talk about them. For example, they may say, "I forgot your check again; guess I should think about what is going on." One good strategy is to make a trial interpretation in the form of a question to test the patient's readiness to address their resistance. Saying "I wonder if your lateness is related to how you feel about coming here today?" or "Your thoughts seem to wander over so many different topics today; I wonder if that reflects your feeling about our work together" gives the patient a way out without having to be put on the defensive. Let's look at this example:

> *Ms F is a relatively new patient who came to treatment looking for help managing distress related to her job. As she talks about her problems at work, you become worried that she might be fired. She consistently arrives for her sessions 15 minutes late and says this is because she is anxious about being seen leaving work early.*

Although you reflect that her lateness could be a resistance, the surface content, her affect, and your countertransference all steer you away from focusing on her lateness as a resistance at this time. On the other hand, if Ms F were an established patient with a strong alliance, a predilection for lateness in other parts of her life, and a solid record at work, you might be more comfortable choosing to focus on the lateness as resistance.

Patients with persistently weakened functioning may rarely, if ever, be able to use confrontation of resistance productively:

> *Mr G is a 38-year-old man with a history of undiagnosed learning disabilities from childhood, who pursues therapy for persistent problems at work. He consistently comes 15 minutes late to sessions, and responds to any suggestions that this could be related to the treatment with demoralization and self-criticism.*

While the therapist might think that his lateness is resistance, Mr G may not be able to use discussion of this in order to learn more about himself and his difficulties.

Is it resistance?

Finally, it is important to consider whether a behavior that you think is a resistance really is one. For example, with Mr G, a man with lifelong executive function problems, his lateness could represent persistent struggles with time management. If this were the case, a discussion of how he gets to appointments and manages his schedule might be more productive than a discussion of resistance. Or consider silence in a temperamentally shy person who rarely talks much in any situation. In addition, the behavior could be both something with which the person has persistently struggled *and* a resistance. Just because a behavior keeps the patient from using therapy doesn't necessarily make it a resistance – you have to consider each patient and each circumstance to make that determination. It's also possible that you and the patient will work differently with the behavior early and later in the treatment:

> Ms H is a 45-year-old woman who regularly missed sessions without calling. Early in treatment, her therapist thought of this as resistance and confronted it, leading Ms H to feel angry and defensive. With a supervisor's help, the therapist asked more about this behavior and discovered that Ms H had organizational problems in multiple areas of life. The therapist and Ms H began to spend more time on these issues, resulting in improvement in executive function and self-esteem. Later in the treatment, they also recognized that Ms H had used her persistent organizational problems to avoid things throughout life.

Intervening

Basic interventions

As with affect, **psychoeducation**, **questions**, **direction**, and **empathy** can all set the stage for further work. Since your first goal is to get to know the resistance, questions designed to get details are key:

> Patient   I had a fight with my wife last night. There's not much to say about it.
>
> Therapist   Well, perhaps you could tell me more about the fight. How did it begin?

Reminding the patient of the need to say whatever comes to mind without censoring can also be helpful. This can encourage the patient, particularly at the onset of treatment. Direction in the form of mild prompts can also be helpful, such as asking the patient to comment on what they are thinking or feeling during periods of silence:

> Mr I is a 40-year-old executive who just lost his job and presents with anxious worry about employment, insomnia, and a general feeling of professional inadequacy. After completing the evaluation and setting the frame, Mr I has trouble getting started in sessions.
>
> Mr I   I'm not sure where to start. I liked it when you were asking me questions.
>
> Therapist   It's fine just to say what comes to mind about what is going on in your life, or about how you are feeling. Wherever you'd like to start is OK.
>
> Mr I   I feel funny just talking about random things.
>
> Therapist   It can sometimes be awkward at first for people, but you can just start wherever you like.

In this case, the therapist **empathizes** with Mr I's experience of being a new patient and offers some **direction** to help him begin more effectively.

Asking for associations to the resistance can also help understand more about it:

> Patient #1   I'm sorry I forgot to pay you today.
>
> Therapist   Does anything come to mind about not paying me?

> Patient #2   *I know that I had a dream but I can't remember it. I'm having a hard time remembering any dreams.*
>
> Therapist   *What are your thoughts about that?*

These calls for associations are designed to help focus the patient on the resistance in order to begin the deepening process.

Supporting interventions

We choose supporting interventions when we elect to leave a resistance in place because, at least at that moment, dislodging it might undermine the patient's functioning. Supporting interventions can help the patient to:

- use more adaptive resistances, and
- lessen the potential of the resistance to derail therapeutic goals.

For patients who are challenged in basic areas of function, such as self-esteem regulation or impulse control, we still listen to the flow of associations; however, our immediate aim is generally not to bring unconscious material into awareness. Instead, the patient's free associations help us understand unconscious processes that guide our decisions about what needs support:

> *A 20-year-old woman who was sexually assaulted as a young girl is now starting to date men. As she talks about dating in her sessions, you notice that she changes the subject rather than admit to any sexual attraction. While you recognize this as a resistance, you also understand that it is remarkable that she is able to talk about this at all. Thus, you decide not to disrupt her new-found comfort by focusing her attention on the resistance. Rather, you decide to accept the resistance as an aspect of how she copes with the trauma while engaging in ongoing relationships with men.*

Certain patients may use resistances such as acting out, missing sessions, not paying bills, or concealing aspects of their thoughts and behaviors to a degree that makes it hard to work with them. Some resistances may jeopardize the treatment or limit the potential for effectiveness. In this case, **directions** and **suggestions** may be helpful. For example, in response to a patient who missed a series of sessions, you might say:

> *I see that you are struggling with coming on time, but arriving late gives us very little time to work. If you could come on time we'd really be able to do more.*

Practical **suggestions** can also be helpful in this situation, such as:

> *I wonder if it makes more sense to take a taxi to session on the days when you leave work 15 minutes before we are scheduled to meet.*

Your aim in the moment is *not* necessarily to "pave the way" for future exploration of the resistances, but simply to strengthen function by helping people to find less costly and less destructive ways of defending themselves. However, it may well be that, with certain patients, these supporting comments could productively be followed by an interpretive intervention at another point in time, or even later in the very same session.

Uncovering interventions

We select uncovering interventions when our aim is to understand the meaning of a resistance, elucidate unconscious elements at work, and ultimately lessen the effect of the resistance on blocking the forward motion of treatment.

Confrontation

As with affect, we start an interpretive exploration with a **confrontation**. In this case, confrontation is calling the patient's attention to the resistance. Your job is to make the patient as curious about the resistance as you are. For example, in response to a patient who comes into the room and does not talk, you might wait and then say, "You are not saying much today." This is a simple confrontation – you are just calling the patient's attention to his silence and then waiting to see if he can talk more about it.

When resistance takes the form of shifting topics, confrontations can help to interest patients in potential connections between them:

> Ms J   *Jim and I had a great dinner out – we talked the whole time, including the cab ride home. We had a good time. When we got home, the dishes were still in the sink from lunch. We argued about who would take out the garbage and went to sleep without having sex. (pause) Anyway, that's what happened last night. Did I ever tell you that my mother used to punish me with long time-outs? Sometimes I'd even miss dinner.*
>
> Therapist *It's interesting – you were telling me about the argument and going to sleep without having sex and then thought back to the time-outs. Do you think that the two might be connected?*

In this example, your comment is a confrontation of the missing link in the patient's train of associations.

Clarification

Clarification helps bring the unconscious into focus by linking similar phenomena. One clarification technique is to bring together multiple examples. This is especially helpful when you begin to see connections between seemingly unrelated forms of resistance. For example, if a patient

- forgets about Tuesday's session saying that he "lost track of time at work"
- forgets to bring his checkbook to pay last month's bill, and
- forgets the details of the dream he had last night

you might say:

> *It seems that a lot of things aren't working as you planned. You missed the last session, forgot your checkbook, and can't remember your dream. I wonder if these things might be related.*

Linking behaviors encourages patients to wonder if there might be an unconscious motivation underlying their behavior. Remember that your tone should be curious, not punitive:

> Mr K, a 50-year-old schoolteacher who sought therapy for "general feelings of disappointment in life," talks at length about being bored at work and his concerns that "today's kids" are more interested in grades than learning. While the sessions seem helpful, you note that he never talks about his wife, and you begin to wonder whether talking about work might be a resistance against exploring more problematic areas. You confront the potential resistance, saying, "While we are making progress in exploring your concerns about work, I am struck that we hardly ever talk about your wife." This comment surprises him, and he becomes curious about this unconscious omission. In a subsequent session, when Mr K talks about his father, you realize that you know very little about his mother. This feels similar to his omissions about his wife, allowing you to make a **clarification** that links the two: "Today, I notice that you're leaving out any mention of your mother, just like the other day when you left out any mention of your wife."

This is a clarification, linking similar resistances and suggesting that they might have a common unconscious source. Again, this is not said as a criticism; the resistance of neglecting a topic just pointed you in the right direction. One point never makes a line – when patients can link seemingly disparate resistances, the pursuit of unconscious motivations becomes more compelling.

Interpretation

When we think we have found an unconscious motive for a resistance, we can make an **interpretation**. Let's think again about the patient who forgot the session, the payment, and the dream. Here's the part of the session in which he forgot his dream:

Patient	*I know I had a dream last night, but for the life of me I can't remember anything about it. It's so frustrating.*
Therapist	*Do you have any thoughts about forgetting it?* (**confrontation**)
Patient	*No, but it feels like it was important, like it would have shed light on how I'm feeling.*
Therapist	*It's interesting – you've forgotten a few things in the last few weeks, like your session on Tuesday and your checkbook last time. It also occurs to me that you haven't talked much about the fact that I'm going on vacation next week – it's kind of like you've "forgotten" to talk about that, too. I wonder if these things are related in some way.* (**clarification**)
Patient	*Maybe, but it's fine that you're going away – you work hard and need a break. (pause) I just had this totally weird fantasy that you would send me a postcard. Not that I want you to, so I don't know why I thought that.*
Therapist	*What comes to mind about the postcard?* (**call for associations**)
Patient	*Well, when I went to summer camp, all the kids got postcards from their parents – even letters – like every week. But not me. I think that I got one postcard the whole time.*
Therapist	*You thought that they had forgotten you.* (**empathic statement**)
Patient	*I mean, I know that they didn't, but it felt that way. (becomes tearful)*

Therapist	*Perhaps some of your forgetting in the last few weeks is related to a worry that I'm going to forget you over my vacation, just like you felt your parents did.* (**interpretation, with genetic component**)
Patient	*I mean, I know you won't, but you'll be having fun with your family. You'll probably be glad to be finished with me and my problems for a few weeks.*

In this example, the resistances (forgetting a session, forgetting the checkbook, and forgetting the dream) avoided a strong affect (anxiety about the summer break), a painful memory (not getting letters from his parents at camp), and a frightening fantasy (being forgotten by the therapist). **Confronting** and **clarifying** the resistance allowed the patient to move into deeper territory, revealing affects and fantasies that were affecting him. This is how the process of psychodynamic psychotherapy unfolds. In this example we also got a window into the patient's defensive style. The patient forgot the obligations he had made to the therapist, rather than leaving open the possibility of being forgotten.

Since resistance is protective, interpretation can feel threatening. Remembering this is key to maintaining empathy during the interpretive process. Listen to these two examples in which the therapist interprets lateness as a resistance:

> *Therapist 1: This is the third time this month you've been late. It's clear you're avoiding working more deeply in therapy.*

> *Therapist 2: I've noticed that you've come late three times this month. We've just started to talk about your ambivalent feelings about your girlfriend, and I have a feeling that you might be coming late in order to avoid talking about it. What are your thoughts about that?*

In the first interpretation, Therapist 1 sounds accusatory and punitive. The interpretation comes from "on high" – it is like the therapist is saying, "here's the way it is." In the second interpretation, Therapist 2 empathizes with the difficulty the patient is having talking about a difficult topic. The tone is collaborative and curious. Same resistance, different tone – and likely to get different responses.

$$* \quad * \quad *$$

In this chapter we have explored the ways in which understanding resistance moves us toward understanding the patient's unconscious. It is an expected and welcome part of the process and one that helps us learn about the patient's defensive style. In the next chapter, we will introduce the concept of **transference**, which will help us in many of the same ways.

Suggested activity

Here are two vignettes that involve resistance. Read them and consider the study questions:

> *Your patient is Ms A, a 34-year-old mother of twins who is currently taking care of them and volunteering in her community full time. She is very upset about her marriage because her husband never helps out around the home. She states he has a very traditional view that she should do all the daytime and child-related tasks, since he is working and doesn't want to have to*

pitch in after work. You find Ms A to be highly competent, approaching childrearing as if it were an executive position, referencing child development experts, and reading prolifically. Similarly, she seems to have very high, exacting standards about taking care of her home. You have suggested a few ways that she might ask her husband to help on weekends, but each time she responds by saying he can't perform the task well enough for her to delegate it to him. You begin to feel that she is shooting down every one of your suggestions.

1. Is there evidence of resistance at work? List examples.
2. How might you work in an uncovering, interpretive mode with Ms A? Suggest a possible confrontation, clarification, and interpretation of the resistance.

Comment

Ms A resists by perennially rejecting your suggestions. She avoids making progress in therapy by never trying anything new. A possible confrontation is: "I wonder if you have noticed that you find a reason not to try everything I suggest." A clarification might be: "It seems like your reaction to my suggestions is not unique, as you tend to be critical of the ways your husband does things as well." An interpretation could be: "I wonder if you avoid asking your husband to help you because it might make you feel that you didn't have a real role in the family."

To continue with the example of Ms A, let's say that in an effort to point out her resistance you say, "I am getting the feeling that you are not really interested in my suggestions." Before you even have a chance to add that she could be doing the same thing with her husband, she becomes enraged, stating, "Have you ever had a child? Do you know what is involved here?" Her defensiveness is quite strident and you feel attacked, so you back away from the confrontation.

1. What does Ms A's response to your confrontation suggest?
2. What technique might you use going forward?

Comment

Ms A gets very defensive, suggesting that she is not ready to be curious about her behavior with the therapist or her husband. Going forward you might switch to a supporting approach designed to build her self-esteem. Over time, her increased self-esteem may lessen her defensiveness, improve her functioning in relationships, and make interpretive work more feasible.

Chapter 20: References

1. Auchincloss, E.L., and Samberg, E. (2012) *Psychoanalytic Terms and Concepts*, Yale University Press, New Haven, p. 205–206.
2. Auchincloss, E.L., and Samberg, E. (2012) *Psychoanalytic Terms and Concepts*, Yale University Press, New Haven, p. 89–90.
3. Greenson, R. (1967) *The Technique and Practice of Psychoanalysis*, vol. 1, International Universities Press, New York, p. 32–33.
4. Auchincloss, E.L., and Samberg, E. (2012) *Psychoanalytic Terms and Concepts*, Yale University Press, New Haven, p. 228–230.

5. Greenson, R. (1967) *The Technique and Practice of Psychoanalysis*, vol. **1**, International Universities Press, New York, p. 59–60.
6. Schlesinger, H.J. (1982) Resistance as process, in *Resistance: Psychodynamic and Behavioral Approaches* (ed. P.L. Wachtel), Plenum Press, New York, p. 27.
7. Freud, A. (1949) Bulletin of the International Psycho-Analytical Association, *Bulletin of the International Psycho-Analytic Association*, **20**, 178–208.
8. Greenson, R. (1967) *The Technique and Practice of Psychoanalysis*, vol. **1**, International Universities Press, New York, p. 59–71.
9. Schlesinger, H.J. (2003) *The Texture of Treatment*, Analytic Press, Hillsdale, NJ, p. 83.
10. Sandler, J., Dare, C., and Holder, A. (1973) Resistance, in *The Patient and the Analyst*, International University Press, Madison, p. 71–83.

21 Transference

Key concepts

Transference is the sum of the feelings that a patient has about the therapist.

Understanding the transference in psychodynamic psychotherapy helps us understand how patients think about themselves and how they relate to other people.

In a supporting mode, we use the information that we get from the transference to understand patients without bringing it to their attention. We may also have to limit and contain the transference when we support.

In an uncovering mode, we interpret the transference in order to help patients learn more about themselves and their relationships with others.

Patients can tell us over and over how they feel about their bosses, their partners, and their parents, but when they tell us how they feel about us we have a unique opportunity to see how they really relate to others. Patients inevitably experience the same feelings about the therapist that they experience toward other people in their lives. We call these feelings **transference**.

What is transference?

Transference is the sum of the feelings that a patient has about the therapist. Some of those feelings are about the patient's here-and-now experience of the therapist, while others relate to feelings the person had for people in the past that are now displaced onto the therapist. As discussed in Chapter 1, thinking about the transference is often a focus of psychodynamic psychotherapy.

Why do we care about transference?

In psychodynamic psychotherapy, transference feelings are a way to learn about the important relationships in a patient's life. If patients react to us in certain ways, we can bet that they react that way in other relationships as well. Making these reactions conscious and linking them to early relationships frees people up to make new choices

---

Psychodynamic Psychotherapy: A Clinical Manual, Second Edition. Deborah L. Cabaniss, Sabrina Cherry, Carolyn J. Douglas and Anna Schwartz.
© 2017 John Wiley & Sons, Ltd. Published 2017 by John Wiley & Sons, Ltd.

about how to relate to others. In addition, transference reactions serve as gateways to exploring memories:

> *After a session in which Mr A began to talk about quitting his high-paying job to try his hand at writing fiction, he missed two sessions. When the therapist asked about this, Mr A said he assumed that the therapist would try to talk him out of this idea. As they discussed this, it became clear that Mr A made this assumption because his parents were very dismissive of artistic pursuits, and had convinced him to take a business job rather than trying to make a life as a writer.*

Here, Mr A makes an assumption about the therapist that stems from his feelings about his parents. Helping Mr A to see that this assumption is displaced onto the therapist enables Mr A to understand more about his expectations of people in his current life.

Is it reality or is it transference?

Frequently, therapists get sidetracked trying to decide whether a patient's reaction is "realistic" or "transference." This is not an either/or question – our patients have feelings about us that relate to our real characteristics, to things that really happen in the therapy relationship, and to the characteristics of other people in their lives. For example:

> *After Mr B's mother died, he felt very supported by his therapist, who called him on the phone and was attentive to his feelings of mourning.*

Here, Mr B has warm feelings about things his therapist actually did. He is responding to the therapist's real characteristics.

> *Ms C felt that her therapist's tradition of taking a two-week summer vacation indicated that she was inattentive to her patients' needs.*

Since a two-week vacation is not inappropriate for a therapist, Ms C's feeling that her therapist is inattentive is probably related to expectations established outside of the therapy relationship or in reference to other feelings about the therapist that are displaced onto the vacation.

Talking about the transference is important since "you were there"

A patient's hostile reaction toward us is very different than one toward a bus driver or boyfriend, because we are there and can corroborate the details of what transpires. In general, it is helpful to explore the details of your patient's transference reactions, since you are a direct observer. Sorting out transference feelings within the real therapy relationship can be therapeutic in itself, since it offers the patient an opportunity to become comfortable talking directly about complex feelings while they are happening. It is important to be open and non-defensive about a patient's experience of you, your comments, and your behavior.

Transference related to the current therapeutic relationship

Encouraging patients to describe what they experience in the moment with the therapist, sometimes referred to as "in the here and now," is a technique used to foster the development of **mentalization** [1]. Mentalization is the ability to describe one's subjective experience and the experience of others, and to understand that these might be different. Here is an example of a patient talking about something in the current relationship with the therapist:

> *The therapist apologized at the beginning of the session for having to start a few minutes late. The patient is quiet, and not able to start talking.*
>
> Therapist   *I wonder if you are feeling something about my starting the session late?*
>
> Patient   *I feel that you must have something important to attend to and that I am getting in the way. It feels like you wish I weren't here now and that whatever I might say can't be as important as what you have to do.*
>
> Therapist   *I am glad you were able to tell me what you are feeling. It really helps me understand why you are quiet. Actually, I just was on hold with a pharmacy and couldn't hang up, but I am very glad to be done with that task and have the chance to focus on you now.*

This interaction encourages the patient to identify and share what he feels in the moment, and suggests that his assumptions about the therapist's feelings might not be right. This could help the patient realize that his assumptions about others might not always be correct as well, leading to a general improvement in his relationships.

Describing and understanding transference

It is helpful to categorize transferences into broad subgroups so that we can better understand them, construct formulations about them, and discuss them in supervision and with colleagues. We will discuss three basic transference categories:

- transference related to affect
- transference related to a past relationship
- displaced transference

Transference related to affect

Sometimes our patients feel good about us and sometimes they don't. We call the good feelings the **positive transference** and the bad feelings the **negative transference**.

Positive transferences are those feelings that arise from loving, trusting, tender, passionate, and respectful attitudes toward the therapist. Subtypes of positive transference include:

- **Idealization** of the therapist, which involves perceiving therapists as more intelligent, loving, and perfect than they really are.
- **Erotic transference**, which refers to sexual or loving feelings that patients develop toward therapists, including falling in love with or wishing to be desired by the therapist.
- **Eroticized transference**, which refers to specific kinds of sexual feelings toward the therapist that are aggressive as well as sexual. The eroticized transference often develops more rapidly than the more loving erotic transference. Trying to seduce the therapist to violate boundaries or recounting sexual fantasies in order to try to arouse the therapist are examples of the more aggressive, eroticized transference.

Note: *There is no need to interpret positive transference* – positive transference is the patient's good feelings about the therapist. These are the feelings of trust that support the therapeutic alliance and help the patient and therapist to work together effectively. Unless these feelings get in the way of treatment – as they might if they are overidealized or eroticized – just leave them alone. They're the glue that holds the treatment together.

Negative transference includes feelings toward the therapist of anger, hatred, contempt, envy, and humiliation. It is almost always important to address negative transference in some way, particularly if it threatens the treatment.

Transference related to past relationships

Other transference feelings are reminiscent of relationships from early childhood. To work effectively with these transferences, patients have to understand the "as if" quality of their feelings toward the therapist. That is, patients experience therapists "as if" they were someone from their past:

> *Ms D is a 22-year-old woman in psychotherapy who says she is afraid to tell you shameful things because they could "change her life forever." You inquire further and ask whether revealing secrets ever led to a bad outcome. She remembers that her mother once discovered her playing "doctor" with a young cousin. Her mother "freaked out," took Ms D to the priest to confess, and severed ties with the cousin's part of the family.*

Your patient's fear that reporting a secret will be humiliating and have dire consequences probably relates to this early history. Thus, telling you a potentially shameful secret in therapy makes her experience you *as if* you were the mother of her early childhood.

We categorize transferences as **maternal, paternal,** or **sibling transferences** in order to reference these origins [2]. Although today both mothers and fathers can be primary caregivers, you will still often hear of maternal transferences as expressing longings for care, holding, and containing; paternal transferences as expressing wishes for protection; and sibling transferences as related to competition. All of these transferences can stem from actual or fantasized childhood relationships. Here are two examples that demonstrate the difference:

> *Mr E was abandoned by his mother when he was 5.*

> *Scenario 1: Mr E idealizes his female therapist and tells her she is perfectly attuned to him.*

In this case, Mr E has a maternal transference related to the wished-for relationship with his mother.

> *Scenario 2: Mr E always presumes the therapist will leave him, particularly around vacations.*

In this case, Mr E has a maternal transference related to his actual relationship with his mother.

We can also think of these transferences as being reminiscent of early types of relationships, such as **dyadic** (previously called pre-Oedipal) or **triadic** (previously called Oedipal) transferences [3]. Dyadic relationships are typical of the earliest years of life (0–3 years) and generally relate to the need to be cared for and loved in an exclusive one-on-one relationship. A dyadic maternal transference refers to the early mothering figure who was needed for basic caretaking, need-fulfilling, and confidence-building roles. Alternately, triadic relationships, which tend to originate in middle childhood (3–6 years), occur once children realize that the people in their lives have relationships with each other. They generally relate to early sexual feelings, competition with caregivers, and jealousy. A triadic maternal or paternal transference refers to the caregivers during middle childhood. During this period children tend to be sexually drawn to one parent (the love object) while feeling competitive with the other (the rival). Thus, a heterosexual female patient who is upset because she saw her male therapist talking to a female colleague might be having a triadic transference.

These are some of the developmental labels that psychodynamic therapists use to describe transferences. They involve unconscious fantasy constellations that we will discuss further in the upcoming chapter on unconscious fantasy and conflict (Chapter 23).

Displaced transference

When transference feelings are too immediate or intense to become conscious, patients may experience them as if they were related to someone else. This is called a **displaced transference**. For example:

> *Mr F spends half of his session ranting about a contractor who has delayed beginning renovations on his house. The intensity of his affect makes you wonder whether his reaction might be related to your recent delay in letting him know whether you could reschedule one of his sessions.*

Here's an example that brings together all three transference categories:

> *Ms G is a 34-year-old woman who is not married, has a busy career, and has trouble sustaining long-term friendships. In therapy sessions, she often comes direct from work dressed in designer business attire with a real flair for fashion. She has been talking about how other women dress at work and often makes derogatory comments about their outfits. She comments that they always wear flat shoes, don't*

reapply lipstick after lunch, and wear out-of-date styles. Her female therapist begins to feel self-conscious about her clothes and wonders what Ms G thinks of her outfit. The therapist then realizes that Ms G is talking about her in the displacement and wonders if the patient is having a transference reaction.

We might call this transference

- displaced
- negative
- maternal
- triadic

since it is derogatory and about competition with a woman.

Transference and resistance

As mentioned in the chapter on resistance, re-experiencing the past in the therapeutic relationship is, among other things, a resistance to remembering the original feelings. In addition, many patients resist acknowledging transference feelings. Alternately, patients sometimes resist accepting that they are having transference feelings at all and prefer to see their feelings only as "real." We call this **resistance to the awareness of the transference** [4]. It sometimes sounds like this:

Patient	*I never get any help from my boss. You know, you expect certain things from the people who are supposed to help you in life, and you never get them.*
Therapist	*I wonder if you could be talking about me, too.*
Patient	*Oh no – I'm just talking about my boss. This doesn't have to do with you.*

Transferences are also layered, with one feeling blocking awareness of another. For example, loving feelings toward the therapist can sometimes block awareness of more negative, competitive feelings, and vice versa.

Technique

Listening

Listening for transference, as with affect and resistance, generally involves consciously looking for it.

Listen for "off-the-cuff" remarks

Transference is often embedded in seemingly innocuous comments such as "Your office is really nice and warm," or "I'll bet your feet hurt at the end of the day wearing shoes that high." In regular conversation they're throwaway lines – in therapy they're clues to the transference. Register these remarks and remember them for future reference.

Tune into the beginning and end of the session

You can often find transference clues outside of the formal structure of the session, for example as patients enter or leave sessions. Comments like, "I always get going just as we near the end" or "It's so hard to get to your office in the rain," may signal the presence of transference. As with affect and resistance, these clues are often in the form of behaviors rather than spoken language, such as coming late to the first session of the week, scanning the materials on your desk, or starting a new topic as you are both standing up to end the session.

Listen for comments about other people – the displaced transference

Another common way to hear transference is as stories about friends, significant others, or co-workers. If these stories are filled with affect or if they remind us of something that is happening in therapy, think about whether they represent displaced transference. In this case, it is helpful to listen for clues that the feelings may also relate to you:

> A few months into treatment, Mr H, a graduate student, begins to discuss a teaching assistant who was unfamiliar with two of Derrida's main essays. Mr H is quite upset about whether he can work with this person given her "scholarly deficits." While listening, you are reminded of your own anxiety about never having read any Derrida and of having wondered whether you should read some in order to better understand this patient.

Here, the patient's fears about whether you can help him are displaced onto feelings about the teaching assistant. While these fears may well relate to real issues with the teaching assistant, they may also be displaced transference, and exploring them can help elucidate his feelings about you and his expectations of others in general.

Listen to your patient's general patterns of relating to others

Listening carefully to the details of your patient's relationships with other people can help you anticipate transference feelings that might arise. For example, if your patient describes a history of being very sensitive to rejection or of having trouble expressing anger, this will likely happen with you as well; or if your patient often has short relationships that end precipitously after a disappointment, be alert to the possibility that this may unfold in the transference. Listen for these as potential scripts that could be repeated in the relationship with you, while filing them away for future reference.

Listen to your countertransference

Although we will discuss countertransference more thoroughly in Chapter 22, it's important to note that one of the best ways to understand your patients' feelings about *you* is to be aware of your feelings about *them*. For example:

> *Although Mr I was very quiet during his last few sessions, his therapist felt a sense of loss.*

Attending to his own feelings helped the therapist to become aware of transference feelings against which the patient was protecting himself. This can be one of the best ways to become aware of displaced or avoided transference feelings.

Reflecting

Once you have noticed a theme, a set of behaviors, or a series of comments that signal a transference feeling, the next step is to consider whether to focus the patient's attention on it at this time. Remember the "three choosing principles" and the "three readiness principles" and consider the following:

Is the patient ready and willing to work with transference?

It is helpful to make trial inquiries about the transference and to monitor the patient's willingness to work with it in treatment. Some patients are not able or ready, in which case you don't want to badger them or sound like a cartoon psychoanalyst from the *New Yorker*. Transference inquiries such as "Did you have any feelings about what I said?" sometimes fall on deaf ears, or patients respond concretely, both of which suggest that they are not ready to work in this mode. Sometimes people say "I don't understand – I thought I wasn't supposed to have thoughts about you since you won't tell me anything." This comment invites **psychoeducation**, which we discuss below. Remember to be on the look-out for *non-verbal* signals that your inquiry has in some way upset or offended patients, for example if they fall silent, purse their lips, shift uneasily, cross their arms, look embarrassed, become anxious, or avoid eye contact.

Is the transference on the surface and the most affect-laden material in the session?

While transference is always operating, that does not mean that it is always the place to focus the patient's attention. For example, if a patient tells you that her son just had a serious bicycle accident and then asks you if you have children, you would focus initially on her son rather than on the transference. It might be possible to explore her transference later in the session, but it would be unfeeling not to inquire about her son at the outset. You could say "Maybe we can come back to that in a minute, but . . ." or "We can certainly talk about that if you like, but . . . I'm so sorry to hear about your son. How is he now?"

Sometimes the most important themes to explore occur out of the office. A frequent misconception about psychodynamic psychotherapy is that the transference should always be given priority. For example:

> Ms J is a 50-year-old woman who experiences her therapist as a warm, benevolent caretaker. One day she comes in crying after an airport customs official suspected her of trying to conceal items she purchased abroad. Through her tears she says that she is relieved to see the therapist and then goes on to talk about the humiliation she experienced at the airport.

Following the affect, the therapist should explore Ms J's experience with the airport official before asking her more about her transference feelings.

Should I interpret the transference?

In Chapter 4, we noted that people who have difficulty with self-esteem regulation, maintaining relationships, or impulse control generally need more support, while people who function well in these areas can tolerate and benefit from uncovering unconscious thoughts and fantasies. In general, this is a good rule of thumb to follow when deciding whether or not to interpret the transference. Patients who are challenged in these basic areas, whether at baseline or in response to a life crisis, generally require supporting interventions when they express feelings about the therapist, while patients who exhibit strength in these areas can often benefit from an uncovering, interpretive approach to the transference.

Studies conducted in the last decade, however, have challenged this traditional view. One study randomized 100 patients to two types of therapy, one with moderate use of transference interpretations and one with no transference interpretations. While there were no measurable differences in treatment outcome based on this variable, patients with poorer interpersonal relationship functioning were found to benefit more from therapy that included transference interpretations than from therapy without transference interpretations [5]. The authors hypothesized that since patients with relationship difficulties also struggle with building and maintaining a strong therapeutic alliance, feelings about the therapist that are not made a focus of interpretation could disrupt an already tenuous treatment and lead to drop-out and treatment failures [6]. "Here-and-now" transference interpretations may also help patients relate better to other people in their lives.

Should I interpret the transference now or let it evolve further?

It is important to understand transference feelings as fully as possible before making interpretations. As with resistance, you want to *live alongside the transference* for a while to get to know it better (Chapter 20).

Should I stay in the displacement or direct attention to the transference?

It often makes sense to explore transference feelings in the displacement before confronting them. This allows you to learn more about the feelings while patients talk about them in a more comfortable sphere. Remember that good work can be done discussing the displaced transference – it's not just treading water. Wait until the transference is very close to the surface before bringing it to the patient's attention.

Should I encourage mentalization or explore the transference?

As with any question related to "should I uncover or support?" the answer lies in knowing your aim. In general:

- *Encourage mentalization* when you think that patients *are not able to* think about their own and/or your thoughts and feelings and your aim is to enable them to do so.
- *Explore the transference* when you think that patients can think about their own and/or your thoughts and feelings and that uncovering them will help you understand their feelings about themselves and others.

Consider this:

> You unexpectedly start a session 10 minutes late because you were on an emergency call. Here is how two patients react to the same situation.

- Patient #1, a 24-year-old woman with a history of chaotic relationships and difficulty trusting others, says, "I know that you are starting the session 10 minutes late because you are angry that I stopped taking the medication two weeks ago."
- Patient #2, a 55-year-old man with a history of stable relationships but conflicts related to self-esteem, says, "No problem. I know that you are busy – but it's a shame because I had a lot to talk about today."

It sounds like Patient #1 has difficulty mentalizing – she is sure she knows what you are thinking and doesn't consider other possibilities. Your aim would be to encourage mentalization by saying something like: "I'm so sorry that I'm late and I hear what you are saying. Do you imagine that there might be any other reason why I started so late today?" On the other hand, Patient #2 seems to be able to mentalize, but has conflicts about whether he is worthy of your time and whether he can be angry with you. Your aim here is to explore his transference fantasies in order to better understand his sense of self and relationships to others by saying something like: "Can you tell me more about your feelings about starting late today?"

Can the patient appreciate the value of exploring the transference?

Working in the transference requires the patient to be able to

- experience feelings toward you, and
- step back and reflect on transferential feelings

Some patients are not able to work with the transference in this way and react to the therapist without being able to identify and express their feelings. In response to this, you can try psychoeducation or use some of the supportive strategies outlined later in this chapter.

Is the transference too intense?

Some patients form early, rapid, intense transference reactions. This can also happen later in the treatment. A "transference storm" – essentially, too much transference – can get in the way of treatment and may threaten the therapeutic alliance. Some patients have problems managing their transference feelings and will view the therapist as the embodiment of hostile or abusive people from their past. This can erupt in treatment as an intense paranoid, hostile, or devaluing transference. It is important to identify when patients are not able to manage their transference affects and to assess whether:

- they have lost reality testing
- they are able to mentalize their experiences
- they have acted out self-destructively based on these affects, and
- the treatment is directly threatened.

This will guide your choice of intervention.

Intervening

Basic interventions

Most patients have to be taught about transference and how to identify it. Some also have to be convinced that talking about transference is worthwhile, as it is often difficult to do and can bring up unsettling feelings. The process of helping patients talk comfortably about transference is an important way to intervene in psychodynamic psychotherapy. Note that it can take a while and may not happen with all patients. Here are some useful interventions:

Psychoeducation

This is a crucial first step in the process. It is helpful to tell people the following at the beginning of a psychodynamic therapy:

> *In this type of psychotherapy, we can learn a lot about you and your relationships with other people by discussing your thoughts and feelings about me.*

This statement can be included when you instruct patients to say whatever comes to mind, as discussed in the chapter on free association (Chapter 20). **Empathizing** with the awkwardness of the task and **explaining** how it can be helpful are key. It is important to realize that even if you explain this at the beginning of treatment, you may have to repeat it as these feelings arise over time. After a few repetitions, you can begin to interpret the patient's discomfort in discussing the transference as a resistance. It is also helpful to **encourage** patients by explaining the utility of discussing feelings about the therapist.

Questions

In order to understand transference feelings, you have to learn about them. Asking questions such as "What was your experience of talking about that yesterday?" or "What were your feelings about my canceling that session?" will give you valuable information about the transference.

Supporting interventions

When our patients have difficulties with functions such as self-esteem regulation, relationships, and reflective capacity, our goals in dealing with the transference are generally to

- help them to feel less overwhelmed by their perceptions and feelings about the therapist, and
- improve and preserve the therapeutic alliance.

Learning from the transference without focusing on it

Understanding the transference is always useful for the therapist – however, it may sometimes overwhelm patients with poor reflective capacity or impulse control. With these patients, we listen for the transference, reflect on it, and learn from it; however, we do not necessarily uncover it. Notwithstanding reports by Hogland mentioned earlier in this chapter, when patients have compromised mental and emotional function, the general rule of thumb has historically been to try to work in a climate of a moderately positive transference and not to focus on transference – especially early in treatment [7–9]. Here's a good example:

> Mr K sometimes missed the first session after the therapist's vacation. Although Mr K was never able to discuss this, whenever it happened the therapist knew that Mr K had had feelings about the separation.

Talking to patients directly about their behavior in the treatment

With some patients, talking to them about the way they act in treatment can help them improve their relationships with others. Here are two examples:

> I noticed that you tend to come to sessions about 5–10 minutes late – do you do that at work, too? It might be one of the things that makes your boss upset with you.

When you get angry with me, you don't tend to address it until a few weeks later. Talking about it up front sometimes keeps things from escalating. Maybe that would help with your wife as well.

Here, the therapist comments on the transference with the intention of directly improving the patient's relationships, rather than exploring transference feelings and fantasies about the therapist.

Repairing, reducing, and containing the transference

It's all well and good to say "don't focus on the transference" when you're using a supporting mode, but the reality is that people who have problems with basic trust, reality testing, self-esteem, and interpersonal relationships are often the most vulnerable to becoming overwhelmed by intense transferences. Sometimes these feelings can disrupt the treatment from the outset, forcing you to address the therapeutic relationship directly. Healthier patients are generally ready to trust the therapist at the start of treatment, readily shrug off our lapses and mistakes, and weather ruptures without problems. More fragile patients have special sensitivities that make it harder for them to forgive the therapist's real or perceived blunders and empathic failures. Some patients have trouble mentalizing and exploring their subjective experience of the therapeutic relationship – if you ask, "Do you notice that you're criticizing me for the same things you hate in your mother?" the response is apt to be, "Just my luck to get a therapist like my mother!" With these more vulnerable patients, *reducing* negative transference and *repairing* ruptures in the therapeutic relationship are vital to preserving the treatment and may be the major ongoing priority related to the transference [10–14].

There is a specific set of supporting techniques for resolving your patients' intense or hostile transferences to you *without* necessarily helping them understand that these are reactions based on feelings toward important people from earlier years:

- **Naming affects**: Putting feelings into words and accurately registering what patients are feeling can help manage the transference. It can sound like this:

    Maybe you were upset when I didn't return your call . . .

    It sounds like you feel you're not important to me.

    I guess it seems like I don't care.

- **Validating experience**: If patients have feelings about you that are accurate, validating their experience can be very containing. Apologizing for lateness is an example of this:

Patient	*I'm really upset that you started 10 minutes late today.*
Therapist	*That makes sense – you expected to start at a certain time and that didn't happen. I'm sorry about that.*

Often, validating feelings, expressing dismay, and leaving it at that is enough, but if not, you can try to explain the patient's feelings – openly and non-defensively – in terms of things that are actually happening in the treatment:

For reasons relating to the patient's safety, a therapist has had to stay in touch with the spouse of a suicidal patient. When the patient accuses the therapist of "spying" on her, the therapist might say, "You're right – I have been in touch with your husband and I can see that that's made you feel like you're not in control of your own therapy. But to me, the most important thing is your safety, so I need to be in touch with him temporarily so that we can keep you as safe as possible. Let's continue to talk about your feelings about this."

- **Interpreting up**: This can help diffuse strong transference feelings by relating them to things that are occurring in a patient's current life and relationships outside the treatment:

    It must have been especially upsetting not to be able to reach me during this time when your wife is away and your parents are not being very supportive.

- **Gently correcting misperceptions and jointly testing reality**: If the alliance can withstand it, you also can try to gently correct misperceptions and reality-test the person's distortions about you:

Patient	I hate it when you're patronizing!
Therapist	What did I say that sounded patronizing?
Patient	I don't know. It was more your tone.
Therapist	I'm very sorry that what I said made you feel insulted . . . that certainly wasn't my intention.

- **Encouraging mentalization**: As described earlier in this chapter, this is another technique for addressing intense transference reactions. Mentalization techniques aim to assist patients in sorting out their feelings about what is happening in the therapeutic relationship. This straightforward approach includes:
    - Asking patients to describe what they are experiencing in therapy
    - Empathizing with their experience regardless of its accuracy
    - Clarifying and exploring their affect
    - Reflecting on their image of the relationship
    - Focusing their attention on what you might be feeling
    - Sharing some aspect of your experience of the moment to support the idea that you have your own subjective experience
    - Helping them contrast their own perception of themselves with your perception of them [15]

Here is an example:

Because of a death in the family, a therapist has to cancel a session with only one day's notice. When he and the patient meet the following week, the patient is quietly annoyed, sitting with folded arms. The therapist asks her to say what is on her mind, and suggests that she must have had feelings about the cancelation. She talks about how jarring it was, given that the therapist generally gives at least two weeks' notice. While listening and empathizing, the therapist encourages the patient to talk in more detail about what she felt, while the therapist adds that it was also hard for him to have to cancel at the last minute, as he values keeping their appointments.

This exchange supports the patient's ability to **mentalize** her experience and that of the therapist.

If all else fails, stay calm under fire and try not to become angry. Showing patients that you can tolerate their strong feelings without judging them, becoming upset, or rejecting them is a central feature of the **holding function** of psychotherapy. It convinces them that, like the mother of a toddler having a tantrum, you will continue to support them even if they are experiencing strong negative feelings [16]. As their therapist, you may be the first person in their life to offer them this kind of security. Repeatedly experiencing this with the therapist can improve the alliance and, eventually, their other relationships. Remember that strains in the alliance are inevitable along the way in any psychotherapy. In fact, research has shown that the course of the alliance in *good outcome* psychotherapy cases is always characterized by a series of ruptures and repairs [16].

Uncovering interventions

We select uncovering interventions when we want to explore the transference in order to uncover unconscious thoughts and feelings.

Confrontation

The first step in uncovering is **confrontation**. We confront when we want to call the patient's attention to the transference. Here are some confrontations of the transference:

> *You got very quiet after the last comment I made. Did you have some feelings about it?*
>
> *Sounds like you're angry about my vacation. Can you say more about that?*

Here's an example in which a confrontation of the transference is used:

> *Mr L is a 26-year-old philosophy graduate student who frequently disparages people who don't understand his area of interest. You wonder if he is talking about you, but you initially explore this in the displacement. During the first session back after your week-long spring vacation, you see him glance at a brochure sitting on your desk from the Walt Disney cruise you just took. While he doesn't refer to it directly, he begins to talk condescendingly about his younger brother's fraternity and the crude "road trip" they went on to Florida. You think his feelings about you are near the surface but, because he is not mentioning them directly, you decide to confront the transference, saying, "You are thinking about how people spend their vacations, but you haven't mentioned thoughts about mine." He then says that he saw the brochure and was embarrassed that you took such a "plebeian" trip.*

The confrontation enables the patient to deepen his discussion of the transference.

Clarification

Clarifications of the transference link situations in which the patient has similar reactions to you:

> *You're very quiet today – and it's the last day before my vacation. This happened the last time I went away, too.*

> *Every time you talk about your wife you're sure that I'll be judgmental.*

> *Although for a while you thought I understood what you were feeling, for the last few weeks you haven't had that feeling at all.*

Clarifications help people have conviction about their transference feelings because they see that these have occurred in several different situations.

Interpretation

There are two basic types of **transference interpretations**. In one, the therapist interprets the patient's behavior as the result of unconscious transference feelings:

> *I think you've been late for the last two sessions because you're worried that I'm angry with you.*

In the other type of transference interpretation, the therapist interprets the transference as being the result of a distortion related to a past relationship:

> *I think you're worried that I might be angry with you because your mother was always upset when you made decisions on your own.*

Both types of interpretations help patients understand themselves and their relationships to others. Here's an example of interpretive work related to the transference:

> Ms M is a 34-year-old woman who works as a school nutritionist and who has been in therapy for two years. She is heterosexual but not married. She has a good alliance with Dr Z, her female therapist, whom she tends to idealize. She has many friends for whom she does too much, generally prioritizing the needs of others. This has been a major focus of the therapeutic work, and Ms M is beginning to assert her own needs. As a child, her father wasn't around and she had a younger brother with cerebral palsy who took up much of her mother's time. Although it seems to the therapist that the mother neglected Ms M, Ms M has generally pitied her mother and tried to do everything in her power to make her life easier. In the week prior to the following session, the therapist told Ms M that she was going to have to miss one of their twice-weekly sessions the next week. This is the session prior to the session that would be missed:

> | Patient | So, the weekend – I had invited my co-worker Yvette and her new husband over for lunch, but they couldn't come at the last minute. I had all this food – but was alone as usual. |
> |---|---|
> | Therapist | That sounds very disappointing. (**empathic remark**) |
> | Patient | Well, I had a lot to do – and it allowed me to catch up on work. She always cancels, so I should know better than to invite them without other people. |
> | Therapist | It sounds like it's a little hard to feel upset about it. (**confrontation**) |

Patient	*Upset? It's just lunch – it's not like it was my wedding or something.*
Therapist	*Maybe weddings are on your mind – like Yvette's wedding.* (**confrontation**)
Patient	*(one tear runs down her face) Yvette was the last one – we were together in "singlehood" – now she has someone and better things to do. But what good does it do to cry about it? It's not going to make her more likely to show up at lunch. Maybe that lunch wasn't very important to her, but it was the center of my weekend. And she canceled at the last minute, like she didn't even care.*
Therapist	*You're talking about your friend today, but I canceled at the last minute too. Maybe you're focusing on her because it's hard to get upset with me.* (**interpretation**)
Patient	*You have a life – you have things to do. I'm not the center of your life.*
Therapist	*Maybe you wish you were.* (**interpretation**)
Patient	*(crying) I wish that I were the center of someone's life. Yvette has Rodney, you have your family – my mother was always taking care of my brother. I don't think that I'll ever be someone's number one priority.*

In this session, the therapist stays in the displacement for a while, since the patient is expressing affect and moving into new emotional territory. **Confrontations** help to decrease the patient's resistance to admitting how upset she is. Once it becomes clear that the feelings about Yvette are nearly identical to those that she has about the therapist, Dr Z connects the displaced feelings and the transference. Ultimately, the patient links her friend, her therapist, and her mother – none of whom, she feels, puts her needs first. Recognizing these feelings is her first step toward understanding how she defensively subjugates her own needs in order to stave off disappointment and anger.

Now that we've explored transference, it's on to the therapist's feelings – **countertransference**.

Suggested activity

Here are three vignettes that involve transference. Read them and consider the study questions:

1. It is the third visit with a new patient, a 25-year-old single musician who had abruptly ended his prior treatment when his therapist told him she could not have sessions at the local coffee shop. He says he could not work with the prior therapist because she was very rigid and recounts how she would not have coffee with him, often ended the sessions even if he was in the middle of an important topic, and seemed not to be interested in dreams. He says he hopes that you can be more helpful and flexible.
   a. Is the patient exhibiting a transference to you?
   b. What type of transference did he have to the prior therapist?
   c. What interventions might you make now?
   d. What interventions might you make at a later point in the treatment?

Comment

The patient is hopeful that you will be a "good mother" and is exhibiting a positive maternal transference at the moment. He had a negative maternal transference to his prior therapist when he ended the treatment. In listening, you wonder if he is using splitting to see you as potentially all good and the old therapist as all bad. Since this is a new patient, you might register the transference, but make sure he understands the treatment frame. This could involve both **demonstrating understanding** and **psychoeducation**:

> It sounds like you have mixed feelings about your former therapist that are important to talk about – but it's also important to know that most therapists wouldn't have coffee with their patients, because the treatment only happens during sessions in the office. I'm glad you brought it up because it's important to be clear about that at the beginning of therapy.

If the issue arose later, for example at a moment when he felt you were frustrating him, you could **interpret** the displacement, saying:

> I think it's easier to evoke memories of your frustrations with your former therapist than it is to talk about your current frustrations with me.

2. You are treating a 32-year-old woman who sought help just over a year ago, complaining of longstanding unhappiness in her marriage and feeling trapped by the relationship. She fears that she may have married the wrong man, but is terrified that if she ends the marriage she will never have children. She has been seeing you twice weekly and feels very engaged in treatment. A year into therapy she gets an ideal job offer; however, she will have to move one of her sessions and you cannot accommodate her scheduling needs. She is very upset and feels that you are making her choose between the perfect job opportunity and therapy. She feels trapped by the relationship with you, and fears that you could possibly stand in her way of taking this job. She says, "If it weren't for you, I would be happily moving ahead in my career. Now I have to either compromise my therapy or not take the perfect job."
   a. Is the patient exhibiting a transference to you?
   b. What type of transference is this?
   c. What interventions might you make if she has weakened function?
   d. What interventions might you make if she is able to do uncovering work?

Comment

The patient sees you as standing in the way of her progress. This could be a competitive triadic maternal transference; that is, she could be experiencing you as if you were a mother who holds her daughter back to prevent her from winning the affection of her father. It could also be a negative maternal dyadic transference related to an envious mother. A supporting intervention might be to **correct misperceptions** by pointing out that you are trying to accommodate her. You could then discuss the idea that she tends to feel trapped when arrangements don't go her way, just like in her relationship. An **interpretive** intervention might include a **confrontation** about her affective experience of feeling trapped, such as:

> What comes to mind about feeling trapped?

You could follow up with a **clarification** about the similarity between her feelings about her husband and you:

> *It's interesting that you're feeling trapped by both me and by your husband – do you have thoughts about that?*

An **interpretation** could ultimately point out that she feels trapped because she both needs you and experiences you as if you were standing in the way of her progress:

> *You're upset with me because you feel conflicted – on the one hand you feel you need me, but on the other hand you feel that I'm keeping you from moving forward.*

Having uncovered this conflict, you might be able to learn more about her feelings about this, and/or about how it related to her early relationships.

3. A 65-year-old retired salesman just had back surgery and is struggling with how to engage in the next stage of his life. When he returns from surgery and you ask him about whether he is still taking any medication, he starts to yell, saying, "What is your problem? You are just like everyone else who just wants to accuse me of being an addict." He continues to scowl, and looks as if he might leave the room.
   a. Is the patient exhibiting a transference to you?
   b. What type of transference is this?
   c. What approach might help in getting through this rupture?

Comment

The patient experiences you as accusing him of abusing pain medication. He is having a paranoid negative transference. This strong, angry transference reaction could threaten the treatment. This is a good time to encourage the patient to describe what he is feeling and encourage him to **mentalize**, by saying, "Can you tell me what you are feeling about my having asked that question?" If he calms down and can reflect on his assumption about you, you could also disclose that you ask this question of all your patients who return from surgery. This discussion should help to repair the alliance, and illustrate the patient's tendency to jump to false conclusions about the experience of others when he feels defensive.

Chapter 21: References

1. Auchincloss, E.L., and Samberg, E. (1990) *Psychoanalytic Terms and Concepts*, Yale University Press, New Haven, p. 151–153.
2. Greenson, R.R. (1967) *The Technique and Practice of Psychoanalysis*, International Universities Press, New York, p. 238–240.
3. Moore, B.E., and Fine, B.D. (1990) *Psychoanalytic Terms and Concepts*, Yale University Press, New Haven, p. 134–135.
4. Gabbard, G.O. (2009) *Textbook of Psychotherapeutic Treatments*, American Psychiatric Publishing, Washington, DC, p. 58.
5. Hoglend, P., Amlo, S., Marble, A., *et al.* (2006) Analysis of the patient-therapist relationship in dynamic psychotherapy: An experimental study of transference interpretations. *American Journal of Psychiatry*, **163**, 1739–1746.

6. Hoglend, P. (2014) Exploration of the patient-therapist relationship in psychotherapy. *American Journal of Psychiatry*, **171**, 1056–1066.

7. Hoglend, P. (2008) Transference interpretations in dynamic psychotherapy: Do they really yield sustained effects? *American Journal of Psychiatry*, **165**, 763.

8. Levy, K.N., Meehan, K.B., Kelly, K.M., *et al.* (2006) Change in attachment patterns and reflective function in a randomized control trial of transference-focused psychotherapy for borderline personality disorder. *Journal of Consulting and Clinical Psychology*, **74** (6), 1027–1040.

9. Gabbard, G.O., and Horowitz, M. (2009) Insight, transference, interpretation and therapeutic change in the dynamic psychotherapy of borderline personality disorder. *American Journal of Psychiatry*, **166** (5), 517–521.

10. Safran, J.D., Muran, J.C., and Proskurov, B. (2009) Alliance, negotiation, and rupture resolution, in *Handbook of Evidence-Based Psychodynamic Psychotherapy* (eds R.A. Levy and J.S. Ablon), Humana Press, New York, p. 201–225.

11. Pinsker, H. (1997) *A Primer of Supportive Psychotherapy*, Analytic Press, Hillsdale, NJ.

12. Winston, A., Rosenthal, R.N., and Pinsker, H. (2004) *Introduction to Supportive Psychotherapy*, American Psychiatric Publishing, Washington, DC.

13. Kernberg, O.F., and Philadelphia, J.B. (1982) Supportive psychotherapy with borderline conditions, in *Critical Problems in Psychiatry* (eds J.O. Cavenar and H.K. Brodie), J.B. Lippincott, New York, p. 195–197.

14. Appelbaum, A.H. (2006) Supportive psychoanalytic psychotherapy for borderline patients: An empirical approach. *American Journal of Psychoanalysis*, **66** (4), 317–332.

15. Bateman, A., and Fonagy, P. (2015) Borderline personality disorder and mood disorders: Mentalizing as a framework for integrated treatment. *Journal of Clinical Psychology*, **71**, 792–804.

16. Safran, J.D., and Kraus, J. (2014) Alliance ruptures, impasses, and enactments: A relational perspective. *Psychotherapy*, **51** (3), 381–387.

22 Countertransference

Key concepts

Countertransference is the sum of the therapist's feelings toward the patient. It includes both conscious and unconscious feelings.

Countertransference is ubiquitous. Far from being something to avoid, it informs our work with patients in many ways.

Understanding countertransference is important because

- being aware of our feelings toward patients makes it less likely that we will act on them
- feelings that we have about our patients help us make assessments, formulate treatment recommendations, and conduct the treatment
- countertransference helps us learn about the important relationships in our patients' lives
- countertransference feelings help us learn about ourselves and our reactions to patients

Countertransference informs our understanding of the patient and our interventions, but is generally not shared directly with patients.

When our countertransference toward a patient is felt toward a supervisor, it is called **parallel process**.

When we inadvertently say or do something with the patient in response to our countertransference, it is called an **enactment**.

When two people sit in a room and talk to each other week after week, they *both* have feelings about *each other*. In the same way that patients have feelings about their therapists, which we call transference, therapists have feelings about their patients, which we call *counter*transference. Although early analysts thought that therapists were supposed to be free of feelings about their patients, we now know that our countertransference feelings help us conduct psychodynamic psychotherapy in many ways [1].

What is countertransference?

As we began to discuss in Chapter 12, countertransference is the sum of the feelings therapists have about their patients. It includes both conscious and unconscious feelings.

Psychodynamic Psychotherapy: A Clinical Manual, Second Edition. Deborah L. Cabaniss, Sabrina Cherry, Carolyn J. Douglas and Anna Schwartz.
© 2017 John Wiley & Sons, Ltd. Published 2017 by John Wiley & Sons, Ltd.

There are two types of countertransference reactions – those that originate in the patient and those that originate in the therapist. In the first type, we have feelings about a patient because of something he or she feels or does:

> *After Ms A forgot to pay her bill for three months in a row, her therapist felt very angry with her. He did not, however, feel angry with his other patients.*

> *Mr B's risky sexual practices made his therapist quite anxious. The therapist realized that Mr B was projecting his anxiety onto her in order to remain in denial about the amount of danger he was placing himself in.*

In the second type, we have feelings when a patient (or patients) reminds us of something in our own life, such as a symptom, a trauma, or a relationship:

> *When Mr C described his father's death, the therapist, whose own father had just died, felt tearful.*

> *Dr Z's early experiences make her feel protective of young patients who have stern mothers.*

One good way to tell the difference is to ask yourself whether you only have the reaction to *this* patient, which suggests that it originated in the patient, or whether you have the reaction to *many* patients, which suggests that it originated within you.

Why do we care about countertransference?

Understanding our countertransference is important for many reasons:

- **Acknowledging and understanding our feelings about patients decreases the chances that we will act on those feelings:** It is inevitable that in the course of working with patients we will have a range of feelings toward them, including anger, irritation, affection, and boredom. The more aware we are of these feelings and of the potential reasons for them, the less likely we are to unconsciously act on them. Consider these two situations:

  > *Therapist #1 fights against acknowledging his boredom with his patient and begins to consistently fall asleep in sessions.*

  > *Therapist #2 acknowledges his boredom with his patient. He discusses this with a supervisor and realizes that it is related to a resistance preventing the patient from engaging with him. The therapist becomes more attentive in sessions as he reflects on the patient's conflict.*

- **Countertransference helps us to diagnose, assess, and treat our patients:** Having very strong positive or negative feelings about patients helps us to recognize the predominance of splitting-based defenses. Understanding our feelings about patients during sessions helps us to recognize many aspects of our patients' functioning, including defenses and their ways of relating to other people.

- **Countertransference helps guide our interventions in a moment-to-moment way by helping us recognize what is important in the session:** As discussed in the chapter on reflecting, understanding countertransference can be one of the best ways to understand when and how to intervene.

- **Countertransference helps us learn more about ourselves as we work with different patients:** Do you always become hopeless when patients reveal that they have an eating disorder? Do you tend to feel depressed when you talk to patients who have substance abuse problems? Do you dread seeing patients who are taking medications? Acknowledging your reactions to patients will help you understand yourself as a therapist and make career decisions that will enable you to do the work you most enjoy.

Is it bad to have countertransference?

As we've mentioned, countertransference used to be thought of as something that interfered with treatment and needed to be eliminated. We no longer believe this, and now accept that countertransference is a useful element in our work with patients. Countertransference is only harmful to a treatment when it is unacknowledged by the therapist or when it is acted on in ways that violate the therapeutic frame (see Chapter 8).

Types of countertransference

In the course of a treatment, it is common to empathize or identify with patients. This is called **concordant countertransference**:

> *Ms D is a 32-year-old woman with an eight-month-old baby. Since having the baby, she has missed many sessions. When she does come, she is often late, arriving breathless and describing how much difficulty she has timing her nursing schedule so that that she has enough time to get to your office. You feel it really is too difficult for her to manage both being in therapy and being a new mother, and you therefore tolerate her lateness and missed sessions without asking her if there is something else she is feeling about you that might contribute to her lateness. You realize that this is not your usual approach to patients when they are late and miss a lot of sessions, and thus that you are having a* **concordant countertransference** *reaction.*

At other times your identification might be with people with whom your patient has (or has had) relationships. This is called **complementary countertransference**:

> *With Ms D, you might become frustrated and angry that she is not making therapy a priority. You might become aware that your anger at her is stronger than what you usually feel toward patients who are acting out by missing sessions. As you think about this more, you recall that she told you that her mother was very exacting, with no room for error, even when the patient was sick or had a crisis. You realize that you are feeling the way the patient's mother did – thus you are having a* **complementary countertransference**.

Both concordant and complementary countertransferences help us learn about our patients and their relationships [2].

What happens if I am not aware of my countertransference?

Our feelings about our patients may be unconscious. Sometimes, we become aware of them during supervision. At other times, they are reflected in how we feel toward a supervisor. When transference/countertransference feelings from a treatment enter into a supervision, we call it **parallel process** [3]. It is important to think about how you feel in supervision and reflect on whether something about the patient is being displaced onto the supervisory relationship.

> Dr Y felt that his psychotherapy supervisor did not think he was doing good work, even though the supervisor had been encouraging and written strong evaluations. When Dr Y thought more about this, he realized that his patient unconsciously felt he was not being a good patient. This was a concordant countertransference displaced onto the supervision.

When our countertransference remains out of our awareness, it can lead us to act on it with our patients. When this happens it is called an **enactment** [4]. Problematic enactments, which involve boundary violations, generally require supervision or consultation. But benign enactments happen all the time and, once understood, can help to elucidate what's happening in the treatment – particularly with regard to the therapeutic relationship:

> Ms E gets frustrated about her lack of progress in therapy and demands that Dr X offer more insight. The therapist, feeling pressured to come up with something brilliant, says more than is needed about the patient's dynamics. Feeling overwhelmed, the patient cancels the next session.

In this enactment, the patient's demands led Dr X to feel pressured and insecure. Acting on these feelings, she changed her technique and ended up overwhelming the patient. If the therapist allows herself to explore her countertransference, she will learn about an important way in which the patient interacts with people. This is sometimes called a **transference–countertransference paradigm**. Since enactments are a regular part of therapy, the point is not to avoid them; rather, the trick is to notice them after the fact and to use them to deepen understanding. Supervision is often helpful in recognizing enactments. If you notice that you're behaving in an uncharacteristic way with a patient, chances are that you're in an enactment. If she is working in an uncovering mode, Dr X could discuss this with Ms E:

> I wonder if you might have missed the last session because you felt overwhelmed by my comments. I noticed that I was talking more than usual, and, in thinking about it afterward, I realized that I felt pressure from you to say a lot because you were disappointed in your progress. That's something that happened between us – you got frustrated and it affected me. Does that feel familiar?

Talking about enactments allows therapist and patient jointly to examine their interaction and elucidate both the therapist's and patient's experience [5]. In this way, understanding enactments can lead to insights about other relationships in the patient's life. Sometimes enactments lead to insights about early relationships and sometimes they simply reflect current interactions in therapy. In both cases, discussion of enactments enhances communication skills, mentalization, and understanding of relationship dynamics.

Technique

Listening

How do you know if you're having countertransference? Here are some thoughts about how to figure this out:

- **Think about how you feel towards the patient:** For beginning therapists, it often takes time to learn to identify feelings toward patients. To start, develop the habit of asking yourself, "How do I feel about this patient?" You can do this right after sessions or even later in the day. Ask yourself this question in a general way as well as in reaction to particular moments in sessions. Often these thoughts randomly enter your awareness and, when they do, pay attention to them and begin to identify them more precisely.

  It is helpful to talk to someone about your patient to help understand your counter-transference. If you're a trainee, you can discuss cases with a supervisor. If you're no longer a trainee, you may still find it useful to have a supervisor, even on an as-needed basis. Many psychodynamic psychotherapists also discuss cases with colleagues, omitting any potentially identifying data. This can occur as a consultation, in an ongoing supervisory relationship, or on an ad hoc basis.

- **Think about your behavior in relation to the patient:** In addition to exploring your feelings, you can also think about your behavior regarding the patient before, during, and between sessions. Some examples include:

  - dressing in a particular way when you see a patient
  - deviating from your usual therapy technique (such as talking less or more)
  - dreaming about a patient
  - having a strong feeling (such as anxiety) in anticipation of seeing a patient
  - changing aspects of the frame with a patient, such as forgetting to mention a vacation or not charging for a missed session

  If you find yourself preoccupied with patients outside of sessions, behaving differently because of your relationship with them, or acting atypically in sessions, think through potential reasons for these behaviors.

  A common example of this type of countertransference is anxiety that a patient will leave treatment. Sometimes these feelings impede therapists from confronting transference anger, or from following through on a cancelation policy. This limits the patient's opportunity to explore the negative transference. Therapists are especially vulnerable to this anxiety if they depend on the patient for course credit or to fill practice hours.

- **Listen for similarities between the way you feel toward patients and what they describe happening in other relationships:** Sometimes you may notice yourself identifying with a set of feelings that patients describe, either in themselves or in another relationship:

    A patient describes feeling that her mother never worried about her. While she is talking, you realize that you have never worried about her either, even though you have often worried about other patients.

    If you allow yourself to notice this sudden countertransference reaction, it will undoubtedly help you understand the patient. For example, the patient may have induced this guilty reaction in you because she thinks that this is the only way that you will take care of her.

- **Listen to your feelings about any supervision you are involved in regarding each case:** As already discussed, feelings you have about a supervisor may be closely related to feelings about the patient.

Reflecting

Once you have identified feelings or behaviors as countertransference, the next step is to reflect on them to understand how they can be used to deepen the treatment. Here are some questions that you can ask yourself in this process:

- Is my countertransference informing me about an affect that the patient feels? You might have a feeling that:
    - the patient consciously feels (concordant)
    - the patient is repressing (concordant)
    - someone in the patient's life might feel toward the patient (complementary)
- Is my countertransference related to a resistance that I had not been aware of until now? For example, the patient may be talking away, but your boredom or distraction in a session could reveal to you that the patient is avoiding something.
- Is my countertransference related to my own history or emotional experience? If so, how is it related to the current treatment?

Countertransference helps us to decide when and how to intervene. "Attend to the countertransference" (Chapter 17) is one of the choosing principles because understanding our feelings about patients is one of the best tools we have to help us decide when and how to intervene. Particularly when a resistance is operative, we may know what the patient is feeling well before they do. Our anxiety level can signal our patients' underlying unconscious affect, or the tenuousness of the therapeutic alliance:

    Ms F is a new patient who seems motivated for treatment and starts off talking about a variety of topics. She arrives 15 minutes late for her first two sessions. The therapist, Ms W, thinks this is probably a resistance related to her ambivalence about treatment. When Ms W thinks about saying this to the patient, she becomes anxious and realizes she fears that it will make Ms F very angry. The therapist decides to wait to confront the resistance.

Here the therapist's countertransference picked up on the patient's anxiety before it was consciously communicated to her. This helped the therapist decide what was on the surface, as well as how and when to intervene.

Intervening

Do you ever tell the patient about your countertransference?

Generally, we do not directly share our countertransference with patients. Instead, we use it to develop ideas about what is most affectively rich and ready for interpretation. Our private feelings of anger, irritation, and affection are best left for our own reflection and discussions with supervisors. We do, however, sometimes tell patients how we feel. Here are some of those circumstances:

- **In response to a socially appropriate cue:** When important things happen to our patients, such as a death in the family, a child's graduation, or the arrival of new baby, we respond. It's fine to say "I'm so sorry" or "Congratulations" – in fact, if we don't, our patients might find it odd. This type of response is often critical for the ongoing therapeutic alliance. In a supporting mode, the intervention might stop there; when uncovering, we ultimately want to understand the patient's feelings about the intervention.

- **When we have a strong opinion:** "I'm worried about your depression and think that you should have a consultation for medication" or "I'm concerned about your safety – I'd like to call your husband to make sure he can stay with you" – both convey feelings that you have about the patient. These disclosures are essential to providing optimal treatment.

- **To help elucidate a repressed affect:** When used judiciously, disclosure of the therapist's affect can help the patient connect to repressed feeling. For example, the therapist who tells her patient "It's interesting – your bar exam is coming up in two weeks and I seem more anxious about it than you do – what do you make of that?" helps the patient understand feelings that she is unconsciously communicating to the therapist.

- **To assist with mentalization:** Patients who have difficulty mentalizing can't imagine that the therapist's perception could be different from their own. Particularly when working in a primarily supporting mode, thoughtfully disclosing feelings can help foster mentalization. Consider this exchange:

  Ms G   *The guy I went out with last week never called back. Now you're thinking, "she's such a loser."*

  Therapist   *Actually I was thinking how disappointed you must have been.*

Asking patients to imagine your feelings

Patients can often learn about how their behavior affects other people by trying to imagine how it affects us [6,7]. For example, we might encourage a patient who skips sessions and is late but never calls to imagine their emotional effect on us by asking something like, "What do you imagine I felt when you did not come to session or call me?" (See the discussion of encouraging mentalization in Chapter 18.)

Validating the patient's experience of the countertransference

Sometimes, patients intuit what we feel toward them. They might say, "I know you are angry with me, don't deny it." While in an uncovering mode, you might say, "Let's imagine you're right – do you have any thoughts about that?" In a supporting mode you might try to use that information to teach the person about their effect on others by saying, "It sounds like you understand that you have been trying to get me to feel angry at you. Does that happen with other people?"

Understanding an enactment in the treatment

As already discussed, enactments are exchanges or events in which therapists unconsciously react to patients or the transference. When this happens, it is important to validate the patient's experiences of what happened and help them imagine, or mentalize, your experience. It is important, however, to do this without revealing too much personal information that could burden the patient and close off avenues of exploration:

> *Your patient has been talking about her mother's breast cancer and is very anxious about a potential recurrence that is under evaluation. She says talking about this is "making it worse," and she does not want to think about it any more. You empathize with how hard it is hard for her not to give up hope. She seems to appreciate your empathic response, and you end the session. After she leaves, you look at your schedule and realize you ended the session 15 minutes early!*

As you think about why you ended the session early, you realize that you empathized with her concern and worried that making her talk about feelings might make her feel worse. You also felt anxious since you were about to have a routine diagnostic procedure later that week. On reflection, you realize that you have a concordant countertransference, identifying with the patient's desire to avoid feeling distressed. This is in part related both to your own anxiety about your upcoming procedure and to your patient's desire to avoid her anxiety about her mother. You discuss with your supervisor how you might handle this in the next session.

> *The following week, your patient arrives and launches into a discussion about her work as if nothing unusual happened the week before. After some time, you decide to address what happened:*

Therapist	*I was thinking about our session last week, and wondered if you noticed that I made an error and ended our session early?* (**confrontation, acknowledging reality**)
Patient	*I wasn't going to say anything, but I did wonder what happened since you never do that.*
Therapist	*I am happy to tell you, but first I wondered what your feelings about it were?* (**confrontation of transference**)
Patient	*Well, to be honest, I was a little put off when I realized, but also relieved since it was so hard to talk about my mother's recurrence and work-up.*
Therapist	*Yes, I think you are right, I was also concerned about your mother's situation and perhaps I ended early because I unconsciously felt your desire to finish talking about it.* (**countertransference disclosure**) *I am sorry about that, and we can make up the missed time at some point if you like.*

In this case, you have to say something to account for your error, but just enough not to burden the patient with more information than necessary. Understanding the enactment helps the patient mentalize that you can have your own reactions. It also models that therapists make mistakes and can take responsibility for acknowledging them.

Talking to your supervisor about your experience in supervision

If you become aware of feelings toward your supervisor, or about the supervision, and wonder if they could relate to your patient, you might explore the possibility that there might be a parallel process:

> Dr V feels that his supervisor is canceling supervision more often than usual, and wonders if he is a bad supervisee. He wonders if this relates to something about the patient he is discussing, who was abandoned by her father at an early age. In supervision, Dr V mentions the supervisor's frequent cancelations and wonders if it could be a parallel process. The therapist and supervisor begin to explore whether this might be correct.

Countertransference can inform our choice of supporting or uncovering approaches

"Attending to the countertransference" (Chapter 17) not only helps us to know when and how to intervene, it also helps us to choose whether a basic, supporting, or uncovering intervention will be most effective at any given moment:

> Mr H is a 32-year-old chef whose sensitivity to perceived slights has resulted in his abruptly leaving jobs. On occasion, Mr H has called his therapist to reschedule when he was running late. Early in the treatment, the therapist generally changed his time if her schedule permitted because she worried that if she didn't he might leave treatment. In the course of therapy, Mr H has developed a strong alliance and has been able to understand his vulnerability and its origins. Later in the treatment, Mr H's requests for scheduling changes make the therapist feel irritated at his sense of entitlement. The therapist notes to herself that as the patient has improved, her

countertransference has shifted. She uses her new-found understanding of the shift in her countertransference to begin to confront the patient's behavior, saying, "I have often been able to make these scheduling shifts in the past, but I wonder what it would feel like if I couldn't accommodate you and you had to pay for the cancelation."

Thus, the countertransference informed her initial choice of a supportive approach to his requests and the shift in the countertransference signaled that he might be able to tolerate a more uncovering type of intervention.

Now that we have reviewed the fundamental elements of psychodynamic therapy – affect, free association, resistance, transference, and countertransference – we are ready to combine these elements in understanding how to approach **unconscious conflict** and **fantasy**.

Suggested activity

Consider these vignettes and questions:

1. *Ms A is talking about her reaction to the September 11 attack on the World Trade Center and tells her therapist that she had been at home that morning, getting ready for work, and happened to listen to the radio and hear about the events. She quickly thought about whether she knew anyone in or near the towers and couldn't think of any one at risk. She talked about having felt sadness and loss for all those directly affected by the event. As she talks, the therapist realizes that she has been feeling guilty that her dog is home alone and is unable to go out for a walk until she gets home.*

   a. What is the countertransference?

   b. Is it concordant or complementary?

   c. How might the therapist intervene?

Comment

In the countertransference, the therapist associated to her dog, who was also alone in her apartment, and she experienced his helpless dependence on her. Her countertransference informed her that there was a connection between the patient's affect and the dog's imagined experience. Thus, her associations reflected a countertransference attunement to her patient's unexplored affect. This is a concordant countertransference. It could help her to realize that the patient felt lost and alone. If the therapist is working in a predominantly supporting mode, she could help the patient to **name her emotions** by saying something like:

> *I wonder if you felt helpless in the face of this crisis?*

If the therapist is working in a more uncovering mode, she might choose to begin by **confronting** the resistance to the affect:

> *You remember thinking about the feelings of others, but not about your own feelings.*

2. *Mr B, a 66-year-old retired widower, is having difficulty with the transition to this stage of life. He has sought psychotherapy for help with insomnia, feelings of worthlessness, and passive suicidal thoughts. After a few weeks of psychotherapy, his depression lifts, but he is still struggling with how to spend his time. The therapist notices that he himself is bored and sleepy during the sessions.*

   a. What is the countertransference?

   b. What questions might the therapist ask himself to better understand the countertransference?

   c. What could the therapist say if the patient suddenly comments, "Hey, Doc, I feel like I am boring you"?

Comment

Boredom and fatigue are the countertransference reactions. The therapist might ask himself why he is having this reaction to Mr B. He could consider whether his boredom is a concordant identification with the patient's boredom in retirement, a complementary identification with an important person from the patient's early life, a projective identification in which the patient has unconsciously projected his boredom and emptiness into the therapist, a sign that he is uncomfortable with something the patient is experiencing, or a sign that he is having difficulty empathizing with the patient. If Mr B asked the therapist about his boredom, the therapist could **confront** this by saying, "Tell me more about your feeling that you are boring me," or "I wonder if your thought that I am bored is telling us something about what you are feeling."

3. *Ms C is a 39-year-old married woman who has struggled with infertility over the last five years. Nine months ago, a second round of in-vitro fertilization was successful and the patient became pregnant with twins. Her therapist has been delighted to watch this pregnancy evolve. As the due date approaches, the patient becomes excited, but also worries about how to maintain her boundaries with her overly involved mother. She fears that her mother's level of involvement will interfere with feeling that she has started a family of her own. As she is walking out the door from the last session before her scheduled C-section, Ms C casually says, "I'll keep you posted." Weeks pass, and the therapist realizes she has not heard from the patient. She starts to worry about whether everything went well and wonders how to find out. After considering a few options, she finds herself mindlessly looking at her patient's social media pages and sees photos of the patient's new babies. She is thrilled, and decides to call Ms C to congratulate her. Ms C thanks the therapist for her kind wishes, but then asks how she found out about the birth.*

   a. Is the patient exhibiting a transference?

   b. How would you describe the patient's transference?

   c. Is the therapist exhibiting a countertransference?

   d. What would we call what transpired in the treatment?

   e. How might we work with this in psychotherapy?

Comment

Not informing the therapist of the birth of her twins was probably an acting-out of the negative, maternal transference (wanting to keep the therapist at arm's length as she does with her mother). This triggered a countertransference anxiety in the therapist, who felt left out and overly curious. The therapist acted outside the usual treatment frame by looking the patient up on the internet and initiating the phone call. Once spoken to, the patient feels intruded on, since she remembered that she did not tell the therapist about the birth. This is an **enactment**; that is, both patient and therapist are acting something out in the transference/countertransference relationship. When the patient returns to therapy it would be a good idea to talk through the patient's feelings at length, encourage **mentalization** of both the patient's and the therapist's experience, and draw genetic links to the patient's fears about her mother. In addition, talking about how the patient contributed to this enactment by giving the therapist the impression that she would be "kept posted" would be an important dimension of helping the patient see how she contributed to setting up this dynamic.

Chapter 22: References

1. Gabbard, G.O. (2010) *Long-Term Psychodynamic Psychotherapy: A Basic Text*, 2nd ed., American Psychiatric Publishing, Washington, DC, p. 11–12.
2. Racker, H. (1957) The meaning and uses of countertransference. *Psychoanalytic Quarterly*, **26**, 303–357.
3. Searles H. (1995) The informational value of the supervisor's emotional experiences. *Psychiatry*, **18**, 135–146.
4. Auchincloss, E.L., and Samberg, E. (1990) *Psychoanalytic Terms and Concepts*, Yale University Press, New Haven, p. 76–77.
5. Safran, J.D., and Muran, J.C. (2000) *Negotiating the Therapeutic Alliance: A Relational Treatment Guide*, Guilford Press, New York.
6. Bateman, A., Fonagy, P., and Allen, J.G. (2009) Theory and practice of mentalization-based therapy, in *Textbook of Psychotherapeutic Treatments* (ed. G.O. Gabbard), American Psychiatric Publishing, Washington, DC, p. 775–776.
7. Bateman, A., and Fonagy, P. (2007) The use of transference in dynamic psychotherapy. *American Journal of Psychiatry*, **164**, 4 (letter to the editor).

23 Unconscious Conflict and Defense

Key concepts

An **unconscious fantasy** is a wish or fear that pervades a person's unconscious, driving behavior and shaping characteristic defenses.

Clusters of linked unconscious fantasies are called **complexes**.

Unconscious conflict happens when opposing unconscious fantasies collide. This produces anxiety and triggers defenses to decrease the anxiety.

Primary gain is the decrease in anxiety that happens when a defense successfully diminishes unconscious conflict.

Secondary gain is the advantage that the defense or symptom gives the person in their life.

Listening for anxiety, affect, parapraxes (slips), incongruities, and nodal points is the best way to detect the presence of unconscious conflict.

In a supporting mode, we identify and reinforce healthy defenses to help patients adopt new, more adaptive ways of dealing with anxiety.

In an uncovering mode, we help patients become conscious of their conflicts and the defenses they use to enable them to make more adaptive defensive choices.

Imagine you're the fire warden for a vast, northern forest. Your job is to search for fires in thousands of acres of silent trees. You have a watchtower and a helicopter. Where do you start? How do you know where the trouble is? You look and smell for smoke. Why? Because you know that where there's smoke, there's fire. It's your only clue.

The same is true for psychodynamic psychotherapists who look for unconscious conflict. The mind is vast and conflict is hidden (unconscious). There's no map. Where to look? Well, where there's smoke, there's fire. Here the smoke is **anxiety**. When you rub two sticks together you get heat; when you rub two opposing unconscious fantasies together you get anxiety. Of course, some people are hard-wired for more anxiety than others and not all anxiety is caused by intra-psychic conflict, but it's a good bet that some kind of intra-psychic conflict is behind a lot of the anxiety you will come across.

Psychodynamic Psychotherapy: A Clinical Manual, Second Edition. Deborah L. Cabaniss, Sabrina Cherry, Carolyn J. Douglas and Anna Schwartz.
© 2017 John Wiley & Sons, Ltd. Published 2017 by John Wiley & Sons, Ltd.

What is intra-psychic conflict?

Intra-psychic conflict is what happens when two opposing unconscious fantasies collide [1]. An unconscious fantasy is an unconscious wish or fear that exists in a person's mind. Some people think that fantasies are always things we want – we can help our patients learn that fantasies can be things we want or things we fear. One way to think about unconscious fantasies is that they are the sentences or stories that populate our unconscious minds. "Father" is just a word – in itself it is not an unconscious fantasy. "I want my father to love me" is an unconscious fantasy if it is out of awareness. Here are some other common examples of unconscious fantasies, although there are as many unconscious fantasies as there are minds:

> *I want to be taken care of.*
>
> *I don't want to be abandoned.*
>
> *I love to be adored.*
>
> *I want to be powerful.*
>
> *I don't feel whole without another person.*
>
> *I fear having to be in control.*
>
> *Being taken care of makes me feel loved.*
>
> *Having to take care of myself makes me feel alone.*

Complexes

Clusters of related unconscious fantasies are called **complexes**. One of the most famous complexes, traditionally called the Oedipus complex, occurs in middle childhood (ages 3–6) [2]. It's nothing more than a cluster of related unconscious fantasies. For the heterosexual little girl, it goes something like this:

> *I love my father and want him all for myself. My mother has my father. I wish I could get rid of my mother so I could have my father. But if I try to attack my mother she'll counterattack and I could be in danger. Plus, I also love and need my mother. (Opposite for the heterosexual boy; same-sex longings for homosexual children.)*

Freud thought that all people have this complex. These unconscious conflicts do seem potent for most people. There are some unconscious fantasies that seem to be quite common. However, all people also have unconscious fantasies and complexes that are unique. By the time most people are adults, their fantasies and complexes are fairly fixed – they might develop new ones and drop old ones, but there are core unconscious complexes that remain relatively stable for people over time. We know this intuitively; when we say that one person is driven by abandonment issues while another is consumed with power, we're talking about stable, core fantasies. *Understanding these fantasies is central for our understanding of how a person operates in terms of defenses, relationships with others, and self-perceptions.*

One thing about fantasies – they collide and then there's trouble:

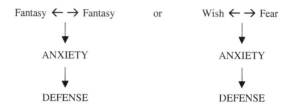

For example, one person might have the following two fantasies: "I feel loved when I'm taken care of," and "I feel like a strong man when I don't need anyone." These are two powerful fantasies that are about as far apart as they can get – 180 degrees, if you will. People are not one-dimensional – they want lots of things that are not necessarily compatible. This person wants to feel both strong and loved and his fantasies about these wishes are seemingly completely incompatible. If both fantasies are dormant or if they aren't active at the same time, things might be OK for a while. But problems arise if they are both active at the same time.

For example, let's say that these two fantasies belong to Mr A:

> *Mr A is a 28-year-old gay man whose father left the family when he was a young boy. While on vacation he meets B, a 32-year-old gay man, with whom he falls in love and has a relationship. His lover is caring and solicitous and Mr A feels wonderful and loved. Unconscious fantasy #1 ("I feel loved when I'm taken care of") is in full force. However, Mr A and his boyfriend live in different cities and after the vacation they return home. Despite frequent emails and calls, Mr A feels that B is less attentive than he is and begins to get angry when B goes a day without making contact. He feels anxious and has insomnia. He becomes irritable with B when he calls, acts aloof, decides he's too busy to have a relationship, and ultimately breaks up with B. Now back at work, he is glad he doesn't have to take time to be involved in a relationship.*

What happened? In the face of growing dependence on B, unconscious fantasy #2 ("I feel like a strong man when I don't need anyone") kicked into gear, making Mr A feel weak for needing B's attention and care. Since this was not in Mr A's awareness, the conflict was *unconscious* and the result was *anxiety*.

Notice that something else happened after the anxiety – Mr A became aloof and decided he was too busy for a relationship. This means that Mr A mounted a **defense** or a set of defenses (some combination of **reaction formation** and **rationalization**). When anxiety is generated by unconscious conflict, the mind mounts defenses. As with unconscious fantasies, defenses become characteristic. In other words, people tend to use the same set of defenses repeatedly over time. In the case of Mr A, when the care that made him feel loved seemed threatened, his feelings of dependency caused him to feel weak and anxiety was generated. Not everyone would have a conflict about this – perhaps Mr A's early abandonment makes him particularly vulnerable to feeling weak when he notices that he needs care. The conflict leads to anxiety, and the anxiety triggers defenses.

The particular defenses that Mr A uses give him both primary and secondary gains [3]. **Primary gain** is the decrease in anxiety that happens when a defense successfully diminishes unconscious conflict. The primary gain is that he no longer has as much anxiety because he is **repressing** his feelings of dependency in order to feel strong. Thus, the conflict is sapped of strength and not as much anxiety is generated. **Secondary gain** is the advantage that the defense or symptom gives the person – in this case, the secondary gain is that Mr A feels that he can work more efficiently because he is relationship free. Note that the unconscious fantasies continue to exist in Mr A, but in the absence of the relationship they are not activated and the conflict is dormant.

So, unconscious fantasies collide, cause unconscious conflict, generate anxiety, and (unconsciously) lead to the use of defense. The defenses decrease anxiety, *but at a price*. Mr A has difficulty with relationships unless he is 100% assured of the care of his lover – which is a hefty price if you're interested in being with real people.

We can help patients to "pay a smaller price" in one of two ways. For high-functioning individuals, bringing their unconscious fantasies, conflicts, and defenses to light can help them develop more flexible defensives, improved relationships, and better self-esteem management. For people who do not have this capacity, we can use our understanding of their unconscious thought processes to identify and strengthen healthy defenses and to suggest new, more adaptive ways of dealing with anxiety. In psychodynamic psychotherapy, we work backward from anxiety to defense and ultimately to unconscious conflict and fantasies in order to help people recognize what is causing them anxiety, problems, and symptoms.

Technique

Listening

There are many things to listen for here: unconscious fantasy, unconscious conflict, and defenses.

Listening for unconscious fantasy

Just like listening for the dominant affect, the dominant transference, and the dominant countertransference, we listen for the dominant unconscious fantasy in a session. We do this by listening to the stories that patients tell us about their fears, wishes, and relationships, and we start to notice stories that sound similar. When we listen for affect, we think, "What does this patient feel right now?" When we listen for unconscious fantasy, we think, "What does this patient want or fear right now?" To hear what is unconscious, listen for *hidden stories* – that is, the stories behind the stories. It's like an optical illusion – when you look at it one way you see one picture, but when you focus on it in a different way you see another, hidden scene.

Our patients tell lots of stories, but the stories that are unconscious fantasies are short and child-like. For patients who have weaker functioning these stories are often on the surface, but for patients who have stronger functioning these stories are generally hidden. These higher-functioning patients are embarrassed and ashamed by their child-like wants and fears, but the fantasies are still there. When you hear something that sounds child-like from an adult, you are likely hearing an unconscious fantasy:

> *A 28-year-old woman tells her therapist, "I don't know why I feel so angry with my father for getting remarried so quickly after Mom died. He's a great guy and he deserves all the happiness he can get after taking care of Mom for so long. And Marsha's pretty nice. But I hoped that they'd plan the wedding for after the baby was born – I don't know why that makes such a difference to me, but it does. It's ridiculous – it's not like they're going to help me take care of it or anything."*

Here, the conscious story is that a 28-year-old woman wants her father to be happy and is confused by her anger at him. Yet the hidden story is that she wants to be her father's first (or only) priority. The patient has repressed this story (put it out of awareness – made it unconscious) because it's a child-like wish about which she is ashamed. Why should a grown woman who is having her own baby want her father all to herself? Why should she want her dad to take care of her instead of taking care of himself? Why indeed – because we all have wishes that persist from childhood. If those wishes were not well gratified when we were young, they may be persistent and **unresolved**. A wish that was perfectly appropriate in childhood but causes shame when it persists into adulthood is said to be unresolved, and can wreak havoc on an adult's efforts to navigate the world. Psychodynamic psychotherapy is designed to help with that.

Listening for unconscious conflict

Like the warden looking for fires, we listen to conscious material for evidence of defenses and the unconscious conflicts that underlie them. This mostly involves listening for anxiety, new affects, and incongruities – hints that there is conflict beneath the surface.

- **Listen for anxiety:** Remember that when we listen for anxiety we listen for:
  - overt statements about anxiety
  - anxious behavior in the room – such as fidgeting, irritability, watching the clock
  - anxious behavior outside of therapy – such as eating and sleeping problems, irritability, procrastination, difficulty concentrating, impulsivity, impaired judgment
  - anxiety dreams
- **Listen for affects:** Any change in affect can be a clue that there is anxiety. Irritability, depressed mood, or even a precipitously elevated mood can indicate the presence of anxiety and conflict.
- **Listen for incongruities:** It makes sense that conflicts produce incongruities. Two active things oppose each other – this will produce all sorts of mismatches. Examples include affects that don't match experience (such as crying at one's birthday party), affects that don't match thoughts (such as feeling depressed when thinking about a loved one), and thoughts that don't match each other (such as being sure that inviting

both sets of in-laws to Thanksgiving is a good idea even though you know they always end up fighting).

- **Listen for parapraxes:** Parapraxes (slips of the tongue) occur when repressed thoughts or feelings inadvertently "pop out" in speech (see Chapter 16). They are good clues to the presence of unconscious conflict. For example, a man who is having trouble with his boss says:

  Yesterday, when I was on the phone with my father – I mean, my boss.

  This parapraxis suggests that something about the difficulty with the boss relates to unconscious fantasies and conflicts involving the man's father.

- **Listen for dreams** Anxiety dreams often signal the presence of anxiety and unconscious conflict. Interpretation of these dreams can help us understand dominant fantasies and their attendant conflicts.

Listening for defenses

Since resistance is defense in the treatment, the presence of resistance means we're listening to a defense. Blocking, silence, lateness – all of these are good clues. It may be hard to know which thoughts and behaviors are defensive at the beginning of treatment, but this becomes easier as you learn a patient's patterns. For example, when a patient becomes irritable before you go on vacation for the first time in treatment, you might not recognize this as defense, but when this happens time and time again the defensive nature of the irritability becomes clear.

Reflecting

Once we've tuned into the patient's unconscious frequency, we can then begin to identify dominant unconscious fantasies, components of unconscious conflicts, and dominant defenses. We do this by thinking about what we're hearing most frequently and what is most connected to the dominant affect. We should be able to put the dominant unconscious fantasies into one or two sentences. We have to think about which type of fantasy is most prominent; for example, it could be a wish, a fear, or a way of thinking about oneself. We begin to deconstruct the unconscious conflicts as we identify the opposing fantasies. And finally we identify the prominent defenses.

A man who has recently immigrated to this country presents with difficulty sleeping and vague stomach complaints. He tells you:

  "All I want is for my children to do well. That's it. That's why I came here. My daughter is very smart. I hope that she'll get into a wonderful college. That's why I'm driving a cab – you know, I'm trained as an engineer in my country, but it's fine. I'd rather be here, doing this, than be back in my country being an engineer. I don't care about my own career. But if I'm sick, I won't be able to work at all and then the whole move will be for nothing."

The surface story is about a man who has sacrificed his own career for the good of his children. However, the repetitive nature of his insistence that he doesn't care suggests the presence of unconscious conflict. His fantasies, conflicts, and defenses might sound something like this:

- **Unconscious fantasies**: I want to be successful. I want to be recognized and admired for my intelligence.
- **Unconscious conflict**: I want these things for myself, but I can't have *both* what I want for myself *and* what I want for my children.
- **Defenses**: Reaction formation, somatization.

Now, what to do with all of this? Often, we hear lots of unconscious material but it is deep beneath the surface. Remember the choosing and readiness principles from Chapter 17. It's important to remember that *just because we hear unconscious material doesn't mean we can use it.* We remember it and wait for it to become closer to the surface, but if it's deep our interventions won't touch it. Worse still, they could increase resistance, causing the unconscious material to be even less accessible to consciousness. As before, *we let the dominant affect guide us toward the surface.* We want to pick the unconscious element that is just below the surface – the one that we can gently nudge into consciousness. Here's an example that illustrates this layering of unconscious material:

> A 38-year-old woman whose father had many affairs presents because she wants to have a baby and has become panicked about her fertility. When you ask about whether this is something she has been worried about for a while, she realizes that her fear escalated after a friend was found to be in premature menopause. She sobs in your office, saying she is afraid to go to the doctor to get checked out because she is sure that she will have the same problem since she has always had irregular periods. She acknowledges that she is frequently phobic about going to the doctor. When you ask about her relationships, she says that she is very much in love with her boyfriend, a wealthy 50-year-old man who is married and whose wife lives in another state. She says it is practically a done deal that he will leave his wife. She becomes irritable when you ask about her previous relationships, but nevertheless tells you that her last boyfriend was married as well.

Reflection: There are many unconscious fantasies, unconscious conflicts, and defenses operating here.

- On the *surface*, she has a symptom, which is her fear of going to the doctor. This comes with attendant anxiety, which is the dominant affect. An early intervention – a question – brings an unconscious connection (her friend's premature menopause) into awareness. This is a clue that this is close to the surface and ready to be dealt with.
- On a *deeper* level, her fear of not being able to have a baby could be related to denial about the likelihood that her 50-year-old married boyfriend would leave his wife to start a family with her. You might wonder whether the panic about the friend's infertility is in fact a defense against her fear that her boyfriend won't leave his wife. The unconscious conflict could be her wish for her boyfriend to choose her versus her

anger at him for not leaving soon enough for her to conceive a child before she is too old. This might be producing anxiety, and her defense could be shifting the anxiety by identifying with her friend. If the problem is that she's infertile, then not having a baby would be her fault (her body's fault) rather than her boyfriend's. This defense allows her to keep her rage at her boyfriend out of awareness. This formulation might be true, but the patient's defensiveness makes it clear that it is not on the surface.

- At the *deepest* level, conflicts about her philandering father and defenses against awareness of them might be resulting in her choosing boyfriends who are just like him. You might think of this immediately, but it is too deep to address now.

In this way, we reflect on the unconscious elements we hear in order to choose those that are closest to the surface. As before, we cautiously use our past experiences, our theories, and our understanding of the therapeutic alliance and the patient's phase of treatment to guide us. For example, once there is a high degree of trust between patient and therapist, the therapist needn't be put off by a bit of defensiveness on the part of the patient, and can go deeper than the patient's comfort level might have allowed at first.

Intervening

Basic interventions

As we've said, defenses are in place for a reason – they protect against frightening or shame-filled feelings that are often very deep. This means that we have to be very respectful as we begin intervening. Starting slowly is the name of the game, and basic interventions help with this. **Questions**, **calls for associations**, and **empathic remarks** help to get your patients talking about the details of their lives that contain the clues to their unconscious fantasies, conflicts, and defenses. Here are some examples:

Patient #1	*I don't know whether to take this new job or to stay where I am.*
Therapist	*Can you tell me more about the new offer? What seems attractive about it?*
Patient #2	*I really like Clara, but I can't seem to get myself to call her.*
Therapist	*When did you last think about calling her?*
Patient #2	*Last night.*
Therapist	*Can you go back to that moment in your mind? What were your thoughts?*

In both of these situations, the therapist hears something that sounds like it might be connected to an unconscious fantasy or conflict. The first interventions should be open-ended questions, designed to get the patient to say more.

Supporting techniques

We choose supporting techniques when we want to strengthen adaptive defenses and suggest alternatives to maladaptive ones. When we suspect that patients' functioning is persistently or temporarily compromised, we generally do not encourage exploration of unconscious fantasy or conflict, since this is likely to increase their anxiety and disorganization.

All defenses serve to protect people from uncomfortable affects and associated conflicts, but they differ in the degree to which they ignore the realities of the outside world, squelch feelings, or disrupt relationships [4]. Defenses are most adaptive when they allow some expression and gratification of wishes and needs while taking into account the realistic constraints of the environment and minimizing any negative social consequences. Consider the following example:

> *Mr C yearns to be loved and cared for, but fears that people will ignore him. There are a range of defenses he might use to protect himself from the uncomfortable feelings of hurt, anger, and unworthiness associated with this conflict.*

- He could **devalue** others ("Who needs them? I can take care of myself!"), but then other people would see him as having a "chip on his shoulder" and steer clear of him.
- He could bury the anger along with the yearnings for love (**isolation of affect**), but then his wishes to be cared for would remain ungratified.
- He could redirect the hurt at a smaller annoyance, for example by upbraiding the barista who screws up his coffee order (**displacement**).
- He could channel his anger into football, becoming the star quarterback on his football team and the focus of adulation from his peers (**sublimation**), even if he still can't seem to get the girl.
- He could decide to go to social work school and dedicate himself to caring for others (**altruism**), which would allow him to enjoy the experience – if only vicariously – and boost his self-esteem.

Each of these solutions has a different "adaptive" value. In working supportively with this man, you *listen* for the clues about the unconscious fantasies and conflicts at work, *reflect* on the defenses he uses to manage uncomfortable affects, and *intervene* if necessary to help him find more adaptive ways of defending himself.

Intervening supportively with defenses is a three-part process:

1. **Identify the defense**: Direct the patient's attention, gently and tactfully, to the problematic behavior that needs to be addressed.
2. **Identify the "cost"**: Demonstrate the negative consequences for the patient in the behavior.
3. **Identify alternatives**: Encourage healthier, less "costly" behaviors.

Depending on the patient's needs in the moment, we can use either supplying and/ or assisting interventions for each of the three steps outlined here. To illustrate this, consider Mr C, the man who yearns to be cared for but fears that others will ignore him:

> Mr C often feels slighted, hurt, and angered by perceived interpersonal disappointments, but has trouble acknowledging or tolerating these emotions, much less the yearning that lies beneath them. He defends against his anger by **projecting** it and, as a result, often feels unfairly attacked by other people, including you. His peevish, blaming behavior irritates co-workers and actually provokes them into mocking him, which makes him feel even more ostracized and bitter. Here is a segment taken from a session early in therapy:

Mr C	I went into the employee lounge this morning to get a cup of coffee, and Jim and Karen were there talking. They gave me this look that really pissed me off. I mean, they didn't say it but it was obvious they wanted me to get lost. Everyone knows they have a thing for each other.
Therapist	I suppose it's true that two people who are dating like to be alone, but I find it's hard to know for sure what someone else is thinking, especially if they haven't said anything directly. Can you think of other reasons why they might have looked up at that moment? (**validation, psychoeducation, reality testing**)
Mr C	(shrugs) I don't know.
Therapist	Maybe they just wanted to see who came in. Does that seem plausible? (**reality testing**)
Mr C	Yeah, I guess it's possible.
Therapist	So then what happened? (**question**)
Mr C	I figured they wanted me to leave, so I said kind of loudly, "Am I interrupting anything?" Except I said it sort of sarcastically, and told them, "The lounge is for everyone, you know." I wasn't going to be pushed around. So Jim said, "Lighten up, will you? We're just having a cup of coffee." And Karen sort of shook her head and snickered at me, like I was crazy.
Therapist	It seems like your first instinct was a good one – to ask if you were interrupting – but things might have gone more smoothly if you had left out the sarcasm. These are problems we could work on together so you won't feel so hurt and angry. Maybe you don't have to suffer so much. (**praising, advising, explicitly joining, empathizing**)
Mr C	OK – I'm not 100% sure you're right, but it's worth a try.

In this example, the therapist hears the disavowed yearning to be acknowledged and cared for. She also hears the unconscious conviction that others will ignore him or, worse still, that he is not worthy of their affection. These unconscious wishes and fears generate feelings of anger, envy, unworthiness, and despair that Mr C finds intolerable. The therapist infers this from the defenses – principally maladaptive projection – that Mr C has marshaled against these affects. Using these defenses, Mr C protects himself against rejection and betrayal by other people – but at the great cost of ending up alone and shunned. Note that the therapist is careful *not* to confront Mr C with these feelings, fantasies, and conflicts that are out of his awareness. The treatment is young, the therapeutic alliance is tenuous, and Mr C has not yet developed a capacity for observing himself or tolerating the powerful feelings that might emerge if his defenses were interpreted. The therapist wisely selects the most "maladaptive" of Mr C's defenses to address first – his tendency to project anger – as this seems most disruptive of his relationships. Then, using a mix of supplying and assisting interventions, the therapist gently focuses Mr C's attention on the behavior, **reality-tests** his misperceptions, and **suggests** more adaptive alternatives, all the while offering direct support in the form of **empathy** and **praise**.

Uncovering techniques

We choose uncovering techniques when we want to make people aware of their unconscious fantasies, conflicts, and defenses in order to free them up to make more adaptive choices.

We have several goals when we intervene to uncover this material:

- **Uncovering unconscious fantasies**: Doing this in a safe environment helps patients understand them, have less shame about them, and be able to make choices without being enslaved by them.
- **Uncovering unconscious conflicts**: Unconscious conflicts paralyze people. If unresolved, they lead to tremendous morbidity caused by anxiety and stasis. They activate more "costly" defense mechanisms that decrease anxiety at the heavy price of problematic behavior patterns and unsatisfactory relationships. Interpreting unconscious conflicts (making people aware of them) helps resolve them, allowing people to use more flexible, adaptive defense mechanisms.
- **Uncovering unconscious defenses**: Unconscious defenses tend to be inflexible and problematic. When they are brought to the surface, people can use secondary process thinking to alter their characteristic defense patterns, leading to healthier functioning and more satisfying interpersonal relationships.

Uncovering unconscious fantasies and defenses in order to promote more adaptive defensive functioning is an essential part of psychodynamic psychotherapy, but it's important to remember that we have to do it very slowly and carefully. There's a reason that these conflicts and fantasies are unconscious – they cause anxiety and uncomfortable affects. Defenses are not bad; in fact, they're necessary. They help us modulate anxiety and protect ourselves in myriad ways. We interpret not to eliminate defenses, but rather because we think that patients could protect themselves in ways that would exact a lesser price.

Knowing that we have to have respect for defenses and for the shame connected to unconscious fantasy, we forge ahead. Once we choose material that is close enough to the surface (choosing principles) and we think the patient is able to handle the inevitable anxiety of learning about unconscious material (readiness principles), we begin the interpretive process (**confrontation, clarification, interpretation**). Early in treatment, much of what we do is to ask questions, confront, and clarify until we really have something to translate into consciousness. Don't worry about not interpreting quickly – it probably means that you're being careful, respectful, and trying to learn about your patient's unique unconscious material. Plus, each interpretive sequence is not an end in itself – it will be repeated and repeated in **working through** in order for real change to occur (see Chapter 29).

Here are some examples. For the sake of illustration, they are compact. In the real world, the interpretive process could extend over many sessions as unconscious material comes more clearly into focus.

Interpretation of unconscious fantasy

> *The patient is a 32-year-old woman who has been living with her 33-year-old boyfriend for three years.*

Patient	*Marcus took me out to a wonderful restaurant last night for my birthday. I've wanted to go there for months. It's great – very romantic. I looked good – wore that new dress I just bought – it was all perfect – but that night in bed I just started to cry. I felt so stupid – the whole evening was lovely, and he was so nice and I know that he loves me.*
Therapist	*Can you tell me more about the dinner or what happened afterword?* (**question**)
Patient	*(exasperated) Nothing happened! That's what was so weird. We walked home – stopped and had a coffee at that nice café that opened on our block. When we got home there was a wrapped package on the coffee table – I don't even know how he got it there – it was a cashmere sweater – and that was so thoughtful of him – he's not a shopper and I know he hates going into all of those cutesy shops I love – but he did it and it was really thoughtful. He's such a great guy – I'm really lucky – so why am I so upset?*
Therapist	*You said the gift was thoughtful – but you didn't say you liked it.* (**confrontation**)
Patient	*How could I not like it? He got it for me and I know he took time to pick it out and everything – it's selfish for me to think about whether I liked it or not (tearful) But you know, two weeks ago, we were at the mall and we went by this store and I saw this other sweater I loved – it was too expensive to just go in and buy for no reason and I sort of oohed and aahed over it – and, I don't know, I was just hoping he'd get me that one – and he didn't. The one he bought is fine, but the color is sort of off for me. He kind of doesn't get it when it comes to shopping, style – he tries so hard, but it's not his thing. Cliff (her old boyfriend) had such a flair – he always guessed exactly what I wanted – it was like magic – it would just appear. I never had any anxiety before birthdays – he just knew what to get. But he was a jerk in so many other ways.*
Therapist	*If you really wanted the other sweater, you could have asked for it.* (**confrontation**)
Patient	*But it's no good that way. That's not a present. It's like when I had to nag him to read my manuscript – he did it and was helpful, but he should just want to do it.*
Therapist	*So in both cases – with the sweater and with the manuscript – you got upset when he didn't figure it out himself.* (**clarification**)
Patient	*Yes – that's it – but that's so unfair – he did read the manuscript and he gave me this lovely birthday and he's so great – but it makes me uneasy – like does he really get me like Cliff did? (more tearful)*
Therapist	*Having him be able to read your mind makes you feel loved – if you have to ask, you don't feel well loved.* (**interpretation**)
Patient	*It's true but it sounds so silly. No one can read minds. My mother never could – she always got us what she wanted for herself.*

In this example, the patient has an unconscious fantasy that goes something like this: "If someone loves you, they know what you want and give it to you without your having to ask for it." She is a grown woman and knows that people can't read minds, and that someone can love you without anticipating all of your wishes, but this is a **core fantasy**. Despite her seemingly good relationship with Marcus, this fantasy kicks in and ruins what would have been a perfectly lovely evening. His "mistake" with the gift makes her feel "misread" and the unconscious fantasy leads her to feel less well loved. In terms of the therapist's technique, the first clues that an unconscious fantasy is at play are the patient's *anxiety* and *incongruous affect* (upset about a lovely birthday). The therapist wants to know more and asks a **question** – this helps indicate what's closest to the surface. Remember, getting details is key. The therapist **confronts** the incongruities twice, then when the patient remembers another similar instance, the therapist brings things into focus with a **clarification**. Once the patient's affect indicates that the unconscious fantasy is close to the surface, the therapist tries an interpretation. We know that this is an interpretation because we can write it as a "because schematic":

You didn't ask for what you wanted and were thus disappointed	– because –	You only feel well loved if the person can read your mind

The patient has more affect, and adds a deep, genetic association indicating that the interpretation was well timed and aimed at the right level. The hope is that revealing this fantasy in the safety of the therapeutic relationship will help her feel less shame about it, own it, understand it, have more control over it in the future, and potentially even resolve it.

Interpretation of unconscious conflict

> *The patient is a 35-year-old man who has just been offered a large promotion. He has been in treatment for two years with a 50-year-old male therapist:*

Patient   *So I'll be a vice president before the age of 40. Ha! My father was never a vice president. He wanted the corner office so badly he could taste it. He was so bitter about that. I don't know how the other guys will take it – they don't seem to like me much. So much of my doing well at work has to do with my work here with you. It means much more money as well. I always feel weird telling you about money – I don't know how much you make and if you make more or less than I do.*

Therapist   *What are your thoughts about that?* (**question, call for associations**)

Patient   *Oh I don't know – I think that people in my field make more than people in your field – you're a professional, you know that, so what's the big deal.*

Therapist   *But it sounds like you had some anxiety telling me that you were going to make more money.* (**confrontation**)

Patient   *Well sure – people don't talk about this in ordinary conversation. I know, I know, this isn't ordinary conversation – but still, we're two guys, and you're older – you might feel bad or something.*

Therapist   *Can you say more about what you think my feelings might be?* (**question**)

Patient	*(frustrated) What am I supposed to say? Yeah, OK, I'm a little worried that if I tell you I'm making more money you'll raise my fee. I feel bad saying that because you've been very helpful to me, but I've got lots of things besides therapy I want to spend this extra money on.*
Therapist	*Part of you wants to tell me about your good fortune, but part of you wants to hide it from me.* (**confrontation of unconscious conflict**)
Patient	*I guess so – I can't tell my dad about the money either – not the amount. He'd totally flip out – and they're having financial problems now – I worry that I'll have to support them and then all that work down the drain.*
Therapist	*So although you hope I'll be happy for you, you also fear I'll hurt you by taking your money, just like you fear your father will – perhaps because you think I'm envious of your success.* (**interpretation**)
Patient	*I know you won't – you've always been very fair with me – but the fear is there. It makes me guarded with you and a little afraid.*

In this example, the patient has an unconscious conflict that makes it difficult for him to work well with and trust other men, including the therapist. He has one fantasy that the therapist will be happy for him and another opposing fantasy that therapist will attack and injure him (take his money) out of envy. The patient worries about the therapist's reaction, then takes it back – this incongruity signals the **conflict** that the therapist **confronts**. Finally, the therapist **interprets the unconscious conflict**: here it is in the "because schematic":

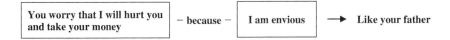

This is both a transference interpretation and a genetic interpretation, since it includes a hypothesis about how an early relationship plays a part in the etiology of the conflict.

Interpretation of defense (defense analysis)

> *The patient is a 68-year-old man who has been in therapy for three years with a 39-year-old female therapist. This is the first session back after a two-week summer break:*

Patient	*Once again I was fine during your vacation. It was nice to have a break from therapy and my accountant approves of the decreased expense. I don't know why I always think that it will be hard. I kept taking the medication and wasn't as anxious as I thought I'd be.*
Therapist	*Of course you were fine – we talked about that before I left – the days of crisis are over.* (**validation, confrontation**)
Patient	*So why do I keep coming here twice a week? I was thinking during the break that maybe I should just come once a week. You've been very helpful to me. I know there are plenty of things we could talk about – there were no blow-ups this summer, but it's not like Janet (his wife) and I were perfect – still no sex since her operation – is this forever? But what's the use of talking about my feelings about it.*
Therapist	*Can you say more about what's happening with your wife?* (**question**)

Patient	*Don't try to change the subject – I'm talking about therapy and my appointments. I remember feeling the same way last year – sort of tired – am I going to start again? We're old – Janet and I – what's the use?*
Therapist	*It's true that you felt this way last year after my vacation as well – do you have any other feelings about that?* (**clarification**)
Patient	*It's hard to be away and then to have to slog through all of those weeks with you – getting to trust you all over again – sometimes I feel like I'm too old for this, give it a rest – it's too difficult.*
Therapist	*Because it's hard to get back into the relationship with me after the break, your inclination is to pull away, put distance between us so the breaks are less painful.* (**interpretation**)
Patient	*If you were just, say, writing the prescriptions, yeah, it would be easier. It's hard for me when you go. You should have a vacation, but I've really come to rely on this room . . .*
Therapist	*And on me.* (**interpretation**)
Patient	*That's harder to say.*

In this example, the patient has an unconscious conflict. He relies on the therapist and has strong feelings about her, but feels that the dependency may be too painful to tolerate. This causes anxiety, which he defends against using some combination of denial of affect, rationalization, and acting out: "I don't need her, that would be less expensive, and I should pull away by decreasing to once a week." The defense first rears its head when the patient says he doesn't actually need the therapist in order not to fall apart – the therapist **confronts** this incongruity by reminding him that she had previously agreed with this. When the patient remembers that he felt the same way last year, the therapist is able to make a **clarification**. Once the patient expresses affect, she feels the patient is ready for an **interpretation of the defense**. The patient acknowledges the defense, but still uses it when he distances from the therapist, saying "this room" rather than "you." Note that her next intervention, "And on me," is short but is nonetheless a **defense interpretation** – it's a short cut between people who know each other well. See if you can put these interpretations in the **because schematic**.

Comparing supporting and uncovering work with defenses

To summarize the *key differences* between supporting and uncovering goals in addressing defenses:

- When we *support*, we identify and encourage adaptive defenses while suggesting alternatives to problematic ones. We may also choose to respect "healthy enough" defenses that do no great harm.

- When we *uncover*, we help patients gradually make defenses conscious in order to uncover underlying fantasies and conflicts and make more adaptive choices.

Another way to pursue unconscious fantasies and conflicts is through the exploration of **dreams**, which is the topic of our next chapter.

Suggested activities

1. Defenses

What defenses is this man using? What would be a goal for helping him with defenses? What might you say if you were primarily supporting? What might you say if you were primarily uncovering?

> I'm sorry I'm late. I don't know why I couldn't get it together to come in on time because I really wanted to come today to talk to you about breaking up with Cindy. It was definitely the right thing to do. Definitely. Once I found that letter that she wrote to Bob – that was the clincher. Definitely the right thing to do. I'm relieved – I really am. Thank goodness I found out now. Phew. Look what happened to my Mom – she didn't know what my Dad was like until too late – until after they had kids. My stomach is acting up again – that IBS stuff. Do you think it's serious? I keep wondering if I have Crohn's disease. I watched TV alone last night. It's great to just be able to watch sports again – no more of that Food Network junk that she always had on.

Comment

Defenses   Avoidance (coming late to the session)
               Rationalization (convincing himself it was the right thing to do despite
                   ambivalence)
               Somatization (experiencing his feelings in terms of bodily symptoms)

Goal – Supporting – normalize having feelings about a break-up in order to diminish somatic worries: "I'm glad you feel good about your decision, but, even if you feel you did the right thing, break-ups are stressful. Maybe that's why your stomach has been so upset."

Uncovering – confront the way defenses might cover conflict about the decision, leading to symptoms: "When you say you're sure so many times it makes me wonder if you might have other feelings that are harder to talk about. Maybe that's one of the reasons you came late today – on some level, you didn't want to talk about more ambivalent feelings."

2. Unconscious fantasy

Read this opening monologue of a session and write three unconscious fantasies that could be operative for this 32-year-old man:

> I have an image of my wife sleeping – when I left this morning she was asleep with a smile on her face. I felt like we were nesting – like she's taken care of – safe – bundled up in the bed with the dog at her feet. I had to leave early to get here – I took my bike – I practically took the whole bike apart this weekend, but I fixed it – I had a great sense of accomplishment – now I know I can fix it myself. I was thinking about our last session – what you said about my mother – that I was dealing with her differently. I realized I didn't feel defensive about your saying that. I thought, "That's cool," like, "Oh, you're pointing something out that's helpful." But then I thought, "Maybe that's your technique" – to tell me that I'm making progress so that I know you're helping me.

Comment

A few possible unconscious fantasies include:

I feel good when I'm taking care of my family.

I feel good when I feel masculine.

People don't usually say nice things unless they have an ulterior motive.

Maybe you only care about me because you're my therapist.

Chapter 23: References

1. Brenner, C. (1982) *The Mind in Conflict*, International Universities Press, New York, p. 55–71.
2. Freud, S. (1916) Introductory lectures on psycho-analysis, in *The Standard Edition of the Complete Psychological Works of Sigmund Freud (1915–1916), Introductory lectures on psycho-analysis (Parts I and II), Vol. XV*, Hogarth Press, London, p. 207.
3. Freud, S. (1917) Introductory lectures on psycho-analysis, in *The Standard Edition of the Complete Psychological Works of Sigmund Freud (1916–1917): Introductory Lectures on Psycho-Analysis (Part III), Vol. 16*, Hogarth Press, London, p. 384.
4. Vaillant, G.E. (1977) *Adaptation to Life*, Little, Brown, Boston.

24 Dreams

Key concepts

Clinical experience indicates that dreams offer us a window into the unconscious.

The **dream story** is what the patient remembers and reports; the **dream associations** help link the dream story to related unconscious elements.

We think of everything a person says just before and after telling a dream as associations to the dream.

Dreams can be thought of as being composed of elements from the dreamer's recent past that become linked to related memories and unconscious fantasies.

When working in a predominantly supporting mode, we generally do not encourage our patients to report dreams. If they bring them up spontaneously, we use the dream story to help them learn about issues and concerns at the surface of their mental life.

When working in a predominantly uncovering mode, we use material in the dream to help patients learn more about their unconscious minds, including affects, transferences, fantasies, relationships, and self-perceptions.

There is nothing in the technique of psychodynamic psychotherapy that sounds more daunting or romantic than "dream interpretation." But don't be afraid to work with dreams. Dreams and their related associations are just productions of the patient's mind. They are interesting, fun, and generally closer to unconscious material than other things patients say. Trainees often feel that they have to "know" what dreams mean in order to talk about them with patients. Actually, it's a distortion to think that we ever "know" what a dream means; all we know is that dreams emerge from the unconscious mind and can help us learn about thoughts and feelings that are out of awareness.

Dreams occupy a special place in the history of psychodynamic theory. *The Interpretation of Dreams* (1900), considered by many to be Freud's *magnum opus*, was his attempt to explain the workings of the mind via dream exploration [1]. When Freud called dreams "the royal road to the unconscious," he meant that listening to dreams offered a direct route to unconscious material. He believed that all dreams – even anxiety dreams – were dreamt to fulfill unconscious wishes. In Freud's model, the unconscious wish "hitches a ride" into consciousness on something that happened in the 24–48 hours before the dream. This was called the **day residue** [2], which could be a perception, an impression, a feeling, or a thought. The day residue was thought to act like a magnet, pulling related unconscious material that had been inadmissible to consciousness (**the latent dream**) into the dream. The **dream work** was thought to be

---

Psychodynamic Psychotherapy: A Clinical Manual, Second Edition. Deborah L. Cabaniss, Sabrina Cherry, Carolyn J. Douglas and Anna Schwartz.
© 2017 John Wiley & Sons, Ltd. Published 2017 by John Wiley & Sons, Ltd.

the process that transformed the latent dream into a story **(the manifest dream)** using the properties of primary process – condensation, displacement, and symbolization (see Chapter 2). Interpreting the dream thus involved understanding the dream work in order to work back to unconscious material [3]:

> *A 36-year-old man, who is still financially dependent on his parents, cannot allow himself to consciously acknowledge angry feelings toward his father. He sees a movie in which a young lawyer has a screaming match with one of the firm's elders. That night, he dreams he is having a fight with the actor who played the older man. In therapy, he links the dream to feelings about his father that were previously inadmissible to consciousness.*

In this example the movie, which is the day residue, presents a situation related to the patient's anger at his father. This finds its way into the dream via displacement. In therapy, he works backward to link his feelings to his relationship with his father.

Today, most psychodynamic psychotherapists do not believe that dreams are wish fulfillments, nor do they believe that dreams are caused by unconscious wishes. Some neurobiologists believe that dreams are used in the service of consolidating memories, but the truth is that the etiology of dreams remains opaque [4]. Nevertheless, dreams seem to be composed of elements from deep in our mind, and clinical experience indicates that working with dreams helps us as therapists learn about patients and their unconscious thoughts, feelings, and fantasies [5]. Since we are trying to get to unconscious material, dreams offer a unique window into the unconscious, and thus working with dreams remains a cornerstone of the technique of psychodynamic psychotherapy.

In this chapter, we will talk about two aspects of dreams:

- **The dream story**, which is what the patient remembers and reports
- **The dream associations**, which link the dream story to related unconscious elements

Both are important in our work with dreams.

Technique

Listening

As with anything else patients tell us, we listen to dreams in order to learn about the unconscious. We listen both to the **dream story** as the patient tells it, and to the **dream associations** to learn about related unconscious elements.

Listening to the dream story

First, we let the dream story wash over us without focusing using **ambient listening**. Then, we **filter** and **focus** our listening on particular elements of the dream.

Listening for mood and affect in the dream

This gives us good information about which part of the dream is closest to the surface, guiding our choices about how and when to intervene. If patients don't spontaneously report their mood in the dream, it's a good idea to ask:

> *A young woman dreamed that she was in a forest pursued by wild animals. The therapist thought this was likely to be a frightening dream but, rather than assuming this, asked about the patient's feeling in the dream. Contrary to the therapist's expectation, the patient said that it seemed exciting and freeing. The therapist then asked more about this feeling, wondering if fear might be less accessible to awareness.*

Listening for points of clarity

Dream stories are generally vague and jumbled: "I had this weird dream . . . I can't really remember it . . . maybe it was in a castle . . . I don't know . . ." But often there are often clear elements that catch our attention:

> *I had this dream, I don't know where it was but there was this enormous blue bird, circling overhead. I can't remember much else, but I can still see that bird.*

These elements are important to listen for, as they often help the patient to associate to deeper material.

Listening to the story itself

Don't forget to listen to the dream story itself. Is it about flying? Taking a trip? An anxious situation? A romantic theme? Although the patient might not understand the story, it probably relates to a similar story in their current or past experience. For example, if early in therapy a patient dreams of starting a journey, this may relate to beginning the "journey" of the treatment. This can also help you listen for the dream's **dominant theme**.

Listening to dream associations

When dreams were thought to be divinely produced and predictive of future events, dream books that gave explanations of dream elements were common. Think of Joseph's interpretation of Pharaoh's prophetic dream. Using the ancient method of "decoding," associations were not necessary – the symbols gave the meaning. In *The Interpretation of Dreams*, Freud refuted this idea, suggesting instead that the meaning of the dream was to be found in the associations. Paying close attention to the associations remains good technical advice when listening to dreams. The same element can represent vastly different things in the dreams of two people – only the associations tell us what it means to each of them. Consider these examples:

> *A 23-year-old woman in psychotherapy with a 35-year-old female therapist reports the following dream:*

"We were here in your office but it wasn't your office – it was more like a living room and we were having coffee. It was a nice feeling, like we were chatting, more than like we were having a session."

Associations – The patient notes that she felt good that the therapist offered her a few moments to compose herself after a very emotional session the day before. This prolonged the session by a few minutes and the patient felt this indicated that the therapist cared about her.

A 19-year-old man who is in psychotherapy with a 35-year-old female therapist had the following dream:

"I came to your office but it was different – I think it was your house. You said, 'We don't have to talk about the session,' and you started to talk about a movie you had just seen. I also think there was someone else there, but I'm not sure."

Associations – The patient had recently noticed that the therapist was pregnant, and worried that her concern about the baby would detract from the therapy.

The stories of these dreams are similar – in each, the patient is in a more casual setting with the therapist. However, in the first the symbolic change represents a feeling of closeness, while in the second it represents a feeling of distance.

Although the dream itself is a discrete narrative, we have to think of everything the patient said just before and after the dream as associations to it. Consider this dream and associations:

I'm sorry I forgot to bring your check today – I'll bring it next week. Oh, I forgot, I had a dream last night. It was completely random – I have no idea what it means. I was in a car, I think in the back seat and the doors were all closed – someone came into the front seat and started the car, but I had no idea where we were going. Whatever that was about. Anyway, I don't want to talk about that – I need to talk to you about work. My boss is giving me such a pain in the neck . . . my old boss gave me a long leash and now I feel like I have no independence . . .

Despite the patient's protestations, the material that comes directly after the dream is about being controlled, and the dream is about not being in control – so the dominant theme of the dream and the immediate associations are linked. Similarly, the transference material that precedes the dream might be related to this theme as well – could forgetting the check relate to feeling controlled by the therapist? We learn the most about a dream when we listen to all of the material around it as if it were linked to the dream in some way.

Listen for connections and nodal points

In addition to the associations, we are aided by listening for connections to other material such as:

- the point in the session when the dream was reported
- words in the dream that seem related to surrounding material

- themes in the dream that seem related to surrounding material
- concepts in the dream that seemed related to surrounding material

As before, the technique for listening to nodal points involves listening for words and symbols that get repeated, as well as for points of clarity.

Reflecting

Once we let the dream wash over us, we reflect on it to try to understand how it might be connected to unconscious material. This will guide our therapeutic strategy for intervening. Our idea is that elements in the dream represent and/or are connected to unconscious feelings, fears, and fantasies. As always, we use the choosing principles to think about what's on the surface and what's deep while trying to identify nodal points and dominant themes. Our best guides for this are affect and repetitive, clear elements. The readiness principles help us with the timing of interventions.

Understanding primary process

Although we no longer think about "decoding" dreams, dream material is difficult to understand because it's organized by **primary process** thinking (see Chapter 2). Understanding how primary process works is key to thinking about what dream elements might represent. Here's a review of the three basic characteristics of primary process thinking as they relate to dreams:

Condensation

Two related unconscious elements combine to form a single dream element:

> *"I had a dream about a woman. She looked like my ex-girlfriend, but she also sort of looked like this picture of my mother in college."*

The "mother/ex-girlfriend" combination is a condensation that suggests that these two people are linked in the dreamer's mind.

Displacement

An element in the story of the dream stands for something unconscious:

> *A 50-year-old man on the eve of a biopsy reports the following dream: "I had a dream last night about being late for my bar exam."*

Here, the anxiety about a "test" in his future is displaced by the story of a "test" in his past.

Symbolization

An element in the story of the dream symbolizes something unconscious, such as a person, wish, thought, or idea:

> *A woman who was two months away from ending psychotherapy reported this dream: "I dreamt that I was in an airport alone waiting for a plane . . . I felt frightened about the trip."*

In this dream, "taking a trip alone" might symbolize her feelings about her future without her therapist.

Common dream themes

Although each dream is unique, thinking about several common unconscious elements helps to reflect on dreams:

- **Transference themes:** Thoughts and feelings about the therapist are frequently represented in the dreams of psychotherapy patients. If you are a beginner, it may be hard to imagine that you could be "important enough" to show up in a patient's dreams, but you undoubtedly will. As you reflect on a dream, you will often discover references to the transference. You can then use the choosing and readiness principles to decide whether these references are close enough to the surface to pursue with uncovering interventions.

- **Unconscious fantasies:** Although we no longer believe that dreams are produced by unconscious wishes, unconscious fantasies abound in dreams. Think of the person who denies aggressive feelings toward a loved one but dreams of that person's death – while this might reflect a fear, it might also reflect unconscious aggressive fantasies.

- **Representations of relationships:** Dreams often include other people and contain important clues about the patient's relationships with significant others – or at least the patient's *perceptions* about those relationships. When thinking about the way relationships are represented in a dream, pay attention to the potential for displacement – a dream about "my boss" is usually not just about the boss but may be about some earlier, related relationship and the feeling it engenders in the patient.

- **Self-perceptions:** Dreams frequently help us to understand how patients think about themselves. Remember that the dreamer can be anywhere in the dream – don't be fooled if patients don't appear as themselves in the story of the dream. When dreamers do appear in dreams, it's a good bet that this does in fact represent them. Here's an interesting example of a self-perception dream in which the dreamer is represented in a displaced way:

> *A 35-year-old man who had a difficult relationship with his father is in psychodynamic psychotherapy with a 50-year-old male therapist. He reports the following dream: "I dreamt that you and I were painting a house together. You also had a young assistant – a boy – it seemed perfectly natural that he was there with us, too." Although the patient's first associations are to whether the therapist has children, he then talks about the way in which the therapist has helped him feel good about himself as a man in a way his father never did. In reflecting on this association, the therapist wonders whether*

the young assistant is a displacement for the patient himself, and thus symbolizes the patient's wish for the therapist to be his father.

Using the organizing sources

Reflecting on dreams also involves considering the history and formulation. We can also *cautiously* use our own experience of the dreams of others to help guide our reflection:

> *A 38-year-old single woman who steadfastly maintains that she is not interested in having children begins to have dreams in which she is growing unexpectedly fat or in which she has something wrong with her internal organs.*

It is not a leap to imagine that this woman is having unconscious thoughts about having children despite consciously saying the opposite. Caution is the name of the game here – while we can use our past experience with others to help guide our hypotheses, *this can not a substitute for listening to the unique associations of each patient.*

Intervening

Basic interventions

Psychoeducation/teaching about the interpretation of dreams

Generally, the first intervention we make about dreams is to teach patients how to work with them. Many people think that the dream story is the whole dream, and many patients who have not had previous experience with therapy find their dreams confusing and random. Patients frequently tell us that they have "no idea" what their dreams mean and often precede their report of a dream by saying they think it's "not relevant." Early in therapy, we let our patients know the following:

- Dreams help elucidate what is going on out of awareness, so trying to remember and talk about dreams in therapy is very useful.
- Dreams don't have "a" meaning; rather, they help us to learn about related themes that are out of awareness. So it's good to talk about any dream you have, even if you don't know what it "means."
- When trying to understand a dream, the dream story itself is often less important than associating to the various elements of the dream.

For example, consider the following excerpt from the therapy of a 32-year-old woman who has been in treatment for one month:

> Patient   *I had a dream last night but I don't know what it means. I think I was on a boat or something – yeah, a boat – on a lake – and there was some sort of natural disaster happening on the shore – I could see it but I wasn't in it. Maybe it was a tidal wave or an earthquake. Then I was locked in the restroom, trying to figure out if I could climb over the top. That's just weird. Why would I dream about the restroom of a boat?*

Therapist	Well, often the "story" you remember when you wake up in the morning seems strange and disjointed, and it's hard to know what the dream "means." When we work with dreams in psychotherapy, the best way to proceed is to just think about different images or pieces of the dream and to say whatever comes to mind about them. For example, in this dream, I wonder what comes to mind about being on a boat on a lake or being trapped in a bathroom?
Patient	The only boat I remember was my uncle's boat on the bay – I used to like to go on that boat with my cousins – they were very nice, my aunt and uncle – much more relaxed than my parents – and they didn't fight like my parents did. I used to lie in bed at night and wish they would adopt me.

In this example, the fantastic story of the dream disorients the patient; however, once the therapist helps her to associate, the patient is able to deepen the material. Perhaps she symbolically depicted her parents' marriage as the disaster on the shore. After a while, patients begin to associate to the dream elements without being prompted.

Questions and calls for associations

If patients don't immediately associate to a dream, you can prompt them to begin. First ask an open-ended question:

What comes to mind about the dream?

Then you can ask more specifically about their mood or other elements of the dream:

How did you feel in the dream?

What comes to mind about being in Russia?

Any thoughts about dreaming about summer camp?

Even experienced patients will sometimes miss elements that might yield associations. In this case – ask! Not talking about a central element in the dream may be resistance, so it is as important to think about the resistance as it is to think about the associations themselves. Choosing whether to comment on the resistance or the content once again involves the choosing principles. For example, let's say a patient tells a dream about being abandoned in a desert holding only a guitar and then only talks about the guitar. It could be that the associations to the guitar are close to the surface affect, or it could be that the patient is talking about the guitar in order to avoid talking about feelings of abandonment or desolation. We'll talk more about confronting resistance in relation to working with dreams later.

Supporting interventions

We use supporting interventions in our work with dreams when we think that using dream elements to uncover unconscious material could increase anxiety and be potentially disorganizing.

In general, we don't encourage patients with weakened function to report dreams, because we think that uncovering unconscious material may heighten their anxiety rather than helping them understand themselves [6,7]. When these patients report dreams spontaneously, we have to judge whether they are likely to tolerate feelings that might emerge in exploring the dream. For example, a patient with impaired reality testing might find it terrifying to delve into the unconscious fears and fantasies suggested by a dream. Similarly, a person straining to control angry impulses might not be helped by associating to a dream about being at his father's funeral. When patients like these report dreams but then seem disinclined to talk about them, we often choose *not* to confront the resistance, but rather to respect their avoidance by **supportively bypassing** the dream. We can also listen to a dream and reflect on possible connections to a patient's unconscious, but then use the elements of the manifest dream to address conscious concerns:

> *A young man with schizophrenia, committed involuntarily to the hospital the previous night for an acute psychotic break, meets his therapist for the first time:*

Therapist	*I hope you had a reasonably comfortable night. Sometimes it's not easy sleeping in the hospital the first night.* (**nurturing, soothing**)
Patient	*Are you kidding? How can anyone sleep when they play those movies in your head all night?*
Therapist	*That would be very upsetting – and scary. Any chance that it might have been a dream?* (**empathizing, naming emotions, jointly reality testing**)
Patient	*They're messing with me.*
Therapist	*Try telling me about it. Talking about things in the light of day usually makes them less frightening.* (**encouraging, reassuring**)
Patient	*I was locked in a dungeon, no food or water. Guards came to torture me. But I found a gun. I thought I was going to be OK. But when I pulled the trigger, it just clicked, and nothing happened.* (**shudders**)
Therapist	*That sounds awful. You know, for a lot of people, being hospitalized can feel like being put in jail – understandably. There are locks on the door, your stuff is taken away . . .* (**empathizing, validation, interpreting up**)
Patient	*That's how I feel – I can't wait to get out of here. At least you understand.*

Since the patient is ruminating about a dream that frightened him and has become part of his persecutory delusion, the therapist decides to work with it in the interest of establishing an alliance and helping with reality testing. By reflecting on the general affects and themes suggested in the dream, the therapist is able to offer an alternative explanation that links the story of the dream to the patient's fears and concerns about being forcibly hospitalized. Without exploring the dream further, the therapist is able to engage the patient, lessen his anxiety, and organize his experience.

Uncovering interventions

We choose uncovering interventions when we think that patients can use dreams to learn more about their unconscious and themselves. Our uncovering interventions are designed to communicate hypotheses about unconscious elements that might be represented in and/or connected to the dream story.

Confrontations of resistance

Not talking about a reported dream is a common resistance. When a patient tells a dream and does not return to it, you can easily confront the resistance by saying, "I notice you haven't returned to talking about the dream you told me." This may prompt the patient to talk about the dream, but don't forget the resistance – there was undoubtedly a reason for it. Also remember that whatever the patient says after the dream is an association to the dream – so not talking directly about the dream is not always resistance. In general, give the patient some time before confronting the resistance in order to hear useful associations.

Confrontation/clarification/interpretation

Like all interpretations, working with dreams is a process – one that needs a good "set-up" to help patients deepen understanding and affect. This process changes with the phases of treatment. As we develop the therapeutic alliance with patients and accumulate many shared experiences with them, we may be able to jump directly to an interpretation without having to pave the way with as much confrontation and clarification. However, the development of good technique involves practice with confrontation and clarification. We generally do not understand enough about a dream to venture an interpretation until the confrontations and clarifications elucidate the unconscious associations.

As always, **confrontations** are intended to interest patients in their minds. Confrontations in dream interpretation often sound like this:

> *What do you make of the fact that there is a monarch butterfly in the dream?*

We do not know why it's there, either – we're just trying to interest patients in the fact that they dreamt about a particular element.

Clarifications point out that an element of a dream has occurred before and suggest a possible relationship to other unconscious material:

> *You often dream about your grandfather when you're about to go on a trip.*

Finally, **interpretations** offer hypotheses about the unconscious underpinnings of dreams. Here is an example of a reported dream, followed by confrontation, clarification, and interpretation:

> Patient   *All I wanted to do was to get engaged to Fred, but since he's given me the ring I feel all out of sorts. I don't really know why – I love him and I'm not interested in anyone else but I just feel blah – am I having second thoughts? My mother called about starting to make wedding plans and I just wanted to sleep. She's being very nice about it – it's like she's more interested in the wedding than I am. Oh – I had a weird dream last night – it seems irrelevant – I got a kitten for my birthday and was petting it and suddenly it was huge – like ferocious – but also like a house cat too – it was very weird. I think there were other parts but I can't remember them. I wonder if I need to go on medication again – am I getting depressed? My friend needed medication before her wedding – even on the day of the ceremony.*

Therapist	*You've veered away from talking about the dream – does anything else come to mind about it?* (**confrontation of resistance**)
Patient	*Not really – it just seemed like a weird dream. I don't even have a cat. I did, though, I loved my cat – I had it when I was very small. It was my cat – it was a very sweet cat – it slept on my bed – but it scratched the living-room furniture and we had to get rid of it.*
Therapist	*Who made that decision?* (**question**)
Patient	*My mother. I cried and cried. I must have been about 7 years old. We never got another pet. I wonder if Fred would be into getting a cat.*
Therapist	*What was your mood in the dream?* (**question**)
Patient	*Hmmm – I think that I was confused – I couldn't tell. I thought it was a sweet cat and then it was scary. Like it turned on me. Anyway, I've got to get going on the wedding stuff. My mother is on my case – calling all the time. She's right – I've got to do it – she's got all these ideas about places that her friends had their weddings – I mean their kids' weddings – but I think I want to do it in the city.*
Therapist	*You've mentioned your mother a few times in the discussion of this dream – do you have any thoughts about that?* (**clarification**)
Patient	*I know that she means well and she's paying for it after all – but she's sort of driving me crazy. I mean it's my wedding, right? But I feel bad saying that – they had no money when they got married and she had nothing – and they've been fighting recently.*
Therapist	*Perhaps the cat in the dream is sort of like your mother – sweet, but you're afraid it will turn on you. Maybe your blah feeling after getting engaged has to do with your fear that starting to plan the wedding will bring out something scary in your mother that feels dangerous.* (**interpretation**)
Patient	*It's just that she always wants whatever I have – I know that she didn't have all the advantages that I have – but she copies my clothing and my jewelry and I guess I'm afraid that she's going to try to co-opt this wedding. Maybe we should just elope.*

In this sequence, the patient sets up the dream, tells it, and then drifts away because of the difficult content. The therapist doesn't know what this is yet and is just listening. The resistance is the first clue about this difficulty as the therapist begins to reflect. The therapist's **call for associations** produces an early memory that involves conflicted feelings and is linked to the mother. The therapist reflects on this and begins to hear a nodal point – mother. The therapist then makes a **clarification** about the nodal point and the patient deepens the material and affect to the point where the therapist can make an interpretation. The therapist hypothesizes that the cat in the dream symbolizes the patient's mother – seemingly sweet, but able to turn into something ferocious and scary. The ferocious and scary part represents the mother's envy, which the patient senses but hasn't fully allowed into consciousness. Defending against her feelings about her mother's envy has resulted in a symptom – the "blah" feeling and lack of interest in the wedding. The symbol "worked" because it was linked to the mother – a "house" pet, like the mother in the house, and linked to the mother since she gave it away. The interpretation was successful because it produced affect and deepened understanding. We can speculate that the "blah" feeling and apathy about the wedding may be mitigated after this interpretive work, although it may have to be repeated in the **working through** before the understanding is consolidated.

Now that we have discussed supporting and uncovering techniques related to affect, resistance, transference, countertransference, unconscious fantasy and conflict, and dreams, let's look at a whole session and consider the way a therapist listens, reflects, and intervenes.

Suggested activity

Read the following dream and consider the study questions:

> *I had a dream last night. It was about a car – I think I was in it – and we conked out on the side of a small highway. It was dark. After a while another car drove over and gave us a jump-start and the headlights went on.*

What if this were the dream of a 40-year-old woman who was recovering from depression and feeling that psychotherapy wasn't helping her much? What might you think as she told you the dream? What might you say? How might this dream be related to the transference?

Comment

If this were the dream of a 40-year-old woman recovering from depression, perhaps the car might symbolize her – conked out but jump-started by treatment. You might say:

> *I wonder if you feel like the car – when you were depressed you thought you'd never run again, but you feel jump-started by therapy.* (**interpretation**)

The therapist might be the car who gave her the jump-start. Interventions to explore this idea include:

> *There's another car in the dream – any thoughts about who might have been driving it?* (**call for associations**)

If the patient is unable to use uncovering interventions, you might use the symbolism in the dream to help her understand that she was feeling better:

> *Sounds like a pretty positive dream – makes sense, since you're starting to feel better – like you're getting a new start, too.* (**offering optimism, naming emotions**)

Chapter 24: References

1. Freud, S. (1900) The Interpretation of Dreams, in *The Standard Edition of the Complete Psychological Works of Sigmund Freud (1900): The Interpretation of Dreams (First Part)*, Vol. 4, Hogarth Press, London, pp. ix–627.
2. Freud, S. (1905) Jokes and their relation to the unconscious, in *The Standard Edition of the Complete Psychological Works of Sigmund Freud*, Vol. 8, Hogarth Press, London, pp. 1–247, 160.

3. Freud, S. (1916) Introductory lectures on psycho-analysis, in *The Standard Edition of the Complete Psychological Works of Sigmund Freud (1915–1916): Introductory Lectures on Psycho-analysis (Parts I and II), Vol. 15*, Hogarth Press, London, p. 120.

4. Stickgold, R., Hobson, J.A., Fosse, R., *et al.* (2001) Sleep, learning, and dreams: Off-line memory reprocessing. *Science*, **294** (5544), 1052–1057.

5. Schlesinger, H. (2003) *The Texture of Treatment*, Analytic Press, Hillsdale, NJ, p. 109.

6. Werman, D. (1978) The use of dreams in psychotherapy. *Journal of the Canadian Psychiatric Association*, **23**, 153–158.

7. Werman, D. (1984) The place of the dream in supportive psychotherapy, in *The Practice of Supportive Psychotherapy*, Brunner/Mazel, New York, pp. 151–155.

Review Activity for Part Five: The "Microprocess Moment" – Understanding a Moment in Therapy

By this point you've learned a tremendous amount – how to assess a patient, how to listen, reflect, and intervene, and how to work with different themes that emerge in therapy. Along the way, you've done some exercises to help you practice your new skills. They all come together in the ability to analyze the moment-to-moment interactions you have with your patients. Being conscious of everything that is going on is crucial for being able to conduct psychodynamic psychotherapy successfully. For any given moment that you have with your patient(s), you should be able to describe:

- what you heard
- how you reflected on what you heard to choose your therapeutic strategy
- what interventions you used and how you think they worked

You should then be able to identify:

1. the dominant affect
2. the dominant resistance
3. the dominant transference
4. the dominant countertransference
5. the dominant unconscious fantasy
6. your dominant technical mode (uncovering or supporting)
7. your therapeutic strategy and how you think it worked

If you can do this, you're well on your way to becoming a psychodynamic psychotherapist. You can write this in a "Microprocess Moment," which not only tells the story of a moment in therapy, but also describes your listening, reflecting, and intervening process [1]. It should include all of the above elements. See if you can identify elements 1–7 in the following Microprocess Moment:

> *In his third year of treatment with me, Mr B, a 35-year-old married, African-American lawyer, came to his Wednesday 5:45 PM session saying that he hadn't really wanted to come but didn't know why. He said that he usually looked forward to coming to sessions, but today had almost called to cancel. He then shifted and began to describe his latest case in great detail.*

> *As he talked, I realized that I was becoming very bored with the details of the case and that my mind was beginning to wander. Since this patient was usually quite engaging, I wondered why that was and thought he might be resisting talking more about his feelings about treatment. I decided to confront this resistance, saying, "You mentioned not wanting to come to the session, then shifted to talking about the case."*

"The case is on my mind," he replied, "The partner I'm working for is driving me really hard. I'm there on nights and weekends. I even have to go back after the session tonight."

I immediately felt bad, as if I should have been able to offer him a later appointment, although he had my last session. Why did I feel so bad, I wondered? I thought that the wish to not come to the session and his feelings about the partner had something to do with each other – perhaps a displaced transference – but I did not understand the connection. I decided to wait to see what Mr B said next.

After a pause, the patient said, "The thing that's driving me crazy about this case is that there are two of us – two associates – working on it. I'm working my tail off on the research, but I think the other guy is going to get the #2 chair at the trial. It's not fair. I think it might be because he's white."

As soon as he said this, I felt bad again – was it because I'm white, I wondered? I considered whether what he was saying was true, and I had the impulse to empathize with him directly. I recognized that I didn't know enough and that the impulse was the result of a countertransference feeling I didn't fully understand. I thought again about being white and about the idea that his anger at the partners might have to do with me, although I didn't know how.

I decided to go back to the beginning of the session and again confront a potential resistance by saying, "You mentioned needing to go back to work after the session, but I wonder if anything else comes to mind about not wanting to come this evening."

"No, I don't think so," he said. "But you probably don't like working this late either. You work long hours – on Monday I come here early in the morning – and you see patients back to back without a break. You probably want to go home by this time of night."

This was an interesting turn, I thought – why was he suddenly concerned about me? And what did it have to do with my guilt?

Since Mr B was starting to get more specific about things that were going on in the therapy, I opted to call for more associations. "What about my seeing patients back to back?" I asked.

"Well," he said, "when I was seeing my therapist in college, he had two doors – one that you came in through, and one that you went out through. That way I never knew who was ahead of me or behind me. I liked that better. Here, I can always see who's coming out of the office before I go in. If you didn't have your patients so close together, I'd never know."

Then I realized that in the last two weeks, a new patient had started in the session before Mr B – a tall, blond white man around the same age. There was the link to the #2 man at the law firm and my guilty countertransference feeling. He was angry that I was making him see that I was treating this white man.

But was this anger near the surface? Mr B was moderately able to acknowledge his anger at the partner for preferring the white man, but he needed to mitigate his anger with me with concern that I worked too hard. I decided that the anger with me was still too deep to address. Yet I also knew that I should address something about the transference, since it had almost resulted in the patient's skipping the session. Was I ready for an interpretation? There were only 15 more minutes in the session – and he seemed willing to talk about this – so I decided to give it a try. Should I go for the whole interpretation – that he didn't want to come to the session because he didn't want to see the new patient? I decided to start more slowly, confronting his resistance to talking about the new patient.

"Perhaps you have some thoughts about someone you've seen leave the office," I ventured.

He paused, and then said, "I rarely look up in the waiting room. I keep my head in a magazine. But last time I was here, this guy almost trips over me to go to the restroom before he leaves. I had to look up."

Brooks Brothers from head to toe. I know that type – those frat guys from college who used to wait for us after games. And in your office – in this chair!"

He was very close, I thought, so I decided to make the interpretation. "Maybe you didn't want to come today because you didn't want to see that patient."

Looking at the ceiling, he said, "I liked that chubby girl who used to come before me. That was fine. But this guy! And now I'm probably going to have to see him every week."

I knew then that he was jealous and thought I preferred the white "frat guy" to him, just as the partner preferred the other associate. I also realized that my guilty feelings had to do with the idea that seeing these patients back to back was insensitive, and that if I understood this I might learn more about the patient's relationship to his race, to women, to white men, and to me. But time was up – it would have to wait until next week.

Comment

- Dominant affect – anger
- Dominant resistance – thinking of missing the sessions, talking about work
- Dominant transferences – triadic, maternal, erotic
- Dominant countertransference – guilt
- Dominant unconscious fantasy – "As a black man, I will always be passed over for white men."
- Dominant technical mode – uncovering.
- Therapeutic strategy – The therapist uses what she learns from confrontation of resistance and reflection on her own countertransference to uncover transferential thoughts and feelings. This deepens the material and allows the patient to connect to unconscious fantasies and feelings.

See if you can do this with a moment from a therapy you are conducting. The more you allow yourself to understand your own feelings, the better you'll be at this. If you need help, discuss it with a peer, a supervisor, or even a therapist of your own. If you can understand one moment, you can string them together to understand the whole treatment. Once you become good at this, it will happen almost automatically as you and your patients learn about their unconscious thoughts and feelings.

[Note to educators – this is a good method for the evaluation of psychodynamic technique. It can also be done as an interactive video review. Both can be assessed using the Microprocess Assessment Form in Appendix 2. For more on this, see the Guide for Educators in Appendix 1.]

Reference

1. Cabaniss, D.L., Havel, L.K., Berger, S., Deo, A., and Arbuckle, M.R. (2015) The Microprocess Moment: A tool for evaluating skills in psychodynamic psychotherapy. *Academic Psychiatry*, doi: 10.1007/s40596-015-0450-6.

PART SIX: Meeting Therapeutic Goals

Key concepts

The major goals of psychodynamic psychotherapy are:

- improving self-perceptions and self-esteem regulation
- improving relationships with others
- improving ways of adapting to external and internal stimulation
- improving cognitive functions

Both supporting and uncovering strategies are used in meeting these goals.

In the previous sections of this manual you have learned how to:

- assess patients for psychodynamic psychotherapy
- begin the treatment
- listen to patients, reflect on what you've heard, and intervene to both support and uncover

Psychodynamic Psychotherapy: A Clinical Manual, Second Edition. Deborah L. Cabaniss, Sabrina Cherry, Carolyn J. Douglas and Anna Schwartz.
© 2017 John Wiley & Sons, Ltd. Published 2017 by John Wiley & Sons, Ltd.

- use listening, reflecting, and intervening to respond to affect, resistance, transference, countertransference, conflict, fantasy, defenses, and dreams

You are now ready to use these techniques to help patients meet their therapeutic goals. This is the main work of the **middle** of therapy. The next four chapters will help you consolidate what you have learned as we apply the techniques from Part Five to **four major goals of psychodynamic psychotherapy**:

- improving self-perceptions and self-esteem regulation
- improving relationships with others
- improving characteristic ways of adapting
- improving cognitive function

25 Improving Self-Perceptions and Self-Esteem Regulation

Key concepts

Self-perception plays a major role in determining how people function in the world.

Improving self-perceptions and the ability to regulate self-esteem is a major goal of psychodynamic psychotherapy.

Self-perceptions may be unconscious.

Developing more realistic self-perceptions can help people to

- improve self-esteem regulation
- have a better understanding of their capabilities and limitations

Supporting techniques can help patients with weaker function strengthen their sense of self and improve self-esteem regulation.

Uncovering techniques can help patients with stronger function by making unconscious self-perceptions conscious.

Problems with self-appraisal can distort self-perception and can be reworked in psychodynamic psychotherapy.

For our self-esteem, life is a battleground. We are pelted daily with blows – small and large – to our sense of self. Store clerks who ignore us, bosses who critique us, and mirrors that show us aging faces and bulging midriffs, all pummel our ability to feel good about ourselves. The ability to buoy our self-esteem – to right ourselves amidst the blows that buffet us every day as we journey through life – is central to being able to function. If we feel bad about ourselves, we don't function well, either on a persistent or acute basis. We become less able to tolerate affects and anxiety, to make realistic appraisals of our capabilities and weaknesses, to make judgments, to control our impulses, to relax – the list goes on. For some people this happens on a short-term basis, but for others it is a persistent problem. Consider the following examples:

> *Mr A, a successful 30-year-old architect who is well liked and generally has a good feeling about himself, was in a meeting in which he was told his plans were inadequate and had to be redone. He began to have an upset stomach and excused himself to go to the restroom. While there, he looked in the mirror and thought he looked old. That night, he went on a date and had a good time, but worried that the woman wouldn't be interested in him. By the next day he felt back to himself, redrafted the plans, and had a good weekend on a bicycle trip with friends.*

Psychodynamic Psychotherapy: A Clinical Manual, Second Edition. Deborah L. Cabaniss, Sabrina Cherry, Carolyn J. Douglas and Anna Schwartz.
© 2017 John Wiley & Sons, Ltd. Published 2017 by John Wiley & Sons, Ltd.

Ms B, a 50-year-old writer who has published three well-regarded books, had a manuscript rejected by her editor. She refused to return phone calls and began to drink heavily in her house. She decided that she would never write again and plunged into a depression for six months for which she did not seek psychiatric help.

Both Mr A and Ms B derive self-esteem from their careers and received blows to their sense of self. These blows upset their ability to self-regulate – both had altered perceptions of themselves, disruption of their ability to regulate anxiety and affect, and disordered behavior. However, Mr A righted himself quickly – he continued to work and socialize and was back to himself by the next day. In contrast, Ms B was derailed for months with a debilitating depression. A person's reaction to a self-esteem blow depends on two major factors

- the force of the blow
- the person's underlying capacity to regulate self-esteem

For example, a person with a healthy sense of self could suffer tremendous loss of functioning if the blow is catastrophic, as in major physical illness, betrayal in a love relationship, unemployment, or emigration. On the other hand, a person with a fragile sense of self could fall apart in response to a minor blow, such as an insult or an easily repaired physical problem.

A solid sense of self is characterized not only by the ability to feel good about oneself, but also by the ability to realistically assess one's capabilities and limitations and to right oneself after a self-esteem threat [1]. Although we don't know exactly how people develop their perceptions of themselves and their capacity for self-esteem management, it makes sense that it results from a combination of inborn traits and interaction with important early caregivers – nature and nurture [2]. We can't change temperament, but we can offer people the opportunity to reassess their sense of self in the context of a new relationship – that is, with the therapist.

Self-appraisal and self-esteem management

Problems with **self-appraisal** can also contribute to distortions in self-perception and difficulty with self-esteem management [3]. This can go in two directions: some people overappraise their capacities, while others underappraise them. Here are two examples:

Ms C felt guilty if she didn't volunteer for every fundraiser organized by the Parent Teacher Association despite the fact that she didn't have time for these activities. She was consequently exhausted and resentful.

Ms C is overly harsh on herself. This leads to a distorted self-perception that she is lazy if she doesn't overdo things. Psychodynamic psychotherapy can be very effective in helping people who are overly harsh on themselves have a more realistic self-perception:

One year out of film school, Mr D is despondent because he has not being recognized by the major Hollywood movie studios.

Mr D has overappraised his abilities. Psychodynamic psychotherapy can help him to look more realistically at his situation in order to help him regulate self-esteem more effectively.

The goal

As discussed in Chapter 2, helping people develop new ways of thinking about themselves and of regulating self-esteem is a primary goal of psychodynamic psycho-therapy. Depending on the person's functioning, we do this with primarily supporting or uncovering techniques. Our hope is that this will enable our patients to regulate their self-esteem in a more adaptive way, and will improve their work life, social life, and emotional life. In the sections that follow, we will outline:

• How to recognize problems relating to self-perception and self-esteem regulation

• Therapeutic strategies for improving these problems

Recognizing the problem

Some people with difficulties in self-perception and self-esteem regulation scaffold their poor self-image with overblown, grandiose, unrealistic perceptions of themselves, while others have more manifestly poor self-esteem. Consider these examples:

> Ms E considered herself the best salesperson in the store – better, even, than the owners. When she got a lukewarm year-end review, she didn't appear at work for two weeks, wrote enraged emails to her colleagues, and was intermittently suicidal.

> Mr F rarely spoke up at meetings because he considered his opinion to be less valuable than those of others. When he got a lukewarm year-end review, he was depressed and socially withdrawn for weeks, but thought that it was evidence of what he already knew about his performance.

Both of these individuals have maladaptive ways of modulating their self-esteem in response to a blow. However, one does it using grandiosity, while the other sinks into depression. Thus, when we are listening for evidence of distorted self-perceptions, we have to be attuned both to grandiosity and to overtly low self-esteem. Anger, depression, social withdrawal, emotional self-flagellation, and impulsive behaviors are common but maladaptive ways in which people try to buoy their sense of self. "Lording it over" someone else – including the therapist – may transiently make a person feel better in the face of a self-esteem blow, as in this example from a patient in psycho-dynamic psychotherapy:

> My boss is such a jerk. He promoted almost everyone in the department except for me. He couldn't see talent if it hit him between the eyes. By the way, you're out of tissues again. That's really unprofessional – you should really make an effort to keep up your office better than you do.

This patient temporarily increases his sense of self by criticizing his therapist. At the opposite extreme, overidealization of the therapist and others can also signal problems with self-esteem regulation.

We also want to understand whether patients do or do not have a realistic sense of their capabilities and limitations. Having a distorted sense of self can lead to significant impairment and may require people to sustain an emotionally costly "false front" in order to maintain positive self-regard. Here are a few examples of what this can sound like:

> Mr G worked as a high-level executive at his family's business despite the fact that he had not graduated from college and had limited skills as a manager. When his father died, he mismanaged the company and then blamed his staff for the ensuing financial debacle. Although most of his workers became disgruntled and left, Mr G remained unable to admit any responsibility for the company's problems. He was increasingly bitter, angry, and socially isolated.

> Ms H is a 60-year-old single woman who presented for depressed mood in the context of "not getting any good singing gigs." She explained that she has been a gospel singer for 40 years and that she once "cut a record" in her 20s. Since then she has been pursuing a recording contract. "Many were interested," she says bitterly, "but now they aren't looking for talent – they're looking for sex appeal." She has been offered work as a singing coach for an after-school program, but has refused this, saying, "That's for has-beens." She has not sung in public for years and is on the brink of financial ruin, although she refuses to apply for bankruptcy.

> Mr I feels demoralized at his job in advertising. He has many creative ideas, but is too afraid to share them so has been relegated to a supportive, peripheral role.

For these patients, the inability to realistically assess their capabilities and limitations has adversely affected every aspect of their lives – their work life, social life, and emotional life. Listening for this helps us notice distortions in self-perception and difficulty managing self-esteem. Here are some questions you can ask to help screen for these problems:

> How would you describe yourself?

> How do you think other people would describe you?

> Do you think other people would describe you as confident? Underconfident?

> How would you describe your strengths and difficulties to someone else?

> When was the last time that something happened to you that really shook your self-esteem? How did you handle it?

> Do you think your parents are (were) supportive of you? How did they show it? [4]

Distorted self-perceptions can often involve a distorted assessment of body image, intelligence, likability, or work performance. A story about any one of these areas can be mined for information about the way people view themselves.

Therapeutic strategies

How can we help people have more realistic perceptions of themselves? Our hypotheses are as follows:

- Unconscious self-perceptions prevent people from using objective data to think realistically about their capabilities and limitations:

  Ms J, a brilliant student, idealizes her father despite the fact that he always told her that she was the "least intellectual" of all the siblings. She accepts that this is true and consequently believes that she will never be truly successful in academic terms. When she receives an award for the best thesis in the university, she cannot use this to help her reappraise her perception of her capabilities.

- Unrealistic self-perceptions lead people to have difficulty righting themselves when faced with self-esteem blows:

  Mr K was always told that he was an outstanding athlete. He did very well on the high school football team despite being somewhat short. When he didn't make the college team, he was unable to accept that this was because other students were more qualified. Instead, he became enraged at the coach and sure that the coach was playing favorites.

Making people aware of their distorted self-perceptions can help them assess themselves more accurately and regulate their self-esteem more easily. Since we generally think that our sense of self develops early in life, reworking our self-perceptions can be considered a way of **reactivating development**. We can address this with both supporting and uncovering strategies:

Supporting strategies

Self-esteem management often requires support. We choose to support self-esteem directly when we feel that patients either cannot do this themselves or cannot tolerate efforts to explore their distorted perceptions. Both supplying and assisting interventions are helpful. For example, patients with very low self-esteem may regularly need encouraging-type interventions, such as **praise** and **encouragement**. Patients who are overly harsh on themselves may be helped by comments designed to **reduce guilt** and **correct misperceptions**. If patients can do some of this work on their own, **collaborative interventions** that allow therapist and patient to reconsider thought patterns, such as **reality testing**, promote the development of new self-perceptions. Here's an example that uses both supplying and assisting interventions:

  Mr L is a 28-year-old writer who sought psychotherapy saying he was dissatisfied with his career. Mr L calls his job as a staff writer for a magazine the "dream job I had always hoped for," but is plagued by the "terrible" feeling that he is a "fraud." "Basically, my father got me the job," he explains. "If he hadn't made that call, there's no way they would have even looked at my resume." His boss has been "nagging" him to finish assignments on time; Mr L says, "He's really getting on my case." Mr L alternates between agonizing self-doubt and bitter resentment that his boss doesn't take the time to give him more supervision – "It's like he wants me to fail." He feels paralyzed at his computer, and at night smokes pot "just to calm down and sleep." Lately, he has started going out to bars because "I can't stand staying home and staring at a blank screen – it might as well be a neon sign blinking 'Loser.'"

Here's some process from an early evaluation session:

Mr L	*I'm such a screw-up – I just can't write. I keep staring at the screen and nothing comes out. I'll never be a good writer.*
Therapist	*Are you saying you've never written anything you felt good about?* (**confrontation**)
Mr L	*No – I've written some good things – but this guy is really after me.*
Therapist	*Do you think that there's another way to think about your editor's behavior?* (**joint reality testing**)
Mr L	*I said no – I can't write and he's going to fire me.*
Therapist	*I wonder if it would help if we thought about some of the things that could be contributing to your difficulty writing.* (**joint inquiry**)
Mr L	*The sleep problem is huge. I'm exhausted.*
Therapist	*I'll bet – I'm actually wondering if you might be depressed – depression can make it difficult to sleep, to work, and to concentrate. Treating the depression might help you a lot. There's also the issue of your pot smoking – that can also knock out your ability to concentrate.* (**empathizing, validating, psychoeducation**)
Mr L	*I never put those together. What do you suggest?*
Therapist	*I think that treating your depression and cutting out the pot smoking will make a big difference to your ability to write. Many writers also work with a partner, or use a writers' group to help with deadlines. If we can get you writing again, I have a feeling that you'll be able to feel better about your work and about yourself.* (**offering optimism, psychoeducation, suggesting**)
Mr L	*That sounds good – it's definitely worth a try.*

The therapist hears the self-esteem problem – the patient presents himself as a "screw-up" who will never amount to anything. However, the therapist suspects there may be more to the story – it seems implausible that Mr L got his current job at a prestigious magazine solely on the strength of his father's connections. He decides to **confront** this distortion and to **reality-test** the patient's contention that his boss is out to get him. However, the patient is unable to use either of these interventions to begin to think about possible unconscious material. The therapist then shifts tack and uses **empathy** and **psychoeducation** to address some of the difficulties that could be affecting the patient's ability to write at this point. This engages the patient and helps him think about ways to improve his current self-esteem.

In the following example, the therapist responds to a patient's feelings toward her to address self-esteem vulnerability:

Ms M is a 40-year-old nurse who has changed jobs three times in the last four years. Perpetually dissatisfied with her professional and personal life, she feels that her abilities and talents are not appreciated by others, and is highly sensitive to perceived slights and criticism, reacting with anger or icy withdrawal. Of note is that her mother was a concentration camp survivor whom Ms M described as "joyless" and chronically depressed. In an early therapy session, the therapist addresses Ms M's anger at her:

Ms M	(In an angry tone of voice) I was really annoyed by what you said to me last time, about my decision to leave this job. You asked me if I thought I might have done anything to contribute to that fiasco with the nursing supervisor, who's so insecure she can't handle it when someone is clearly smarter than she is.
Therapist	Can you tell me more about how you felt when I asked that question? (**question**)
Ms M	It really made me feel like you don't understand my situation, and that you don't think I'm that smart. Like you're not on my side either. (Becoming tearful) I thought that you were different than those doctors I work with who are such jerks.
Therapist	I'm sorry my question upset you. I can see how it must have felt that I just didn't get it, and was being critical. That's not at all what I intended. (**empathizing, soothing, identifying an empathic failure**)
Ms. M	Then why did you ask if I had done something wrong? I was just doing my job, and it's not my fault if I'm more of a perfectionist than anyone else at work. I graduated first in my class in nursing school, and it's really frustrating to work with people who aren't at my level.
Therapist	Wow, you never told me you were first in your class. That's impressive. I know you have really high standards for yourself, and it's frustrating when people don't appreciate the work that you do. (**praising, empathizing, validating**)
Ms. M	Yeah, it is. I often feel that instead of getting the recognition I deserve, people just think I'm showing off.

The therapist begins by asking the patient more about her reaction to the therapist's last intervention. Ms M reveals feeling not just angry, but misunderstood and unsupported. Sensing that Ms M's sense of self is too shaky right now to benefit from an uncovering strategy, the therapist uses supporting interventions – empathy, praise, validation, and soothing – to help repair the rupture in the therapeutic alliance and bolster Ms M's self-esteem. The therapist relies on a developmental model that posits that Ms M did not receive the kind of empathic admiration and praise from her traumatized mother that she craved. When the therapist supplies these, Ms M is able to be more self-reflective.

Uncovering strategies

We can use all of our uncovering techniques to help patients become more aware of their distorted self-perceptions. This can help them develop a more realistic sense of self. Here are some examples:

Interpreting defenses

Mr N is a 28-year-old writer who sought psychotherapy saying that he was dissatisfied with his career. Working as a staff writer for a magazine, he has co-authored several successful articles with his editor. His co-workers are aware that Mr N wrote these articles almost entirely by himself, and are encouraging him to write an article on his own. When he tries to do this, he is plagued by self-doubt and writer's block. Of note is that Mr N's father is a formerly successful actor who told endless stories of his early triumphs, but had little time to read his son's stories.

Mr N	*I'm such a screw-up – I just can't write. I keep staring at the screen and nothing comes out. I'll never be a good writer.*
Therapist	*It's interesting because when you wrote the article with your editor this wasn't a problem at all.* (**confrontation**)
Mr N	*You're right – that felt so different. Everyone loved that article – though I'm not sure that it was really as good as they thought it was. My editor liked it, but he wasn't effusive. He's won a Pulitzer, you know. He was a major journalist about 20 years ago. And even though everyone else has been encouraging me, he hasn't. I thought well, maybe he's just measured in his response – but a good mentor would do that, right?*
Therapist	*You know, I wonder if you might be having difficulty writing this new piece on your own because you're worried that it might upset your editor.* (**interpretation**)
Mr N	*It's almost funny to think that would upset him – but I have thought it's almost painful to watch him in his office – he looks unhappy. I can picture him as a young writer. Now everyone on staff is young – we hang out – he's just doling out assignments and talking about his Pulitzers.*
Therapist	*Sounds a little bit like your dad.* (**genetic component of the interpretation**)
Mr N	*Yeah, I guess it does. Talking about the old days. But I'd love him to want me to do well, too . . .*

As with Mr L, the therapist hears the self-esteem problem – the patient perceives himself as a "screw-up" who will never amount to anything. However, the therapist knows that the patient is capable of writing and decides to **confront** the incongruity between the patient's perception of his capabilities and the objective evidence. This leads to a break in the resistance – the patient says that he's thought about an alternative way of looking at the situation. He also mentions the editor. The therapist wonders if the patient's problem is related to the editor, and ventures an **interpretation**. Although the patient has difficulty thinking about this alternative way of looking at the situation, his affect and use of humor suggest that this is just beneath the surface. The genetic link is now accessible, and the therapist decides to make a **genetic interpretation**, which further deepens the patient's understanding of the situation.

In this case, we suspect that Mr N's distorted self-image may be *defensive*. Worried that his own success would threaten his father, Mr N may have unconsciously hidden his talents and begun to think of himself as less capable than he actually is. Uncovering this defense could enable Mr N to understand why he does this, and subsequently to feel less afraid of demonstrating his talents. The therapist knows that this uncovering process will continue in future sessions. His hope is that the patient's increased ability to understand his **unconscious fantasy** that the editor/father will only mentor/love him if he denigrates his own abilities will help him gain a more realistic view of his own capabilities and will help him correct the distortion in his self-perception.

Interpretation of the transference

Distorted self-perceptions inevitably come up in the transference, and thus interpretation of the transference is often a very good strategy for reworking ways in which patients think about themselves. As an example, let's consider Ms O:

Ms O consulted a therapist because she had difficulty asserting herself. During therapy, she has generally been very self-reflective and able to discuss her relationship with the therapist. Recently, she canceled a session because of a business meeting and did not ask to reschedule. Here is part of a session from several weeks later:

Ms O   *Oh – I remember that I had a dream last night – I can't remember all of it – I was in a session – it wasn't here – it was your office, but there was a whole group of people here – you knew them. I couldn't tell if we were all patients of yours – but then I thought that maybe it wasn't my session – maybe it was more like a party. That's all I can remember.*

Therapist   *Does anything else come to mind about the dream?* (**call for associations**)

Ms O   *It was weird that there were so many people there. I rarely see anyone here – maybe just the person before me or the person after me. You work incredibly hard – you don't even have a break between patients. I don't know how you do it. You're a very busy person. I'm lucky to be able to schedule two sessions a week with you. I did notice that the patient who comes after me on Mondays is new – at least she hasn't come at that time before. I wonder how many new patients you see each week. I figured that that's why you wouldn't be able to reschedule my session.*

Therapist   *It's interesting – at the time you didn't ask about rescheduling. In fact, I can't remember your ever asking to reschedule. Do you have more thoughts about that?* (**confrontation/clarification**)

Ms O   *No, I never do. I mean, it's my fault that I'm not coming – I'd feel guilty asking you to change your schedule for me.*

Therapist   *But your dream and your thoughts about the dream suggest that you have other feelings about this. Maybe the reason you never ask to reschedule is that you worry that you're not as important to me as other people are.* (**interpretation**)

Ms O   *It seems so unfair – you give me so much – my problems aren't so terrible – maybe that new patient has something really wrong with her. And I've never been in a situation where someone else would go out of their way for me . . . but I guess you're saying that maybe you would.*

The therapist hears the dream and the clear transference references. He notes the breaks in pattern, "It was your office – it wasn't your office – it was my session – it wasn't my session," which hint at conflicting unconscious thoughts and feelings about the therapist. The therapist wonders if the meaning of the resistance (not discussing the missed session) could have something to do with feelings about the therapist. He thinks that uncovering work could begin and starts with a **call for associations** related to the dream. The patient then brings up the missed session and her fantasy that the therapist would be too busy with other patients to offer time to reschedule. The therapist decides that this is close enough to the surface and full of affect, so he chooses to **confront** the fact that the patient had not brought up the wish to reschedule. In addition, he recalls that this has happened before, so he makes a **clarification** that ties these together. The patient resists the confrontation, and the therapist thinks this might be a manifestation of her feeling that she is not worthy of asking the therapist to change her schedule, as well as her tendency to judge herself very harshly. However, the dream and the associations to the dream suggest that the patient has feelings about this, and that she might feel that the therapist favors others over her. The therapist decides that this is close enough to the surface to try an **interpretation**. This enables the patient to uncover new ideas about the therapeutic relationship.

In this vignette, Ms O's self-esteem problems lead to an assumption that others won't go out of their way for her. This prevents her from asking the therapist if she could change the session time and is likely linked to her difficulty asserting herself. This happens in *real time* between therapist and patient. The patient makes an assumption – as she must with most people in her life – that the therapist wouldn't offer her something she asked for. However, when the therapist points out that this is not necessarily an appropriate assumption, the patient is exposed to an alternate way of viewing herself. If our strategy is primarily uncovering, we call this to the patient's attention; if we are using primarily supporting techniques, we might just allow it to happen.

These examples illustrate how we use supporting and uncovering techniques to help improve self-esteem management and self-perceptions. Now let's go on to think about how we use these techniques to improve relationships.

Chapter 25: References

1. Kohut, H., and Wolff, E.S. (1978) The disorders of the self and their treatment, an outline. *International Journal of Psychoanalysis*, **59**, 414.
2. Stern, D. (1985) *The Interpersonal World of the Infant: A View from Psychoanalysis and Developmental Psychology*, Basic Books, New York, p. 3–12.
3. Jacobson, E. (1964) *The Self and the Object World*, International Universities Press, New York, p. 141–155.
4. Herman, J.L. (1992) *Trauma and Recovery*, Basic Books, New York, p. 111.

26 Improving Relationships with Others

Key concepts

For most people, the ability to have meaningful relationships with others is critical to the way they function in the world.

A major goal of psychodynamic psychotherapy is helping people develop mutually satisfying relationships with other people.

Supporting interventions help patients whose difficulty with relationships stems from problems with empathy, mentalization, and reading social cues.

Uncovering techniques help patients whose difficulty with relationships stem from unconscious fantasies about/expectations of others that impair their ability to engage in relationships.

Although some people truly prefer to be alone, most people feel that their lives are richer if they spend them interacting with others. The kinds of relationships we have with romantic partners, colleagues, friends, and family members are all different, but they are all important. People generally want to have people in their lives they care about and who care about them. However, there are many reasons why people are unable to have the mutually satisfying relationships they long for.

The goal

Having difficulty with relationships is one of the major reasons that people seek psychotherapy – and psychodynamic psychotherapy is a good treatment for this. Helping people with problems that cause them to have difficulties with relationships is a major goal of psychodynamic psychotherapy.

Recognizing the problem

Problems with relationships come in all shapes and sizes. Here are some chief complaints that signal the presence of problems with relationships:

I just can't seem to get along with people at work.

There are no good men out there.

Psychodynamic Psychotherapy: A Clinical Manual, Second Edition. Deborah L. Cabaniss, Sabrina Cherry, Carolyn J. Douglas and Anna Schwartz.
© 2017 John Wiley & Sons, Ltd. Published 2017 by John Wiley & Sons, Ltd.

I've been dating her for two years, but I'm not sure I want to get married.

My mother is driving me crazy.

I don't have any close friends.

My daughter won't talk to me any more.

Loneliness, problems with commitment, complaints about loved ones, frequent arguments, and disappointment in others all point to the presence of interpersonal difficulties. Anybody can have difficulty with one person or another, but if a person has consistent difficulties in their relationships we should be alert to the possibility that these problems are due to an ongoing problem with their emotional functioning.

Generally, it is not hard to recognize that a person has interpersonal difficulties. The challenge is to define the problem. Some people are able to have relationships but have difficulty with some of them because of unconscious fantasies and expectations. On the other hand, some people lack the skills required to have any successful relationships. Let's take a look at these two types of problems:

Unconscious expectations of and fantasies about others

As people grow up, their early interactions with important people in their environment make an indelible mark on the way they interact with others throughout their lives. People who are loved and well cared for learn to expect that from others, while people who are abused or neglected learn to expect mistreatment [1]. Even if people are not conscious of these *expectations*, they affect every interaction they have. Consider these examples:

> *Mr A was raised in foster homes – as soon as he became used to one family he was moved. As an adult, he has a pattern of leaving his girlfriends before they break up with him. He presents feeling dissatisfied with his romantic relationships.*

> *Ms B's mother stayed at home and attended to her every need. As a newlywed, Ms B is enraged that her husband wants occasionally to go out alone with friends. She presents with disillusionment about her young marriage.*

The adult relationships of both Mr A and Ms B are affected by their early relationships, albeit in different ways. Mr A expects to be left so has learned to leave first to avoid the pain of separation. Ms B expects that her husband will attend to her in the same way her mother did and is disappointed when he doesn't. Although we may see this clearly, their chief complaints suggest that they are completely unaware of the way their current problems are influenced by their past relationships. Bringing these expectations into awareness can help both of them better understand the problems they are having in the present.

We are affected by what *did* happen to us with people in our past, but we are also affected by what we *hoped* would happen. **Fantasies** about people in our early life can persist in our unconscious and affect the choices we make in our adult relationships. Here are a few examples:

> *Dr C's father was highly critical and rarely praised him. As a young pediatrician, Dr C works 100 hours a week and never asks for help. He presents because his domestic partner is ready to move out because Dr C is never home and is constantly preoccupied with work.*

Ms D's father was a flamboyant sportsman who intermittently took her with him on exciting skiing and hiking trips. Generally, though, Ms D was left with her shy mother, who was disabled by rheumatoid arthritis. Ms D presents with confusion about her engagement – although she loves her fiancé, she worries that he's not "manly" enough.

Both Dr C and Ms D have fantasies about people in their early lives. Dr C has a fantasy about a father/authority figure who will finally praise him. Ms D has a fantasy about a man who possesses the idealized aspects of her otherwise disappointing father. Whether or not they are aware of this, these fantasies affect their choices, their affect, and their behavior with the people in their adult lives.

As with all unconscious fantasies, they remain out of awareness because they cause shame, anxiety, or other strong, uncomfortable feelings. If people are unaware of their unconscious needs, they cannot choose others with whom they will have mutually satisfying relationships. For example, people might consciously wish to be independent and autonomous, but unconsciously wish to be taken care of. Or they might consciously wish to be nurtured, but unconsciously feel undeserving and expect rejection. In either case, they might consistently choose non-nurturing partners who rapidly disappoint them. We can become aware that unconscious expectations and fantasies about others are active when interpersonal expectations seem out of sync with objective data. Two examples are a man who is always afraid that his girlfriend will leave him despite the fact that she keeps hinting about getting married, and a woman who is repeatedly promoted at work but is sure that her boss wants to fire her.

Problems with social functioning

While some people know how to interact with others but are impeded in their ability to do so by unconscious expectations and fantasies, others are unable to have relationships because of gaps in functioning [2]. We consider the ability to have relationships with others an essential dimension of functioning, but there are important subfunctions that are essential for healthy relationships.

Capacity for empathy

As discussed in Chapter 13, empathy can be defined as the ability to see life through someone else's eyes. We have to be able to do this in order to have healthy, mutually satisfying relationships. Without this ability, we cannot understand how other people see the world. Empathy helps us know how to care for our loved ones, how to soothe our friends when they are in distress, and how to solve interpersonal disputes. People who lack empathy are generally self-absorbed, entitled, and emotionally distant. All of these traits impair the ability to engage in relationships with others:

Mr E comes home from work every day and talks endlessly about the politics in his office without asking his wife about her day. He cannot understand why she calls him "insensitive," saying simply that his work is "more stressful than just taking care of the kids all day."

Mr E's lack of empathy renders him unable to understand his wife's experiences, and could jeopardize their relationship.

Ability to read social cues

When people interact, they give each other verbal and non-verbal cues that reflect their level of interest, their preferred physical and emotional distance, and when and how they want to end the interaction. If someone has difficulty reading these cues, they will inevitably have difficulty negotiating relationships:

> *Ms F cannot understand why she does not have more friends at the office. She explains that she is a fabulous friend – as soon as she meets someone she likes, she is "always available," calling them frequently and wanting to get together as much as possible. She says that the people around her seemed "shallow" and that after a few weeks they seemed to "disappear."*

Ms F's inability to understand that she is crowding her new friends makes her unable to sustain meaningful relationships with them.

Temperamental shyness

Although we don't always understand the reasons, some people are more outgoing than others. We may wonder if a person's shyness is the result of inhibitions or an anxiety disorder (like social anxiety disorder), but if the history indicates that the person has been reserved around others since childhood, the reason may be temperamental [3].

> *After transferring schools in the ninth grade, Ms G ate lunch alone for five months before she worked up the nerve to sit with other students. Now, in her 20s, she has the same problem in the corporate cafeteria.*

Therapeutic strategies

One of the most important ways we help our patients improve relationships is by allowing them to form a new relationship with us. Although its boundaries are specified by the frame, the therapeutic relationship is extremely important to our patients. For many, the relationship with the therapist represents something completely new. For the first time, they have a person in their life who is consistently reliable, attentive, non-judgmental, able to contain emotions and withstand negative affect, and motivated to help. The idea that relationships like this exist flies in the face of their expectations of others and opens up the possibility that the situation could be replicated. When working in a supporting mode, the very existence of the relationship can be therapeutic; when working in an uncovering mode, the way in which the new relationship alters existing expectations can be interpreted.

Aside from the therapeutic relationship itself, there are both supporting and uncovering strategies for helping to improve relationships:

Supporting strategies

If we think that a person's relationship problems stem from gaps in social functioning, then our interventions have to be aimed at supplying missing functions or assisting weakened ones.

Supplying interventions for improving relationships

These may include praising, empathizing, nurturing, soothing, validating, and offering hope, but focus on the following:

- **Advising** patients about basic guidelines for interacting with others and understanding social cues:

    If she hasn't returned your call after the third try, chances are she's not interested.

    You're putting a lot of pressure on yourself and on her. You might do better if you give yourself time to get to know each other before you make big decisions about the relationship.

- **Correcting misperceptions** of the behaviors and intentions of others:

    I don't understand why you think you're going to be fired – didn't your boss just give you a raise?

    I think you might be reading too much into what she said.

    There are other explanations for what's going on that make more sense to me – for example, is it possible he wasn't angry at you but was just in a bad mood for some other reason?

- **Reinforcing** adaptive defenses and behaviors:

    Leaving the room when you started to feel steamed was definitely the right way to go.

    That was a great idea to exercise during your lunch hour – I think it's helping you feel less frustrated with your husband when you get home after work.

- **Suggesting** alternatives to maladaptive defenses and behaviors:

    I suppose that a drink after work helps some people unwind, but for you it just seems to take the lid off, and you end up fighting with your wife and kids . . . maybe it would help more if you sat quietly and read the paper when you get home.

    When you have that impulse to yell at your son, I think that you need to reach out to someone – that would be a good time to call a friend.

Assisting weakened functions related to relationships

Modeling: We model how to interact with others by the way we interact with patients:

- **Listening empathetically** and **demonstrating understanding**
- **Mentalizing** – helping patients imagine what the therapist (or others) might be feeling or thinking. Questions like the following can foster this and help with the development of empathy:

    How do you think I/they felt when you did that?

I'm aware of feeling cautious in what I say to you, as if I could easily say or do the wrong thing.

It feels to me like you're withdrawing right now.

- **Apologizing** and accepting responsibility for our behavior:

  I'm sorry if that hurt your feelings.

  I didn't realize that the fact that you called me indicated that you wanted another session – I missed that.

Collaborating: We can collaborate with patients to think through ways in which they can improve their relationships with others. Here are some examples:

- **Jointly exploring alternative ways of thinking about and perceiving interactions**:

  Are you sure he meant to insult you? Is that the only explanation for what's happening?

  You say that Patty and Susan have been giving you the cold shoulder at drop-off, but didn't they ask you to bring your daughter for a play-date twice last week? What does that suggest to you?

- **Jointly thinking through consequences of an intended behavior**:

  If you tell off the boss, how is he likely to respond? Are you prepared to deal with the fall-out? Is there any other, less risky way to approach him about your grievances?

Uncovering strategies

We can uncover our patients' unconscious expectations of others and fantasies about others by talking to them about

- their relationships with people in their lives, and
- their relationships with us

Interpreting aspects of our patients' relationships with others

Patients spend a lot of time discussing their relationships with others. When we think we hear evidence that an unconscious expectation or fantasy is affecting a patient's interpersonal functioning, we can try to uncover that material in order to help the person's relationships:

> *Ms H is a 35-year-old woman who perceived that her father, a famous academic, lost interest in her after she was diagnosed with dyslexia. Over the years, she has often worried that friends and boyfriends will reject her for various "deficiencies." In her 20s, she had one ovary removed because of a large cyst. She has had difficulties maintaining romantic relationships, but is now in a deepening relationship that she hopes will lead to marriage. Ms H describes her boyfriend, Calvin, as attentive and loving, but is "terrified" of telling him that she has only one ovary. Here is a moment in a session when this comes up:*
>
> Ms H   *We had brunch with some of my friends today – they all have kids. Calvin loves kids and is great with them. After, he was particularly loving, and started to talk about baby names he likes. I can't believe I'm actually going to have to tell him that I only have one ovary – he'll probably break up with me when he finds out.*

Therapist	*What makes you think that?* (**confrontation**)
Ms H	*I'm defective (she begins to cry) – why should he have a defective wife when he could have a normally fertile wife?*
Therapist	*But everything you've said about your relationship indicates that he loves you very much – so I wonder if your fear that he'd break up with you might be related to the kinds of worries you've had with other people.* (**reassuring, clarification**)
Ms H	*I know what you're saying and I get that – and who knows if it will even affect my fertility – but I'm hysterical about this and it feels like it will be the end of our relationship.*
Therapist	*I think you're worried because you have the expectation he'll reject you just like your father did. But there doesn't seem to be any evidence of that with Calvin.* (**genetic interpretation, reassuring**)
Ms H	*It's hard for me to think any other way – but the fact is, he's nothing like my father. I'm just so terrified of losing him.*

The therapist hears the pattern break – it sounds like Ms H thinks the relationship is going well and then she suddenly says she thinks it will end. The therapist hears enough affect that he decides to **confront** the incongruity. This produces more feeling in the patient (evidenced by the word "defective"). The therapist suspects that her feeling of being defective is deeply held and would be hard to confront. The therapist also knows that she has worried about being rejected by others. He begins with some **reassurance** that also serves to **test reality**, then makes a **clarification** that ties Ms H's worries about her boyfriend to past fears. The patient is able to consider this clarification and to question her views – despite the continued presence of high affect. Ultimately, the **genetic interpretation** allows Ms H to consider the idea that her fears of losing her boyfriend are related to an unconscious expectation of relationships based on her childhood relationship with her father – rather than on the realities of the current situation.

Interpreting aspects of our patients' relationships with us (transference)

Interpreting transference can be one of the most powerful ways to help people rework their unconscious expectations of others. Patients can tell you as much as they can about their difficulties with other people, but when it happens in therapy you can see it right in front of your eyes. There's much less possibility of misperceiving the situation. Think of the difference between these two situations:

Ms I constantly complains that her boyfriend doesn't pay any attention to her. She describes him as self-absorbed and dismissive.

Ms J tells you she knows that you are inattentive because you glanced at the clock during her session.

Not knowing Ms I's boyfriend, you have no idea what to make of her complaint. But when Ms J complains about you, you know the situation. You can see that her perception of you is out of proportion to what actually happened. Ms J's low threshold for feeling ignored undoubtedly affects her relationships and is likely based on expectations from past relationships. Helping her see the distortion in her expectations of others in order to improve her current relationships is the goal of our work in this area. Here's an example of how we do this:

> *Mr K is a 44-year-old man who presented because he was having difficulties with colleagues at work. A somewhat bitter person, Mr K felt that his co-workers "dumped" on him and he came to expect that they would be unsupportive. In the following session, the therapist uncharacteristically began 5 minutes late. This is a sequence from the last 15 minutes of a 45-minute session:*

Mr K	*I think that that's all I have to say – I feel like I just ran out of gas.*
Therapist	*That's quite unusual for you – I wonder what just happened?* (**confrontation**)
Mr K	*I don't know – I know that the session is almost over and our session is going to be cut short today.*
Therapist	*So you expect that you'll lose time in your session today because I started 5 minutes late.* (**interpretation**)
Mr K	*Yeah, I guess I do – even though you don't usually do things that way. I think I was getting mad, sitting here thinking about it. That's what happens at work, too.*

The therapist registers the resistance of Mr K's having nothing to say and **confronts** it. He hears the patient's expectation that the session will be shorter because of the late start and **interprets** this as the product of an unconscious expectation of others. This deepens the patient's understanding of his unconscious fantasy. Seeing this within the therapeutic relationship helps

- the therapist understand the patient's unconscious expectation, and
- the patient recognize this pattern and begin to imagine that he could realistically have different expectations of people in his environment.

The hope is that Mr K can gradually rework his unconscious expectations of others as he sees that the therapist does not conform to what he generally anticipates from people in his environment. As with changing self-perceptions, this can be conceptualized as **reactivating development**.

Now that we've explored how we use our techniques to improve self-esteem regulation and relationships with others, let's move on to using them to shift characteristic ways of adapting to stress.

Chapter 26: References

1. Herman, J.L. (1992) *Trauma and Recovery*, Basic Books, New York, p. 111.
2. Winston, A., Rosenthal, R., and Pinsker, H. (2004) *Introduction to Supportive Psychotherapy*, American Psychiatric Publishing, Washington, DC, p. 6.
3. Kagan, J., Snidman, N., and Arcus, D. (1995) The role of temperament in social development. *Annals of the New York Academy of Sciences*, **771**, 485–490.

27 Improving Adapting to Stress

Key concepts

Stress is anything that overwhelms our usual way of operating. It can come from inside of us, like anxiety or impulses, or from outside of us, like trauma or financial pressures.

We all have characteristic ways of coping with stress, some of which are more adaptive than others.

We use both conscious and unconscious coping mechanisms to adapt to stress. We call our unconscious coping mechanisms **defenses.**

Improving the ways in which we characteristically adapt to stress is a major goal of psychodynamic psychotherapy.

Stress is anything that overwhelms our usual way of operating. As discussed in Chapter 4, things that put stress on the way we function can come from inside of us (like anxiety or impulses) or from outside of us (like trauma or financial pressures).

Internal stress	External stress
Anxiety	Trauma
Affects	Neglect
Developmental pressures	Relationship problems
Medical illness	Job/financial stress

People can have trouble adapting to stress either because their stress level is very high (for example during mania or because they were fired), or because they have persistent difficulty handling stress (for example because they cannot manage their emotions or have executive function problems). Helping people adapt optimally to stress is a major therapeutic goal of psychodynamic psychotherapy [1–3].

Conscious and unconscious coping mechanisms

Every system has characteristic ways of dealing with stress. Electrical systems are programmed to shut down when things get too hot, animals play dead, and hungry

Psychodynamic Psychotherapy: A Clinical Manual, Second Edition. Deborah L. Cabaniss, Sabrina Cherry, Carolyn J. Douglas and Anna Schwartz.
© 2017 John Wiley & Sons, Ltd. Published 2017 by John Wiley & Sons, Ltd.

infants cry. Our minds have ways of dealing with stress, too, some of which are more adaptive than others.

Our adaptations to stress can be conscious or unconscious. Sometimes, we consciously say to ourselves, "That's too much for me – I can't think about that right now." But more often, these adaptations are unconscious, kicking into action without our awareness. Unconscious adaptations are often called **defense mechanisms** (see Chapters 4 and 23). Defense mechanisms operate out of awareness to protect us from internal anxieties and feelings that threaten to overwhelm us, as well as from external stressors that threaten to overload our capacity to deal with them.

In what ways can defenses be maladaptive?

Often, our characteristic ways of adapting to stress cause morbidity in their own right. For example, people who are anxious in public may characteristically avoid others, leading to chronic loneliness. Or people who have endured severe trauma may frequently dissociate, disrupting their ability to think, feel, and interact with others in a meaningful, ongoing way.

Before trying to change someone's coping strategies, it's critical to remember that defenses causing the adult difficulties were once adaptive to the child [4]. Splitting allows children to maintain good feelings about grossly inadequate parents, and dissociation shields small victims of abuse from overwhelming terror. Keep this in mind while working with defenses: it will help you empathize with the difficulty your patients have in changing these ingrained ways of operating. It's helpful for them to understand this as well – you can experiment with how to explain it:

> *I think it's important for us to work on your tendency to shut down when you're arguing with your husband – this makes him feel that you aren't engaged with him and it's making it difficult for the two of you to work out problems. But this is something you've done since you were a child, and that really helped during your mother's tirades. So what once helped you is now giving you problems.*

This way of thinking about maladaptive defenses will help both you and your patients as you proceed.

That said, there are several ways in which defenses can be maladaptive:

- **Defenses can use up too much mental energy:** Sometimes, the maneuvers we use to prevent ourselves from being overwhelmed by internal or external stress require so much mental energy that we are left with very little ability to use other vital functions. Examples of this include **dissociation** and **projection**.

- **Defenses can impede our ability to have mutually satisfying relationships:** If the only way we can stave off being overwhelmed is to **split** – that is, to see some people as all good and others as all bad – we may decrease our internal stress load at the expense of having satisfying relationships. This can happen with **splitting, idealization, devaluation**, and **projective identification**.

- **Defenses can impede our ability to experience feelings:** Knowing what we are feeling is central to our ability to know ourselves and have relationships with others, so defenses that cut us off from our feelings (like **isolation of affect** and **intellectualization**) and that exaggerate certain feelings to avoid others (like **excessive emotionality**) can cause problems with function in many domains.

- **Defenses can be too rigid:** All systems need to have the ability to shift adaptations on a moment-to-moment basis in response to changes in the environment. The same is true for defenses. Using the same defenses regardless of the situation can be very maladaptive.

- **Defenses can be self-destructive:** The very maneuvers that we use to protect ourselves can often hurt us. Acting-out behaviors, like binging and purging, self-mutilation, and unsafe sex, are examples of this. They may temporarily decrease anxiety or overwhelming affects, but they do it in a way that has the potential to be dangerous or harmful.

- **Defenses can lead to physical distress:** **Somatization** and **conversion** deal with emotional stress by converting it to physical distress, often leading to tremendous morbidity.

The goal

A primary goal of psychodynamic psychotherapy is helping people adapt more effectively to internal and external stressors [5–8]. Again, these adaptations or coping mechanisms can be conscious or unconscious – only when they are unconscious do we call them defenses.

Recognizing the problem

How do we recognize that people are using maladaptive coping mechanisms?

Here are some clues to recognizing this problem:

Symptoms

The presence of symptoms is a sure sign that people are having difficulty adapting. Eating problems, anxiety and mood symptoms, somatic symptoms, and sensory and phobic symptoms are typical examples:

> Mr A complained of not being able to have a relationship, but spent all of his time going from doctor to doctor in search of relief from fatigue that after years of tests seemed to have no somatic basis.

Sometimes these symptoms meet criteria for other treatments, such as medications.

Distress

Subjective feelings of unhappiness and distress often mean that the person is not dealing with stress in an adaptive way:

> *Ms B binged every time her boyfriend failed to call her at night, then cried herself to sleep.*

Problems in relationships

Difficulty with adapting often impairs people's ability to have successful relationships – thus, problems with relationships can be a good clue that characteristic modes of dealing with stress are maladaptive:

> *Mr C was distraught that he couldn't hold down a job that would support his family. He had been fired three times for "insubordination," but couldn't figure out what had happened.*

Countertransference

Significant early feelings toward a patient (positive or negative) can be a very good way to pick up prominent splitting-based defenses during an assessment:

> *In their first session, Ms D told Mr Z that he was the smartest therapist she'd ever consulted. Mr Z initially felt very excited about the prospect of treating Ms D, but after a few hours realized she had overidealized him.*

Therapeutic strategies

Both uncovering and supporting strategies can help improve the ways our patients adapt to stress. The first step is to help patients recognize that adapting is a problem. Telling them that their coping mechanisms are maladaptive is of limited utility; helping them come to that conclusion with you is much more effective. First, look for an opportunity to **confront** a discrepancy or incongruity that might interest them:

> *I know you said you haven't had any problems at work, but you also said that you've been fired three times this year. Do you think something could be tripping you up that's been hard for you to notice?*

Here the therapist juxtaposes "no problems at work" with "three firings in a year" to interest the patient in the possibility that there might be a problem. Here's another example:

> *You said that the new job was easy to handle, but you also said that you've gained 40 pounds since beginning it – do you have any thoughts about that?*

Once you interest a patient in a discrepancy, you can use **collaborative interventions** to look more closely at the situation:

> *So it does seem like something you're doing might be contributing to your difficulty in keeping a relationship going. Let's look at this together – we can start with your last relationship. Can you*

think of anything that you might have done that could have had a hand in some of your arguments?

This fosters the therapeutic alliance, which is crucial at all times but especially when you're encouraging patients to become vulnerable enough to recognize a maladaptive defense. *Remember that defenses are our protection* – they may be maladaptive, but we need them. We don't want to leave patients without any protective coping strategies, and we want to do this work very gently, causing as little pain as possible in the process.

Once patients understand that there is a problem, we can move ahead to improve their ways of dealing with stress. Our aim is to diminish dependence on less adaptive defenses and increase their use of more adaptive ones. Sometimes this involves reinforcing mechanisms that patients are already using, and sometimes it involves helping them come up with and try completely new strategies. Depending on the patient's strengths and difficulties, this can involve either supporting or uncovering.

Supporting strategies

Both supplying and assisting interventions are helpful here. When we supply, we presume that patients cannot come up with new ways of adapting on their own – either on a persistent basis or at the moment. **Discouraging** maladaptive patterns and **reinforcing** adaptive ones can sound like this:

Wow – what a difference it made when you were able to contain your negative comments at the dinner table last night. It sounds like everyone had a better time – including you.

This is also **praise** – although even more overt praise may be necessary for some patients:

You've come such a long way – you've been talking to your son for the better part of this year. That's a real change.

If patients can't come up with new, more adaptive solutions, **suggesting** or **advising** can help:

Why don't you try this – the next time your daughter-in-law starts criticizing your housekeeping, just walk out of the room.

Or consider this exchange with a woman who has difficulty with sensory regulation:

Patient	*Sometimes I just wear earplugs – like if I have to ride the subway. But at the office I need to be able to hear the customers and answer the phone.*
Therapist	*So we'll have to get creative and think of some other ways to make the environment more bearable for you. What about finding a dark and quiet room to lie down for a while? Or maybe taking extra time in the bathroom just to get away from the lights and noise for a few minutes?* (**explicitly joining, suggestion**)

Psychoeducation is often helpful as well:

> *For a lot of people, it's really hard to stop overeating after a stressful day. Many people find it helpful to come up with some other type of activity, like reading or taking a relaxing bath.*

For people who have some capacity to cope with stress more adaptively, assistance may be all that's needed. **Collaborative interventions**, like **joint inquiry** and **thinking through consequences,** can be very effective:

Therapist	*So now we know it drives you crazy when your co-worker starts talking about personal things while you're trying to get things done and we know that yelling at him just makes you unpopular in your department. Let's think together about some other things you could do when he starts that up again.* (**joint inquiry**)
Patient	*What about giving him the cold shoulder?*
Therapist	*That would definitely be less volatile – but how do you think that would work in the long run?* (**thinking through consequences**)

In general, assisting interventions "stick to the ribs" better because patients have a hand in them – so you might start there and then supply if needed.

Here is an example of using support to improve adapting:

> *Mr E is a 55-year-old man who presented with difficulty at work.*

Mr E	*I just know my boss wants to fire me. He's giving me crappy assignments and unrealistic deadlines so that I fail and he can get rid of me.*
Therapist	*Sounds like you are angry with him.* (**confrontation**)
Mr E	*No, I'm fine with him – but he can't stand me.*
Therapist	*Wow, that sounds like a really difficult situation. But didn't he just say that you'd made a good presentation?* (**empathizing, reframing**)
Mr E	*It's true – but maybe that was just to throw me off.*
Therapist	*Just for my sake, let's think together about other ways we could understand how your boss has been acting.* (**jointly exploring alternate ways of thinking**)

Unable to tolerate the strong feelings he is having at work, which could include anger at his boss and anxiety about his workload, Mr E uses projection instead. The therapist tries a confrontation, but then turns to supporting techniques to try to move Mr E toward more adaptive defenses.

Uncovering strategies

The aim of uncovering strategies is to make maladaptive defenses conscious so that patients can

- know what they're doing, and
- begin to deal with overwhelming affect and anxiety in more adaptive ways.

Here's an example that uses uncovering strategies to work with defenses:

> *The patient is a 30-year-old female internist in twice-weekly psychotherapy with a 40-year-old female therapist. She presented with difficulty in relationships. The patient just broke up with her boyfriend.*

Ms F	*I haven't been sleeping well again, so I called in a trazodone prescription for myself over the weekend. I keep thinking about Phil and I can't sleep. I was miserable.*
Therapist	*You called it in?* (**confrontation**)
Ms F	*Yeah – it was Saturday and I didn't want to bother you. I've taken it before. When I did it, I thought – should I call her? But then I thought, I'd call in an antibiotic prescription for myself if I had a sore throat – so why not this? But then I knew that we'd have to talk about it. I just feel like it was such a small thing and you deserve to have your weekend without calls about things like this.*
Therapist	*Can you say more about your thoughts about possibly calling me?* (**confrontation**)
Ms F	*I never want to bother you. I rarely call. Only if I have to cancel. And you only have your office phone number on your machine and I know that you're not in your office on the weekend – at least I think that you're not in the office on the weekend. You're probably with your family then – with your kids – I don't know.*
Therapist	*You're very insistent that you didn't want to bother me, but it sounds like you were very sad this weekend.* (**confrontation**)
Ms F	*I was – very sad – but what could you have done? It's not like I could have called you up and you'd say, "I'll be right over" – we weren't going to hang out. I see you here for 45 minutes twice a week – I understand that.*
Therapist	*But maybe you sometimes wish I were more available than that.* (**confrontation**)
Ms F	*Maybe – but it's not the way it is. And I'm not going to embarrass myself the way my sister does. My mother constantly runs to her – it's always been that way – she's always been a mess. There's just no need for that.*
Therapist	*So even letting me call in a prescription for you makes you feel as needy as your sister.* (**interpretation**)
Ms F	*(sighs) Yeah, I guess that that doesn't make sense. But it does feel that way. I don't need you to do it, but guess it doesn't mean that.*

Ms F longs for care from the therapist, but this wish makes her feel like her needy sister. Thus, she unconsciously uses various defenses to distance herself from feelings that make her uncomfortable. She **acts out** by calling in her own prescription, she **denies** her wish for the therapist to care for her, and she uses **reaction formation** when she insists that she never wants to bother the therapist. By slowly confronting these defenses, the therapist helps Ms F to notice her conflicts and ambivalence. Ultimately, the therapist is able to interpret Ms F's use of maladaptive defenses, allowing her access to difficult feelings and longings. With more access to her feelings, she can allow herself to be more comfortable with her wish to be cared for by others, improving her relationships across the board.

Adapting is an important function that we aim to improve with psychodynamic psychotherapy. Let's go on to consider several other functions in the next chapter.

Chapter 27: References

1. Cohler, B.J. (1987) Adversity, resilience and the study of lives, in *The Invulnerable Child* (eds A. J. Anthony and B. J. Cohler), Guilford Press, New York, p. 372–378.
2. Appelbaum, A. (2005) Supportive psychotherapy. *The American Psychiatric Textbook of Personality Disorders* (eds J.M. Oldham, A.E. Skodol, and D.S. Bender), American Psychiatric Publishing, Washington, DC, p. 335.
3. White, R.W. (1974) Strategies of adaptation: An attempt at systematic description, in *Coping and Adaptation* (eds. G.V. Coelho, D.A. Hamburg, and J.E. Adams), Basic Books, New York.
4. Schlesinger, H. (2003) *The Texture of Treatment*, Analytic Press, Hillsdale, NJ, p. 37.
5. Greenson, R.R. (1967) *The Technique and Practice of Psychoanalysis*, Vol. **1**, International Universities Press, New York, p. 29.
6. Freud, A. (1946) *The Ego and The Mechanisms of Defense*, International Universities Press, New York, p. 45–70.
7. Vaillant, G.E. (1976) Natural history of male psychological health, V: Relation of choice of ego mechanisms of defense to adult adjustment. *Archives of General Psychiatry*, **33**, 535–545.
8. Caligor, E., Kernberg, O.F., and Clarkin, J.F. (2007) *Handbook of Dynamic Psychotherapy for Higher Level Personality Pathology*, American Psychiatric Publishing, Washington, DC, p. 24–31, **76**, 86.

28 Improving Cognitive Function

Key concepts

A major goal of psychodynamic psychotherapy is improving cognitive functions such as reflective capacity, reality testing, managing emotions, judgment/impulse control, problem solving, decision making, and organizing. These are sometimes called **executive functions**.

Both uncovering and supporting strategies can be used.

Determining whether a person "can" or "cannot" perform these functions is essential for choosing whether to uncover or support.

When we think about the goals of psychodynamic psychotherapy, improving self-esteem, relationships, and adapting to stress generally come to mind. But don't forget about cognitive function! How we conceptualize our minds, organize thoughts, and test reality make a huge difference in how we work, love, and play – and psychodynamic psychotherapy can help.

Can they or can't they?

In order to help someone with their cognitive functions, we have to make some judgment as to whether patients generally have the capacity for a specific function but are "blocked" in their ability to use it by unconscious factors, or whether they lack the capacity for that function. Traditionally, this has been thought of as a question of **conflict vs. deficit** – if the person has the capacity to perform the function but is blocked, this was thought of as a problem that is caused by a *conflict*, whereas if the person lacks the capacity to perform the function, this was thought of as a problem caused by a *deficit* [1]. However, we know that unconscious issues other than conflicts, such as affects, fantasies, and defenses, can cause impairment in function, and we know that people who have the capacity for a specific function can sometimes transiently lose their ability to use it due to short-term stress (such as medical illness, psychiatric syndromes, and other circumstances that temporarily overwhelm). Thus, assessing a person's cognitive function in terms of "can they?" or "can't they?" may be a better way to think about these problems:

Psychodynamic Psychotherapy: A Clinical Manual, Second Edition. Deborah L. Cabaniss, Sabrina Cherry, Carolyn J. Douglas and Anna Schwartz.
© 2017 John Wiley & Sons, Ltd. Published 2017 by John Wiley & Sons, Ltd.

Mr A, a 45-year-old successful businessman, presents for therapy shortly after his father's death. He has been appointed executor for the estate, but finds himself unable to organize his father's financial affairs. Before his father died, Mr A had been angry with him for "running his finances into the ground" and putting the burden on his children to organize things. Mr A now worries that he is getting attention deficit disorder and wonders whether he needs a stimulant. When you take the history, you find that he is able to organize financial matters at his job without difficulty and only encounters problems in relation to arranging his father's estate. You hypothesize that he possesses the capacity to be organized about finances, but that unconscious feelings about his father and his father's death are blocking him from being able to do so in this particular situation.

In this example, we know that Mr A *can* organize his finances because

- this has never been an area of difficulty for him in the past, and
- he is currently using organizational skills without apparent difficulty in other aspects of his life.

His unconscious feelings about his father prevent him from being able to use his generally intact ability to organize finances in a circumscribed area of his life. Given this, an uncovering strategy is indicated. Now consider the contrasting example of Mr B:

Mr B, a 45-year-old writer, presents for therapy because he is terrified of losing his home. He has taken out a second mortgage and is unable to make the monthly payments. When you ask him about his budget, it becomes clear that he has never had one and that he has no sense of how much income he needs per month to cover expenses. The history reveals that he has experienced trouble planning ahead in many other ways, including never planning vacations or managing time well on weekends. He thinks he was diagnosed with a learning disability as a child, but is unsure of the specifics.

Mr B *cannot* organize his finances. His history indicates that he has never been able to do this in any aspect of his life, suggesting that this is an area of persistent vulnerability. Supporting strategies are indicated. Finally, consider the situation of Mr C:

Mr C is a 45-year-old high-school principal who presents with symptoms of major depression during a divorce. After a 20-year marriage, his wife has just left him for his best friend. He is devastated and has symptoms of insomnia, anhedonia, and a 15-pound weight loss. Although he is afraid he will lose his children, he has not organized himself to get a lawyer and pay the required retainer. In fact, although he has always been the family money manager, he has not paid any bills for three months and recently had his lights turned off for lack of payment.

This is a much more ambiguous situation. Clearly, Mr C has had the capacity to organize his finances in the past – so what's happening now? Are unconscious thoughts and feelings causing Mr C to be unable to use his fundamentally good capacity for financial organization? Is depression, anxiety, or acute grief impeding his organizational skills? All we know at the moment is that for now, Mr C is unable to use this essential function – and this has put him in a compromised situation. We have to presume that, *for the time being*, Mr C's organizational capacity requires support and that he *cannot* perform certain essential functions.

The goal

Helping people improve their cognitive function is a major goal of psychodynamic psychotherapy. When people have difficulty in this area, we can help them develop new capacities or strengthen weakened ones; when people are unable to mobilize usually intact functions because of unconscious issues, we can help them to "unblock" the capacities that they have.

Recognizing the problem

How can we tell if a person can or cannot function in a particular way? Here are some strategies for parsing this out.

Is the problem global or selective?

This is probably your best guide for determining whether a person can or cannot use a function. Can a patient call everyone back except his mother? Is he able to use good judgment in all situations except when purchasing expensive shoes? Is he able to organize everything except his bachelor party? These situations suggest that the capacity to use these particular functions is present, but that unconscious factors are in the way. Asking the following questions can help you to make this determination:

> *Are there any situations in which this is not a problem for you?*
>
> *Do you find you just can't do this when you're anxious/tired/depressed/with people you don't know?*
>
> *Do you have any strategies that allow you to do this even though it's difficult?*

Is the problem longstanding or recent?

If people have had the problem since childhood or adolescence, it is more likely to be a gap in function than to be caused by unconscious feelings, fantasies, or conflicts. This is true of many problems in the cognitive realm, but may also be true of other functions like impulse control and judgment. Here are two contrasting examples:

> *Mr D is at risk of losing his job because he cannot manage his time properly. Formerly a high-level consultant, he previously was able to manage large, multi-center projects. After Mr D lost his job in a massive layoff sweep, he reluctantly took his current job, which is at a much lower level. He is contemptuous of his boss and feels listless during work hours.*

Mr D has recently been managing his time poorly, but performed well in this area in the past. There is ample evidence that unconscious feelings are impeding his previously intact time-management skills.

> *Mr E is at risk of losing his job because he cannot manage his time properly. He has had difficulty with this since childhood – throughout high school and college, tutors helped him break down long-term projects into manageable tasks. He briefly took stimulants, but felt he had "outgrown" them and*

wanted to "do it on his own." Now in his first job, he cannot manage this for himself and hides from his boss because he knows that he is behind on many projects.

There is strong evidence that Mr E has had difficulty with time management since childhood. His anxiety about not being able to perform certain tasks is well founded, since he has never been able to perform them without assistance. Unfortunately, rather than acknowledging his realistic limitations, using coping skills that served him well in the past, and asking for help, he is using *maladaptive* ways of coping, including denying the need for assistance and avoiding his boss.

Is the problem associated with other kinds of psychiatric symptoms?

No one knows exactly how various functions develop, but it seems clear that problems like mood and anxiety disorders, substance abuse, and other psychiatric syndromes can play a role in both how these capacities develop and also how well they work over time [2]. For example, if a young man develops bipolar disorder in early adolescence – a critical stage during which most teenagers are developing and practicing the capacity to regulate affect and control impulses – he may experience ongoing difficulties in these areas as an adult, even when his mood disorder is under control. Determining whether a patient's apparent difficulties in functioning are exacerbated by or developed in the setting of other psychiatric problems can help you decide if the person basically "can" or "cannot" perform a given function. Here are a few examples:

Ordinarily very decisive, Mr F becomes unable to make choices when he is depressed. This has become a marker that he and his therapist use to pick up early signs of relapse.

Although she is generally a very responsible mother, when Ms G is anxious her judgment about her children is impaired – she forgets to pick them up from school and allows them to stay out later than they should.

Fearing another panic attack, Mr H was unable to stay in an important business meeting and ran out of the room. When he is gripped with fear, his impulse control is impaired.

In these examples, understanding the constellation of symptoms involved is essential to assessing whether the person "can" or "cannot" perform a given function.

Therapeutic strategies

Your therapeutic strategy will differ depending on whether you decide that a person can or cannot perform a given function. In general, uncovering strategies help "unblock" functions when unconscious issues are getting in the way, while supporting strategies assist with faltering functions or supply absent ones.

In this chapter, we will describe these approaches in relation to a number of cognitive functions:

- reflective capacity
- reality testing

- judgment/impulse control (including ethical judgment)
- managing emotions
- organizing, planning, problem solving

As we explore each of these areas, think about these questions to hone your decision making about therapeutic strategies:

- Is the problem in function global or selective?
- Is the problem longstanding or recent?
- Is the problem associated with other kinds of psychiatric symptoms?
- Can patients exercise the function with minimal help from the therapist or do they require the therapist to "supply" or "assist" in exercising the missing capacity?

Reflective capacity

In all psychodynamic psychotherapies – even predominantly supporting treatments – we are always interested in enhancing the patient's self-understanding. However, as discussed in Chapter 3, some people readily conceptualize their minds as having unconscious elements while others do not. Assessing the way in which patients think about their mental functioning is essential for deciding which type of technique is most appropriate. Uncovering techniques require patients to have at least some basic ability to reflect on their inner mental life, while supporting interventions help develop or strengthen this capacity. Here are two examples that relate to reflective capacity:

> *Ms I is a 36-year-old married woman with three children under the age of 10 who has been referred by her internist to be evaluated for possible underlying depression. Ms I launches immediately into a litany of physical complaints, including headaches, back and neck discomfort, and "terrible" premenstrual syndrome, for which she has consulted many specialists. These symptoms began after the birth of her baby a year ago, and now severely limit her ability to take care of her children. This exchange is from the intake:*

Ms I	*My doctor thinks I need an antidepressant.*
Therapist	*What do you think?* (**question**)
Ms I	*I think I'm in pain.*
Therapist	*Sounds like it's been really difficult. Do you notice that there are any situations or times of day when the pain is better or worse?* (**empathizing, question**)
Ms I	*Mornings are the worst – getting breakfast together, sending the kids off to school, all the while holding the baby . . .*
Therapist	*That must send your stress level through the roof . . . As your internist may have already told you, stress can really exacerbate pain by increasing muscle tension and stimulating activity in the sympathetic nervous system.* (**empathizing, validating, informing**)
Ms I	*I didn't realize that. All I feel is pain, but you're right that the stress probably makes it worse.*

The therapist speculates that Ms I's somatic preoccupation may be a defense against unacceptable feelings of resentment generated by the birth of her youngest child. However, he recognizes that, for the time being, Ms I needs help simply labeling her feelings and registering emotional reactions. He begins by "going with" her defense by talking about her difficulties in terms of her physical problems, while trying to help her consider that her pain might be related to stress and emotions. This is a first step to increasing self-awareness.

> *Ms J is a 32-year-old woman who presents saying that she "can't decide" which graduate school to attend. She has gotten two very good offers and is in a "panic" because she apparently has to make a decision in two days. She says that she is usually very good at making decisions, but that this one is "driving her crazy." In your first session she produces reams of papers with "pros and cons" lists written on them. She also tells you that her boyfriend of two years lives in the city that houses one of the programs, but she insists "that isn't an issue." Here's part of a session:*

Ms J	*So the dorms are better in School A, but the stipend is better at School B. Ah! I just keep going around in circles.*
Therapist	*Circles?* (**confrontation**)
Ms J	*Yes – as soon as I feel like I'm going to make a decision, something else comes up and then I'm back to the drawing board. I'm driving my boyfriend crazy with this too – we've spent hours on the phone talking about it.*
Therapist	*Does he have an opinion?* (**question**)
Ms J	*No – he's completely measured – which is good – he's completely committed to making this all about me and what I want. That's the best – I wouldn't want him to weigh in – absolutely not.*
Therapist	*That was a lot of "no's" – is there any possibility you might want him to have an opinion?* (**confrontation**)
Ms J	*I said no because I mean no – I'm an educated, independent woman and my career comes first. Right?*
Therapist	*That's up to you, of course, but I wonder if you might have several different feelings about it. Part of you might want to be completely independent, but part of you might want to feel like he really wants to be with you.* (**confrontation**)
Ms J	*(tearful) Well, I'm 32 years old! I'm not getting younger! It will be at least six years before I get my PhD, then I'll be 38. Maybe he doesn't care about that.*
Therapist	*You mean about having a family?* (**confrontation**)
Ms J	*I hate that it matters to me, but I guess it does.*
Therapist	*Maybe it's been easier to think of this in terms of the "pros and cons" of the programs than to think about how hurt you feel that he's not being more proactive about trying to be together.* (**interpretation**)
Ms J	*(sitting back into her chair) That's hard to swallow, but it makes sense. What do I care about what the dorms are like?*

In this situation, the patient can generally make decisions, so the therapist hypothesizes that something out of awareness is making Ms J think about this situation too concretely. Together, they discover that Ms J's reflective ability was blocked by unconscious thoughts and feelings. Helping her see this brings back her ability to be more reflective about her situation.

Reality testing

You don't have to have a psychotic illness to have impaired reality testing. Patients with personality disorders who are not frankly psychotic may have misperceptions or distortions related to their use of reality-blurring defenses like **denial** or **projection** (see Chapter 4). Such defenses are commonly seen in patients with borderline personality disorder, but may also be used by patients who generally use higher-level defenses. Here are two examples of patients with disturbances in reality testing:

> Mr K is a 37-year-old single, unemployed man with a history of schizophrenia. He is the eldest of four sons, three of whom are physicians. Shortly after learning that his youngest brother had been awarded a prestigious research fellowship, Mr K abruptly stopped his antipsychotic medication and is now admitted to the hospital in a floridly delusional state. Here's a sequence from the inpatient intake:

Therapist	Can you tell me something about why you came to the hospital? (**question**)
Mr K	(glances around nervously, then mutters under his breath) The Tuskegee experiment.
Therapist	I don't know you well enough yet to understand what you mean, but I gather from the doctors in the emergency room that you're afraid that something like the Tuskegee experiment might be happening to you. (**demonstrating interest and understanding, joint inquiry**)
Mr K	They want my brain. I have a very rare disorder. This was my brother's idea. He told the doctors that I wasn't making sense.
Therapist	I guess your brother was concerned that your thinking may have become confused again, after you stopped the medication for your illness. Do you think that might be possible? (**correcting misperceptions, jointly exploring alternate ways of thinking**)
Mr K	What? Oh . . . I don't need it any more . . . Do I?

In this situation, the disturbance in reality testing is most likely caused by an acute exacerbation of a longstanding psychotic illness, triggered by the patient's discontinuation of his medication. The therapist hypothesizes that Mr K's non-compliance with medication may have been motivated by an unconscious reaction to his brother's most recent achievement, and that his paranoid and grandiose delusions about being a "rare" and special research patient may compensate for painful feelings of failure and envy. However, the therapist also reflects that, at least at this moment, Mr K *cannot* discriminate reality from delusion and thus that supporting interventions will be most helpful.

> Ms L is an 18-year-old high-school senior who is just two weeks shy of graduation. She has been in psychotherapy for three years for symptoms of anxiety and depression, intermittent suicidal ideation, and binge eating, all of which typically worsen at the beginning of each new school year. She has a solid alliance with her therapist and, with the help of therapy, has been functioning

very well. During this past year, she had no problems with the transition back to school and sailed through the college application process without apparent difficulty. As recently as a week earlier, she had seemed content and stable, so it was with some surprise and a little anxiety that the therapist received an "emergency" message from her parents, saying that Ms L was "paranoid." After assuring himself that the patient was neither medically ill nor using substances, the therapist has the following exchange with her in the next session:

Ms L   (sobbing) I hate you! I know I made you angry and you've been waiting for your chance to get rid of me!

Therapist   You're obviously really upset with me. Let's slow down for a minute and try to understand what's going on between us. When did you start having these thoughts about me? (**naming emotions, slowing down, explicitly joining, jointly reality testing**)

Ms L   (irritably) I don't know. A couple of days ago. After the prom.

Therapist   The prom – how was it? (**question**)

Ms L   Awful – a complete sham – my date dumped me. On my way home alone, I just got a weird feeling – like I was out of my body – like everyone hated me, particularly you – and that you've just been waiting for all this to happen. (crying) I feel like I'm going crazy.

Therapist   You and I know that when you're under a lot of stress, you can become pretty spaced out, right? Do you remember something like this happening a few years ago, when you were about to go abroad for the summer? You may have forgotten – you talked yourself through it and it didn't last long. Any ideas about what might be stressing you out now? (**clarification, reminding patient of capacities, offering optimism, question**)

Ms L   Everything seems so pointless. The prom was horrible. I was really looking forward to it, but then when I got there, it all seemed so false. Why have a big party, and pretend you're all happy, when everybody is leaving in two weeks?

Therapist   I wonder if things feel unreal to you because something sort of unreal is about to happen to you – you're about to leave home in two months. That means leaving your friends, your family – and me. I think that may be upsetting you more than you're aware of. (**interpretation**)

Ms L   I can't believe that I have to leave here – you – you're what's held me together this year. How am I going to do it without you?

In this example, Ms L does not have a psychotic illness, but she is experiencing difficulty with reality testing in the setting of a number of significant milestones – graduating from high school, moving away from home, ending treatment with her therapist, and starting college. She has had difficulty with transitions and separations like this in the past. Her therapist quickly determines that there has been no recent drug use, medical problem, or other psychiatric problems that might account for her sudden disorganized and paranoid thinking. He feels reasonably certain that her trouble with reality testing is related to unconscious anxiety about separating from her parents and therapist, along with conflicting feelings of humiliation and anger about still needing and depending on them. However, the therapist knows that in order for Ms L to be able to explore these difficult feelings, he first needs to help her feel safe, calm her overwhelming affects, and reduce her paranoid perceptions about him.

Bear in mind that there are degrees to which people can test reality. Mr K cannot test reality at all and needs the therapist to *supply* that capacity; Ms L became paranoid under stress and needs the therapist to *assist* her with reality testing before they can *uncover* the unconscious factors that led to her loss of equilibrium. Note that in both examples, the therapist attempts – gently and tactfully – to help the patients

- recognize they are misperceiving things, and
- consider alternative perspectives in a more flexible way.

Judgment and impulse control

People with good judgment have the capacity to anticipate the consequences of their actions, predict how other people are apt to react and, if necessary, hold themselves in check, shift set, and rethink plans. Thus, sound judgment requires good impulse control, and improving judgment often goes hand in hand with decreasing impulsivity. When impaired judgment and impulse control might lead to a life-threatening situation, we may need to intervene directly (for example, by hospitalizing patients or directing them to use safe-sex precautions; see Chapter 10). However, when impaired judgment and impulse control are not directly endangering the patient, another person, or the treatment, our goals are to help improve these functions using either supporting or uncovering techniques.

Here are two examples of patients with impaired judgment and impulse control problems. In the first example, the therapist uses mostly supporting interventions (supplying and assisting) to strengthen the faltering capacities, while in the second case, the therapist both supports and uncovers:

> Mr M is a 28-year-old radio ad salesman who sought consultation at his father's insistence, saying, "I'm fed up with my job, and my Dad's fed up with paying my rent. I don't know why he cares – he never takes any interest if I'm doing well." Mr M describes a pattern of starting new jobs with great enthusiasm, then becoming quickly bored and quitting or getting himself fired. This is his third job in as many years, and after only a few months he is already "sick of talking to whiney clients on the phone all day." He tells the therapist he nearly quit earlier in the week after his boss pointed out he was well short of his three-month sales goal and had already been late six times that month.

Mr M	I really wanted to tell my boss to take the job and shove it. He's full of criticism but doesn't give me any help.
Therapist	Wow, sounds rough. What's the job market like these days? (**empathizing, question, jointly thinking through consequences**)
Mr M	Terrible. It took me three months and five interviews to get this job.
Therapist	So quitting would put you right back out there. (**continuing to think through consequences**)
Mr M	I never think of that in the moment. It goes out of my mind when I get so frustrated.
Therapist	I get that – let's work together to think of some strategies you can use during those moments. (**joint problem solving**)

The therapist wonders whether the patient might be playing out something with his boss that belongs to his relationship with his father, and thus that unconscious factors might be leading to his poor judgment. However, taking into account the three readiness principles (see Chapter 17) – state of the alliance (so far non-existent), the patient's current functioning (weakened), and the phase of the treatment (first meeting) – as well as the fact that the patient's job may be in jeopardy, the therapist elects to **supportively bypass** these unconscious conflicts to focus on building an alliance and buttressing Mr M's faltering judgment and impulse control.

> Ms N is a 42-year-old married business executive whose husband recently announced he was having an affair and wanted a divorce. Ms N is still in shock and feels too humiliated to tell her friends and family – especially her mother, who never liked her husband and said, "He's a user – just like your father." On her way to the airport for an overseas trip, Ms N shares a cab with the company chief executive and begins flirting with him. Although Ms N says that friends regard her as a cautious person with a tendency to "overthink" decisions, she invites her colleague back to her hotel room for a drink and ends up spending the night with him. After the trip, Ms N calls her former therapist. The following is from their first appointment:
>
> Ms N   This is getting totally out of control! I know I should end it. He's married! But every time I hear his voice, I just can't help myself. Why am I doing this?
>
> Therapist   Do you have any ideas about that? (**confrontation**)
>
> Ms N   He's smart. He's handsome. He makes me feel sexy and desirable.
>
> Therapist   But my guess is that you have more complicated feelings about it. (**question, confrontation**)
>
> Ms N   Yes – it's crazy! Sleeping with the boss? I must be out of my mind – I keep saying to myself, "don't call him" and then before I know it I'm calling him again.
>
> Therapist   This has been a really hard time for you. I know that you're focusing on this relationship, but I haven't seen you since your husband left. (**empathizing, confrontation**)
>
> Ms N   (bursts into tears) I feel totally humiliated! Again!
>
> Therapist   Again? Sounds like this situation is related to feelings you're still having about your husband. (**clarification**)
>
> Ms N   I don't know. You must be thinking, "I can't believe she did it again!"
>
> Therapist   Your husband's betrayal was devastating. Perhaps seducing your boss was a way to feel that **you** were in control – not victimized, like your mother. (**interpretation, with genetic component**)
>
> Ms N   I guess you're saying I can take control of the situation if I want to. It's not just his call.

In the setting of a recent, humiliating blow to her self-esteem, this ordinarily self-controlled woman with impeccable judgment suddenly begins behaving in erratic and risky ways. Her therapist uses a mix of supporting and uncovering interventions to help her begin to understand the way in which her behaviors are linked to unconscious thoughts and feelings that she has been hiding from herself and others.

Ethical judgment, formerly part of what was considered **super-ego function**, can also be worked with in psychodynamic psychotherapy. We can often help patients who are overly moralistic understand the meaning of their rigidly held views, opening them up to better relationships with others and less harshness toward themselves (see Chapter 25). Unfortunately, however, psychodynamic psychotherapy can generally do little to improve weak ethical judgment [3].

Managing emotions

Sometimes, our biggest stressors are our own emotions. Anger, fear, sexual feelings, and shame can overwhelm our ability to handle them, affecting every aspect of our function. The ability to manage emotions is thus critical to the way we think about ourselves and have relationships. As with the other functions we have discussed, managing emotions can be acutely or persistently weakened, and can be impeded in certain circumstances by unconscious factors. Here are two examples demonstrating the use of supporting and uncovering strategies for improving this critical function:

> *Mr O is a 28-year-old man who presented with anger management problems.*

> Mr O   *So I was on the bus at rush hour – it's completely full and I'm holding on to a pole – and this guy behind me starts shoving. I just lose it – zero to 100 – and I turn around and start screaming at him, "You #$%^!" People were looking at me. I was shaking – I scared myself.*

> Therapist   *Well, given how angry you were, it's great that you didn't do anything physical. Let's see if we can think of better ways to deal with situations like that. Were you wearing your headphones?* (**interpreting up, joint problem solving**)

> Mr O   *Oh, no – I forgot to put them on.*

> Therapist   *No problem – but I think that will help – next time you get onto a crowded bus, make sure you're listening to something very soothing.* (**reassuring, suggesting**)

Here, supporting techniques helped to support more adaptive ways of managing emotion. Contrast Ms. P:

> *Ms P is a 45-year-old woman with a 14-year-old daughter.*

> Ms P   *I'm usually on a pretty even keel, but when she puts on that music I just go through the roof!*

> Therapist   *Tell me more about that feeling.* (**confrontation**)

> Ms P   *I actually sort of like her music – it's just that I feel like she's playing it to show me she doesn't have to listen to me.*

> Therapist   *Something about that idea really bothers you.* (**confrontation**)

> Ms P   *Yeah – my brother was like that – he never studied and I did – so he'd play loud music just to distract me from my work. And my mother never said anything.*

With Ms P, the difficulty managing emotions is circumscribed and relates to a particular interpersonal issue, so uncovering can help.

Organizing, planning, decision making, and problem solving

Some patients have lifelong difficulties with basic cognitive functions such as organizing, attention, planning, and decision making. These patients often experience trouble prioritizing, starting and finishing work on time, keeping track of tasks, completing long-term projects, problem solving, and planning for the future [4]. Patients with these kinds of difficulties generally benefit – at least initially – from a more supporting approach aimed at strengthening function. If, however, there is compelling evidence that unconscious feelings are impeding generally intact cognitive skills, a more uncovering approach may be helpful. Here are two examples – the first patient's problems are more global and longstanding, while the second's are more selective and apparently related to unconscious conflict stimulated by recent life stressors:

> Mr Q is an 18-year-old college student who has just been asked to consider taking a leave of absence from his freshman year because of failing grades. His parents brought him in for a consultation hoping to help him "get back on the horse" and finish out the semester. They report that Mr Q is chronically restless and fidgety, talks excessively, and needed the help of tutors in 11th and 12th grades to finish papers and complete college applications on time. Mr Q was very optimistic about his ability to function on his own as he started the school year; however, he is now significantly behind in all of his courses. In the therapist's office, Mr Q is panic stricken, saying he is too overwhelmed to finish out the semester but can't imagine going home "with my tail between my legs." After the therapist takes a full history and assesses all of Mr Q's symptoms, he and the patient have this exchange:

Mr Q	(jiggling his legs nervously and running his hands through his hair) I don't know what to do. I'm stuck.
Therapist	You're stuck? (**confrontation**)
Mr Q	I don't think I can make it through the semester. But if I drop out, what am I going to tell my friends when they come home for winter break? That I'm an epic failure?
Therapist	You can look at it that way, or you can say you've been trying to tell people around you that you need more help than you've been getting. Perhaps we can think about some of the things that are tripping you up with your schoolwork so we come up with the best plan to help you. (**interpreting up**, **explicitly joining**, **joint inquiry**)
Mr Q	(brightening) I guess you're right – what do you suggest?
Therapist	First of all, there's no shame in continuing to need tutors or help with organizing. You'd be surprised how many people need that kind of assistance – and not only students. Sounds like you should also have a consultation to see if you might have attention deficit disorder – you have many of the symptoms, and medication might really help. Then, we can work on honing in on some of the difficulties you're having. Maybe you can start us off . . . what's the last assignment with which you had difficulty? (**reassuring**, **validating**, **universalizing**, **jointly working on a project**)
Mr Q	That history research project really nailed me – that's exactly the kind of thing that makes me crazy. I don't know where to start so I bury it under a pile.
Therapist	Perfect – that's a great place to start. So let's talk about what you do when you first get the assignment . . . (**praise**, **joint inquiry**)

The history obtained from the parents is consistent with the therapist's initial impression of a longstanding undiagnosed attention deficit disorder. The therapist speculates that when faced with the challenges of college-level work – and without his parents' support and guidance – Mr Q was unable to organize a study schedule or manage his time effectively. Instead of marshaling appropriate resources and asking for help, Mr Q avoided his schoolwork. The therapist uses both supplying and assisting techniques to approach the delicate task of addressing Mr Q's problems with organization and time management while simultaneously buttressing his self-esteem.

> Ms R is a 59-year-old recently widowed mother of three grown children who says she is at risk of losing her job because "I can't seem to manage my time properly." Ms R explains that she was formerly a highly sought-after organizational psychology consultant who was able to manage complex multi-faceted responsibilities. However, after losing her job in a massive layoff sweep, she was obliged to accept her current position at a much lower level – and with a considerable pay cut. Ms R feels listless and distracted during work hours, often finds her mind wandering, and is experiencing more difficulty getting reports to her boss on time.

Ms R	A year ago, I could have done this sort of work blindfolded, with one arm tied behind my back. Sometimes I think I'm developing Alzheimer's.
Therapist	I haven't noticed any problems with your memory, but are you having trouble managing your time and staying organized in other areas of your life – keeping up with bills, organizing doctors' appointments, planning vacations, that sort of thing? (**reassuring, question**)
Ms R	Not really. That's what's so weird. I'm OK in my outside life, but when I come into the office it's like a black veil descends.
Therapist	Black veil? (**confrontation**)
Ms R	A black veil . . . like I'm going to my own funeral! (laughs)
Therapist	Well, you've had a lot of losses recently. (**empathizing, clarification**)
Ms R	It's been exactly one year since Jerry died. (becomes tearful) If he were still alive, I wouldn't have to be at this crummy job.
Therapist	You clearly miss him so much. But I think you might also be angry that you have to take care of yourself now. I have a feeling this might be linked to some of the difficulty you're having at work. (**empathizing, naming the emotion, interpretation**)
Ms R	I hate to feel angry with him because I miss him so much, but I wish I had options now, and I just don't.

Ms R's "black veil" metaphor suggests to the therapist that unconscious feelings about her husband's death are related to her current difficulties. After a **confrontation**, the therapist is able to **interpret** the way in which Ms R's unconscious anger is impeding her work function.

Although the vignettes we've presented in these chapters on therapeutic goals are fairly short, it often takes many iterations to lead to lasting change. We call this process **working through**, and it's the topic of our next chapter.

Chapter 28: References

1. Pine, F. (1990) The concept of ego deficit, in *Drive, Ego, Object, Self*, Basic Books, New York, p. 198–231.
2. Bjorklund, P. (2000) Assessing ego strength: Spinning straw into gold. *Perspectives in Psychiatric Care*, **36** (1), 14–23.
3. Gibbon, S., Duggan, C., Stoffers, J., *et al.* (2010) Psychological interventions for antisocial personality disorder. *Cochrane Database of Systematic Reviews* **16** (6): CD007668. doi: 10.1002/14651858.CD007668.pub2
4. Loring, D.W. (ed.) (1999) *INS Dictionary of Neuropsychology*, Oxford University Press, New York, p. 1–2.

PART SEVEN: Working Through and Ending

Key concepts

The later phases of psychodynamic psychotherapy are the **middle** and the **ending**.

During the middle phase, patient and therapist work together to gradually effect lasting change by addressing core problems as they emerge repeatedly in the treatment. This is called **working through**.

Ending, the final phase of psychodynamic psychotherapy, marks the end of the treatment and requires the therapist to use particular techniques suited for this phase.

Just as the beginning of treatment calls for specific techniques, so too do the middle and end phases. Usually the longest phase of the treatment, the middle phase is when patient and therapist have a strong alliance and are working well together. This is the time to address all of the therapeutic goals we discussed in Part Six. Ending is a time of strong feelings, regression, mourning, and consolidation. In the following chapters we will review these phases, with special attention to how and when to modify your technique. Note that the Review Activity for Parts Six and Seven is at the end of Chapter 30.

Psychodynamic Psychotherapy: A Clinical Manual, Second Edition. Deborah L. Cabaniss, Sabrina Cherry, Carolyn J. Douglas and Anna Schwartz.
© 2017 John Wiley & Sons, Ltd. Published 2017 by John Wiley & Sons, Ltd.

29 Working Through

Key concepts

Working through can be thought of as a three-phase process in which people gradually change some aspect of their mental functioning. These phases progress from

- Phase 1: **Limited awareness** of a problem or the cause of a problem, to
- Phase 2: **Increasing awareness and practicing** new ways of functioning, to
- Phase 3: **Lasting change** in thoughts, feelings, or behaviors.

These changes can occur in all domains of function, including sense of self, relationships, adapting to stress, cognitive function, and work/play.

In psychodynamic psychotherapy, we expect that these changes happen slowly over time through a gradual process of working and reworking the same issues until lasting change occurs.

What is working through?

Have you ever tried to change even one aspect of your behavior? Think about all those New Year's resolutions you've made over the years – to eat only health foods and to exercise regularly – most are out the window by the time you go to brunch on January 1st. Imagine, then, people who are trying to change their habitual ways of thinking about themselves, relating to others, and reacting to stress – it's very hard. As adults, we've been perfecting our characteristic patterns of thought and behavior over a lifetime, so trying to change them is daunting at best. Although we still don't know exactly how psychotherapy alters our neural circuitry, it clearly must, and those changes take time [1]. This gradual process is called **working through** and it's a central feature of psychodynamic psychotherapy [2,3].

Whether we're working in a predominantly uncovering or supporting mode, we can think of working through as the way change occurs in psychodynamic psychotherapy. The miraculous psychotherapeutic epiphanies dramatized in films like *Spellbound*, in which people realize why they behave the way they do in one fantastic moment and are changed forever, are just the stuff of movies. Although people do have flashes of insight, these rarely produce lasting change in thought patterns, ways of relating to self and others, or habitual patterns of reacting to stress.

As with resistance, the fact that this is a gradual process is not to be thought of as a hindrance; rather, understanding and accepting its slow pace are essential and

Psychodynamic Psychotherapy: A Clinical Manual, Second Edition. Deborah L. Cabaniss, Sabrina Cherry, Carolyn J. Douglas and Anna Schwartz.
© 2017 John Wiley & Sons, Ltd. Published 2017 by John Wiley & Sons, Ltd.

fundamental to its success. Consider the following exchange between a therapist and her supervisor:

Therapist	*I can't believe Mr A is sabotaging himself at work again! We've discussed this so many times in his treatment. And the frustrating thing is that he sees what he's doing now, but still provokes his boss when he gets anxious. Is this ever going to work?*
Supervisor	*Absolutely. This is the way things move and change in psychodynamic psychotherapy. A few months ago, Mr A wouldn't even have been able to see what he was doing – as this pattern continues to repeat itself, you'll be able to continue to work on it and gradually he'll start to change his behavior as well.*

Rather than signifying failure, this is the way in which the process works. Realizing this is fundamental to learning how to be a therapist. In addition, it helps us with feelings of countertransference frustration that are inevitable in the face of this kind of slow change. A good way to think of it is as *practicing*: no one learns to walk, read, or play a sport well immediately – it takes constant repetitions to get it right. The same is true in psychodynamic psychotherapy. Working on the same issues over and over helps patients practice new ways of thinking and behaving that over time become automatic.

Working through can be thought of as having three phases:

Phase 1	**limited awareness** of the problem or cause of the problem.
Phase 2	**increasing awareness** of the problem or the cause of the problem and/or **practicing** new ways of functioning.
Phase 3	**lasting change** in thought pattern or behavior.

Increase in awareness is sometimes called **insight** and psychodynamic psychotherapy is sometimes called **insight-oriented psychotherapy** [4]. However, looking at working through in this way helps us realize that while insight is helpful, it is really only a way station to lasting change. In addition, some change happens without frank insight. In a more contemporary way of looking at psychodynamic psychotherapy, insight is one thing that can promote change, but so can *experiencing* other aspects of the treatment, such as the relationship with the therapist and the holding function of therapy [5].

We can think of working through as a learning process that occurs continuously throughout psychodynamic psychotherapy – from the first encounter to beyond the ending. Working through different issues occurs at different paces: for example, people might experience lasting and profound change in the way they view themselves, yet lag behind in changing their expectations of others. Our awareness of the phases of working through helps us be attuned to our patients as they try to change patterns of thought and behavior that, until this point, have been fundamental to who they are.

Technique

Listening

What do we hear in the different phases of working through? What are we listening for?

Phase 1: Limited awareness

In this initial phase, people are either unaware that a problem exists or have very limited awareness of its internal causes. How these two situations can sound is explored in what follows:

Limited awareness of the problem

Mr B   *Is it OK if I wait until next month to pay you? I'd really appreciate that because I want to buy a new car and I need all my spare cash for the down payment.*

Therapist   *That request is interesting for two reasons. First, it's not the agreement we made when we started treatment, and second, your difficulty paying bills late is what led to the end of your last therapy.*

Mr B   *That's because my old therapist wasn't flexible – and I guess you're not either.*

Here, the patient threatens the frame of the treatment in a way that clearly recapitulates a problem he has in other aspects of his life. The therapist **confronts** this behavior, but the patient is completely unaware that it is problematic.

Limited awareness of the cause of the problem

Ms C   *Why can't I have a relationship? All my friends are getting married and I can't even get a third date. And I thought that the second date went really well. I'm so frustrated!*

Therapist   *Could you have misperceived how well things were going on that last date?*

Ms C   *Maybe – but I really can't think of why I would do that. Something is clearly wrong, but I haven't the vaguest idea of what it is.*

Unlike Mr B, Ms C knows she has a problem – in this case with relationships – but she doesn't know why. Again, the therapist **confronts** the problem, but Ms C has little ability to deepen her awareness of the cause.

What do we listen for to know that we are in this phase?

- **Affect**: Affects like frustration, anger, hopelessness, and incredulousness are typical of this phase. Patients may also sound stubborn or willful as they seemingly refuse to acknowledge awareness of their difficulties.

- **Limited capacity to associate**: During this phase, our invitations to patients to deepen their associations are often met by shallow responses, such as "What do you mean 'can I say more about that?' What's there to say? My boyfriend is just a jerk."

- **Resistance**: Prominent resistance is the rule during this phase. Since resistance is the mind's way of keeping things out of awareness during therapy, we can think of it as the person's way of staying in Phase 1. Listen for all kinds of resistance, from silence to lateness.

- **Externalization**: A good indication of lack of awareness is the patient's insistence that problems are arising from external sources. "I'm always late because the mass transit system in this country is a mess," "Women are fickle – that's why all of my relationships have failed," and "The problems in my marriage all boil down to my mother-in-law" are examples of this.

- **Countertransference**: Our own frustration, irritation, and hopelessness about our ability to help patients are also potential indications of this phase.

- **Patterns**: Listening for patterns is crucial for this phase of the working-through process:

  > Ms D complained to her therapist that her thesis adviser was unfairly treating her. The therapist recalled that the week before she had complained about the fact that her landlord preferentially fixed leaks in her neighbor's apartment.

Phase 2: Increasing awareness and practicing

Here are clues that patients are gaining increased awareness of their problems and starting to practice new ways of functioning:

- **Insight**: Insight is indicated by increased self-awareness of problems and/or causes. Phrases that start with "I realized that . . . ," "I'm starting to figure out . . . ," and "It's starting to make sense to me that . . . " are all good indications that insight is developing.

- **Continued frustration**: Despite burgeoning insight, this phase is often characterized by a continuation of "old" habitual thought or behavior patterns. In fact, it is the discrepancy between increased insight and continuation of old behaviors that is the *sine qua non* of this phase. Here are some examples:

  > Last night when I was talking to my mother I knew that she was just pushing my buttons, but I still couldn't help myself from getting annoyed with her.

  > When I was flirting with that girl at the bar last night it felt different – this time I knew that she was the wrong kind of person to get involved with, but I just kept it up.

  > When I woke up half an hour late for the session, I knew it was because I was upset about what we talked about yesterday.

  These patients have *insight* but still haven't *changed* their behaviors.

- **Shame and depression**: Increased insight can often provoke shame as patients come face to face with problematic thoughts and behaviors. Far from being signs of regression, these painful affects generally signal that patients are moving forward and allowing themselves to be more aware of unconscious, maladaptive patterns.

  > Mr E became depressed as he realized that his estranged relationship with his brother was the result of his own provocative behavior.

- **Anxiety and fear**: Beginning to try something new always comes with ambivalence, and anxiety is part of that.

- **Excitement**: Increased insight can also produce feelings of excitement and mastery, as patients begin to glimpse the light at the end of the tunnel:

  Ms F looked pleased and proud as she reported to her therapist that their work on goal setting made her realize how much this could help her in other aspects of her life.

- **New and old patterns**: This phase is a mosaic of new and old patterns. Remember that development is not linear – after patients try out new ways of thinking and behaving, they often revert to their tried and true patterns. No need to think of this as regression – forward and backward motion is part and parcel of this phase.

Phase 3: Lasting change in thought and behavior patterns

What can we listen for to know when things have changed?

- **No fanfare**: When change happens, it usually happens quietly. As opposed to the high affect/anxiety states associated with maladaptive patterns of thought and behavior, patients often notice change in hindsight. They are often surprised to realize that they have behaved in a new way, so we have to listen very carefully for it:

  Ms G, who had been obsessively worried about leaving her son with a babysitter for much of the treatment, reported on a wonderful weekend away with her husband. When her therapist asked about whether she had been worried about leaving her son, she realized that, although she had carefully arranged the childcare, she hadn't worried about it at all.

- **Decreased anxiety and affect about previously charged topics**: As above, it's often the *lack* of affect about things that were previously highly charged that we have to listen for.

- **Countertransference**: Noticing that our patients have changed often makes us feel proud. Change that might lead to ending may also induce feelings of loss as we anticipate the impending separation from someone we have worked with for a long time.

Reflecting

When we reflect on working through, we try to think about what phase of the process we're in. Is the anxiety we're hearing indicative of a lack of insight, or the fear that accompanies trying something new? Is the patient tolerating the process of change, or do we need to support their functioning? Would sharing observations about the patient's progress help or hinder the process? As always, the choosing principles can help guide your decision making – staying close to affect, surface material, and your countertransference will help you understand how the patient feels. However, here the readiness principles and your history with the patient will be your best guides. Where are you in the treatment? Is this something that you've been working on for a while? Does the patient's way of talking about it sound new? Does it sound like the level of insight has increased? As always, use your moment-to-moment understanding of the patient's functioning to help you decide whether to support or to uncover. Here are two contrasting examples:

> *Ms H comes to her third psychotherapy session in a state of high anxiety. "Based on what we talked about last week, I realized that my parents really screwed me up and I decided to confront them. They screamed at me and hung up and now I'm a mess."*

In this example, the patient and therapist have very little history with this – or any other – topic. The insight seems premature, as does the action, and it has produced intolerable anxiety for the patient. As the therapist reflects on what he has heard, he decides that the patient is still likely to be in the phase of limited awareness.

> *Mr I, who has been in psychotherapy for three years, comes to his therapy session and says, "I'm feeling anxious today because I realize I was angry with you after the last session. I figured it out once I got home and worried about it, but I thought that after all this time I really should discuss it with you despite the fact that that makes me nervous."*

Here, the therapeutic alliance seems strong, and the history is extensive. The therapist sees that something new has happened – the patient, who was generally loath to discuss negative feelings about the therapist, tries to do so despite attendant anxiety. The therapist decides that the patient is in the phase of increased awareness.

Intervening

Although we will outline specific interventions designed to facilitate working through, one of the most important things the therapist can do to promote this process is to have *patience*. Repeating the interventions described in this book, whether supporting or uncovering, over and over in a way that respects the tremendous difficulties human beings have in altering habitual modes of thought and behavior is what will ultimately help patients achieve lasting change in their functioning. Like a patient parent or coach, the therapist should presume from the outset that these repetitions are part of the process. Thus, they are an expected aspect of therapy, rather than the result of the patient's stubbornness or the therapist's incompetence. This stance not only indicates an understanding of therapeutic action (Chapter 2), it also helps reduce counter-transference frustration and transference shame.

As you read the following examples, think about the best ways to convey the need for repetition to your patients:

> Mr J   *So there I was again, screwing up a job interview. I knew what was happening, but the guy was such a jerk I couldn't help myself.*
>
> Therapist   *That's the third time that's happened since you started therapy – if you keep that up you'll never get a job. We'd better work on that.*

This therapist understands the pattern, but her intervention is borne of frustration. The therapist sounds exasperated and blames the patient for something that may well be out of his control. Here is another possible intervention:

Therapist   *That sounds like it was really frustrating. But it wasn't the same as before because this time you knew what was happening. Why don't you tell me more about the interview so we can learn what happened to help you next time.*

This intervention incorporates basic supporting and uncovering interventions in a non-judgmental way to promote working through. It validates the patient's affective experience, identifies that the patient has done something new, calls for more associations, and invites a collaborative process.

The aim of our interventions in working through can either be to support functioning with the goal of having the patient internalize support over time, or to make unconscious processes increasingly conscious so that new adaptations can become habitual.

Supporting interventions

Encouraging and **praising** the patient's attempts to think and behave in new ways are extremely helpful in this process. These interventions can be quite varied:

It's terrific you were able to stop yourself from binging after your exam this time.

The way you're talking about your mother today is quite new and represents a real shift in your thinking.

Marking ways in which a patient's functioning is changing is useful whether you are supporting or uncovering. Any supplying intervention that promotes this aim can be used. Assisting interventions can also help the process:

I see a real change in the way you went about working on that project. Let's go through how you did it in order to help you understand how new your approach really was.

This is a **collaborative intervention** that helps patients understand their own progress and breaks it into component parts.

Uncovering interventions

Confronting and **clarifying** new ways of thinking and behaving help interest patients in the changes going on in their minds:

Patient   *I wanted to call and call him until he answered, but I didn't.*

Therapist   *You waited – that's new for you.*

Patient   *You're right – I didn't realize that – I just did it. Last year I couldn't have tolerated waiting.*

The therapist's **confrontation** of the new behavior invites associations and promotes uncovering of something new – the realization of change.

Interpretations of many sorts can also aid in this process. Interpretation of resistance to change is often important here, as is interpretation of resistance to recognizing change. Here are two examples. The first highlights resistance to change:

> *It's hard for you to think of yourself as dealing with your boss in a new way because you can't imagine behaving differently from the way you acted with your mother.*

The next interpretation highlights the resistance to the recognition of change:

> *It's hard for you to see the new ways you're behaving with your boss because you worry it's a betrayal of your mother to be different from her.*

All patients need to know that they're progressing. Whether you're uncovering or supporting, it's important to let your patients know both that they're making changes and also that you recognize it. How do you know when enough change has occurred and you're ready to **end?** That's the subject of the next chapter.

Suggested activity

What phase of working through do you think each of the following patients is in and why?

1. *Ms A: I can't believe I fell for my father's bait – again! How many times have we gone over this? Three months ago, he told me he was going to pay for the kids' summer camp – he said he had the money and it was his pleasure – so I signed them up. Am I an idiot? Now they're all excited about it and it's three weeks away and he calls and says that the market is bad and he can't spare the cash. But it really depresses me – still – I stayed in bed all day yesterday – I just can't face the kids and I don't think that my husband and I can pay for it. When am I going to stop this?*

Comment

This sound like Phase 2: Increasing awareness and practicing. Ms A recognizes the pattern she gets into with her father, but is still having difficulty avoiding it, probably because she continues to wish that things would turn out differently. In addition, she still gets very depressed when it occurs.

2. *Ms B: I went on three blind dates in the last two weeks and wasn't asked for a single second date. What's wrong with me? I really felt like I did everything right – they all went well. The guys seemed nice and attentive – I talked and talked and felt really comfortable. They were all incredibly interested in me and seemed interested in what I had to say, so I am completely puzzled. I couldn't help drinking more last night – I was so upset.*

Comment

Ms B is in Phase 1: Limited awareness. She does not recognize patterns, blames others for difficulties, and uses maladaptive coping strategies. Given her comments, she may have limited empathy for others, monopolizing the conversation and showing little interest in her dates, but is unable to recognize that this could contribute to her difficulty in relationships.

3. *Mr C: Jack left for his last year of college today. I'm going to miss him, but the day was fine – I dropped him at the airport and came back and made dinner with Carmen – we had a lovely evening. When we were having a glass of wine, she was remembering what a mess I was when Jack first left. It's funny – I do remember that but it seems a lifetime ago. Carmen and I leave for Puerto Rico on Saturday – we never could have done that in September when the kids were home.*

Comment

Mr C is in Phase 3: Lasting change. After much work on his relationship with his son, Mr C is now able to separate without anxiety. While he can recall the old behavior, it seems part of ancient history. He reports noticing this change without undue fanfare or need for praise.

Chapter 29: References

1. Kandel, E.R. (1979) Psychotherapy and the single synapse: The impact of psychiatric thought on neurobiological research. *New England Journal of Medicine*, **301** (19), 1028–1036.
2. Sandler, J., Dare, C., Holder, A., *et al.* (1973) *The Patient and the Analyst*, International Universities Press, Madison, WI, p. 121–127.
3. Greenson, R.R. (1965) The problem of working through. *Drives, Affects, Behavior* (ed. M. Schur), International Universities Press, Madison, WI, p. 277–314.
4. Moore, B.E., and Fine, B.D. (1990) *Psychoanalytic Terms and Concepts*, American Psychoanalytic Association, New York, p. 99.
5. Gabbard, G.O. (2005) *Psychodynamic Psychiatry in Clinical Practice*, 4th ed., American Psychiatric Publishing, Washington, DC, p. 109–112.

30 Ending

Key concepts

Ending (sometimes called termination) is the final phase of psychodynamic psychotherapy. The major work of ending includes:

- consolidating goals
- reviewing the treatment
- realistically appraising change
- planning for the future (including treatment if necessary)
- taking leave

The ending phase is usually proportional to the length of treatment.
Technique alters during the ending phase, reflecting the wish to "close up" and finish.
Ending can be a time of intense transference and countertransference.

Ending any very intense experience is difficult. Think of graduating from college. After four years of hard work, students and faculty come together in a ritual that involves celebration and sadness, looking forward and looking backward, progression and regression. This tradition is an essential part of the process, and is designed to mark an important moment of passage. The same is true of ending psychodynamic psychotherapy. After two people – patient and therapist – have worked together, week after week, for months and even years, it's time to say goodbye. This period shares many features of a graduation, and it's just as important to mark.

We will talk about several aspects of ending, including:

- How do we decide when or if to end a psychodynamic psychotherapy?
- What happens during the ending phase?
- How do we alter our technique when ending?
- What are some typical transference and countertransference reactions?

Psychodynamic Psychotherapy: A Clinical Manual, Second Edition. Deborah L. Cabaniss, Sabrina Cherry, Carolyn J. Douglas and Anna Schwartz.
© 2017 John Wiley & Sons, Ltd. Published 2017 by John Wiley & Sons, Ltd.

How do we decide when to end a psychodynamic psychotherapy?

Thinking about the goals of psychodynamic psychotherapy is the best way to decide when to end the treatment [1,2]. Although the goals are different for each patient, we generally think about some common aims:

- **Improved symptoms:** It goes without saying that improvement in the symptoms that brought the patient to treatment is important in thinking about when to end. This includes improvements in mood, anxiety, and persistent negative affects. However, note that symptomatic improvement without some of the changes discussed later may not be enough to signal readiness to end.

- **Improved sense of self:** Increased confidence and sense of self are key, as is a consistently realistic appraisal of one's talents and limitations.

- **Improved relationships with others:** This can be evidenced in healthier relationships – inside and outside of the treatment – as well as by shifts in the patient's unconscious expectations of relationships.

- **Improved adapting:** Often a main goal of psychodynamic psychotherapy, this includes use of more adaptive defenses, as well as increased defensive flexibility.

- **Increased reflective capacity:** This used to be the *sine qua non* of readiness for ending – that is, that patients are ready to leave when they are able to interpret themselves. Although we now think that change in psychodynamic psychotherapy is about more than insight, increased capacity for self-observation is still an indication that ending is near.

- **Improved work and play:** Most importantly, we want patients to have better, more satisfying lives. This includes their ability to work and to play. Improved sexual function, enhanced creativity, and an increased ability to relax may all be part of this.

- **Increased feelings of independence:** Many patients, especially more fragile and dependent ones, have the fantasy that any gains made in the therapy will disappear after ending therapy. Accepting their gains as their own rather than as contingent on continued therapy may be a sign of readiness to end.

Either therapist or patient can introduce the subject of ending. When patients bring this up, it is important to understand their motivation for this wish. Early in treatment, it can be a resistance – the desire to leave before there is too much dependency, for example, or the wish to leave to avoid uncovering painful affects. Knowing whether the request for ending is a resistance or whether it is a reasonable time for the patient to finish takes time and experience, however a few rules of thumb are helpful here:

- **How far into the treatment are you?** If this is a few weeks or months into a psychodynamic psychotherapy, consider the possibility that this may represent resistance. Since this treatment often takes time, if you've just gotten started and the patient is talking about ending, try to understand why this is coming up. Patients sometimes have what is called a **"flight into health"** after beginning treatment that makes them feel as if they have solved all their problems. When this happens, we can acknowledge the good feelings while also suggesting that this might just be the beginning of more exploration and change. The prospect of a "long-term treatment" may be exciting at the beginning, but soon the "long" takes over and can feel oppressive to the patient. Think of your excitement at the beginning of a long hike versus the fatigue at hour 6 or 7 – you can empathize with this frustration and remind the patient that lasting change often takes time. Since our goal is generally to change lifelong patterns of behavior, one useful comment is, "You know, it took you 34 years to develop these patterns – we'd be surprised if you could change them so fast!" At the same time, don't forget that occasionally patients are helped in just a few sessions.

- **What is the context of the discussion of ending?** If patients begin to talk about ending right after beginning to explore something painful, or if they start new relationships in the context of the treatment and then want to end, think about resistance.

- **How does the patient talk about the wish to end therapy?** Asking patients their ideas about ending or why they want to end is central to your technique in this situation. Time and money concerns are often at least partially real, but can also hide other fears and anxieties.

- **What is the patient's affect?** Is the patient angry with you? Dismissive? Patients who have worked well with you in a psychodynamic psychotherapy are usually quite ambivalent about ending – they are generally grateful, eager to "try it on their own," but also pretty sure they will miss you. If you don't pick up this kind of three-dimensionality, this might not be the time to end.

- **What is your countertransference?** Are *you* angry with the patient? Are you relieved that he/she doesn't want to continue? Do you feel hurt, or sense that things are being disrupted midstream? If so, there is likely to be more here than just a wish to end. Often, the therapist who has worked well with a patient has complementary ambivalent feelings – pride that things have gone well, accompanied by the anticipation of loss. Think of the parent vacationing with a child who will go off to college in September. If these are not the kinds of feelings you're having, you might consider that the patient is not really ready to end.

Here's how to listen, reflect, and intervene when thinking about ending:

- **Listening:** Listen for affect and ask questions to get more information about thoughts, feelings, and fantasies related to the idea of ending. Often patients have dreams relating to ending that can be helpful. For example, a dream of escaping from something versus a dream of taking a tearful leave of beloved relatives can mean different things about readiness to end.

- **Reflecting:** Process what you've heard to determine what's closest to the surface and what is the dominant affect. Think about whether what you're hearing is defensive and thus related to a resistance against deepening.

- **Intervening:** Tread lightly here – we always want to take the patient's wish to end seriously, and not just "interpret it." If patients are ultimately going to agree that it is not time to end, you want to give them a face-saving way to change their mind. If you think that the wish to end is resistance, then you will ultimately interpret this.

Sometimes, patients want to end before you think they are ready. Perhaps you think there is an active resistance or that the patient has more work to do. You will do best to explore the wish to end, and then gently confront and interpret the resistance:

Patient	*How long will I have to keep coming here twice a week? I feel much better and it's so hard to get here in the morning.*
Therapist	*Things have changed for you, that's clear – but I have a feeling you've been talking more about the wish to stop therapy ever since you started dating Maya.* (**empathic remark, confrontation**)
Patient	*Maybe – I think that I'd rather that she didn't know I was seeing you.*

Here, the therapist acknowledges the good feelings, then connects the patient's wish to end with the potential shame of telling his new girlfriend he's in therapy.

In some cases, the wish to stop treatment is actually an expression of entrenched expectations about people and relationships. For example, a patient who tends to feel that others will trap him or not allow him to do what he wants will often itch to leave as the transference deepens. This can be the crux of the treatment for a patient like this and is very important to understand and potentially interpret:

Patient	*I feel like I'm stuck here – like even if I want to leave you won't let me.*
Therapist	*Let you?* (**confrontation**)
Patient	*Yeah – like I have no control in this situation.*
Therapist	*Of course you know that you can stop therapy any time you like – but I'm struck by the fact that you're having that same feeling about your girlfriend.* (**empathic remark and clarification**)
Patient	*It's all on her terms – ever since we got serious, she makes plans for us all weekend – what if one night I just want to go out with the boys?*
Therapist	*Maybe you're feeling the same way with me too.* (**transference interpretation**)

In this situation, it is clear that the wish to end is analogous to the characteristic expectation that getting close to someone will mean loss of autonomy.

Giving patients some encouragement to stay is not against the rules. If patients are about to leave and you think it's not a good idea, you can tell them you think they should stay as long as you remain consciously aware of transference and countertransference feelings that might be at play. For example, therapists might try to convince patients not to end because they have affectionate feelings for them, or because they feel guilty that they haven't done a good enough job in the therapy. Real-life factors, such as potential loss of income or academic credit, could also fuel the therapist's countertransference in this situation. Staying alert to the possibility that countertransference feelings are informing your ideas about ending is key to handling the situation in the best way possible. Having extremely strong feelings about this or getting into a power struggle with the patient should signal the need for discussion of the case with a supervisor or peer.

It's also important to remember that patients are likely to react strongly – both positively and negatively – when their therapists suggest that they should stay in treatment rather than end. Exploring these feelings can deepen their understanding of the transference:

> *Mr A is a 42 year-old man who never felt his parents cared whether he finished things or not. During sessions in the second year of therapy, he pushes to end. Here is a segment from that time:*

> Mr A   *This is done – I've changed enough and have so much to do in the rest of my life.*

> Therapist   *I'm surprised this is coming up now, because it seems to me you're just starting to get to issues that brought you here to begin with. I think that this is an important time for you in therapy and that it would be helpful for you to continue. Do you have thoughts about that?*

> Mr A   *What do you care? You can just fill the slot with someone else – they might even pay more than I do.*

> Therapist   *I think that you're feeling that I, like your parents, don't care whether you continue or not.*

> Mr A   *You're right – they never did. I quit all sorts of things and they didn't care as long as it didn't upset their tee times.*

Mr A decided to stay in treatment. Here's a segment from a session six months later:

> Mr A   *I had a dream last night that we were finishing the session and you asked me to stay for another 5 minutes.*

> Therapist   *What are your thoughts about that?*

> Mr A   *I thought about it this morning and remembered that session when you said you thought it was important for me to stay in therapy. I almost quit – just at the wrong time. I was surprised you said that.*

> Therapist   *It felt new to you – you always felt your parents were indifferent to whether you quit things or not.*

> Mr A   *Yeah, it made me almost unable to understand that it mattered to you.*

In this case, the way Mr A and his therapist ultimately explored and understood his reaction to the suggestion that he stay in treatment led to an important shift in the transference and in his expectations of others.

If these techniques do not work and patients still want to leave treatment, then let them – provided you think it is a safe choice. There are two types of endings:

- **Bilateral endings:** Therapist and patient agree that the goals have been attained and the treatment is ready to end. In time-limited treatments, this is set at the onset of the treatment; in open-ended treatments, it is decided during the course of the treatment.

- **Unilateral endings:** Therapist or patient ends the treatment for some reason. This could be because a trainee is finishing a training program, or because the patient is moving away [3].

Life and therapy are long – sometimes patients have to leave in order to figure out that they want to come back. If you are respectful of their wishes while demonstrating care and interest, they are more likely to return. Always let them know that your door is open – even if the ending is unilateral.

How long should the ending phase be?

The length of the ending phase should generally be proportional to the length of the treatment. Thus, a seven-year treatment might have an ending phase of a year, while a few months might suffice for a year-long treatment. Planning the ending phase gives the patient adequate time for reviewing, mourning, and leave taking [4]. Working together to choose an actual end date makes the end a clear reality and facilitates this phase.

Technique

Listening during the ending phase

The ending phase begins when therapist and patient decide to end treatment. In the case of unilateral endings, this happens when an imposed deadline (like the end of an academic year for trainees or the patient's graduation from school) requires them to finish. In bilateral endings, it is when they decide it's a good time to end. Regardless of what instigates it, the ending phase is a time for closure. This is very different from the rest of treatment, when our whole technical approach is designed to open things up. While we are always somewhat open-ended, things come up in the ending we don't have time for and thus handle in a different way. Despite this, important work happens during this time.

There are some things that are typical of ending – knowing about them will help your listening during this affect-filled phase:

Regression

Without fail, patients in the ending phase regress to symptoms and transferences that neither patient nor therapist has seen for months or even years. This can derail the inexperienced therapist, who may worry that the patient is not ready to end. On the contrary – it is absolutely characteristic of this phase. Patients who were late during the beginning phase will suddenly start to come late again; patients who hadn't questioned your billing or cancelation policies in years will resume arguing about them. Anticipating regression and the way it may mask other feelings can help you to "hear it" during the ending phase:

> *Ms B, who had been very skeptical of her therapist's interest in her during the first year of treatment, had come to trust him and spent a great deal of time during the ending phase talking about how he was one of the first people who really cared about her. Three months prior to the end of Ms B's treatment, the therapist uncharacteristically picked up a phone call during a session. The therapist was surprised when Ms B became enraged about this, saying his caring was "all a charade" and that perhaps she should just end now. Exploration of this revealed Ms B's fantasy that the therapist was now more interested in other patients, and her jealousy that someone else would have "her time."*

Mourning

Patients often become very sad when ending. Therapists will do well to remember how important they are to their patients – this is often most apparent during ending. Tearfulness and feelings of loss are the norm. Occasionally, a patient will become depressed during this phase – always be on the lookout for the need for medication, though these feelings may also subside on their own. When you think about it, ending is a very strange thing to do; two people develop a very intense, meaningful relationship, and then don't see each other again. Previously, a patient's wish to see the therapist after ending was thought to indicate that the treatment was unfinished; now, however, it is very common for patients to return for "check-ups" during stressful or exciting times in their lives. If patients are on medication and the therapist is also the prescriber, monthly medication checks may continue even after the formal period of therapy concludes. However, even with the possibility of occasional visits in the future, the end of the therapy proper is a loss for patients. It may be that no one has ever listened to them as intensely as the therapist has, or that no one has ever been as regularly interested in their life. Even if new relationships have been found thanks to treatment, the therapist needs to remember that the loss of the therapist is a *real* loss and thus that mourning is natural and expected. In fact, if the patient does not talk about feelings of loss and mourning, the therapist should suspect resistance to these feelings.

Another thing that is mourned during the ending phase is that while some things have changed, others have not [3]. The loss of the fantasy of endless possibilities is often very difficult. The end of therapy is generally a time when people come to terms with their capabilities *and* their limitations. The fact that they still have difficult parents, or that the person they married during therapy is not as empathic as they would have imagined, can bring on feelings of resignation. This is true of unconscious fantasies as well – there may be disappointment that therapy did not completely cure their shyness or that a symptom still emerges in times of stress. This can also be very difficult for therapists, particularly if they have their own fantasies about how they wanted to optimally help their patient. Exploring these fantasies in our patients and in ourselves is the best technique at this point – along with acknowledging the affect and attendant disappointment. Remember that therapy, like mothering, need only be "good enough" – so disappointments are inevitable. Just as children's disappointment with the good-enough mother helps them to develop, so too do patients' disappointment with their therapist. Our job is to help them see the therapist more realistically and to separate during the ending phase.

Finding a replacement relationship

It makes sense that people anticipating a loss might want to find a replacement – and the therapist is wise to listen for this. As in the beginning of treatment, it is common for patients to find new friends and lovers during the ending phase. Listening for and anticipating this can help therapists point out the connection between new relation-ships and the loss of the therapist. This does not necessarily negate the worth of the new relationships, although understanding the connection can help patients more objec-tively evaluate their nature.

Reflecting during the ending phase

As with listening, reflecting during the ending phase is aided by knowing that this phase has distinct characteristics. We still use the choosing principles and the readiness principles to think about where to focus, but during this time we pay special attention to the *phase of treatment.* Just as we filter most things that we hear at the beginning of treatment through the lens of beginning, we now filter what we hear through the lens of ending and think about everything we hear as if it might relate to this. How might this affect be related to ending the treatment? How might this dream relate to feelings about ending? How might this new relationship be compensating for loss of the therapist? How might this symptom be a recapitulation of an old symptom in the context of the regression of ending? Although we might not comment on this every time it occurs, we give priority to ending-related themes during this time in order to help patients make sense of their feelings and fantasies related to ending treatment:

> During the ending phase, Mr C has a dream that he is an astronaut who is about to go on the first manned mission to Mars. His associations are to excitement about the trip, but as he is strapped into the rocket, he realizes with a start that he is alone. The therapist's reflection about this dream is that it relates to the ambivalence of ending – the excitement of new possibilities, alongside the anxiety of "going it alone."

Intervening during the ending phase

We use basic, supporting, and uncovering interventions during the ending phase. Since a goal of ending is to close the treatment, we try to limit our interpretive comments to related themes. When patients open up new areas during this time, we generally limit exploration, trying always to relate them to familiar themes and to the work of ending. Consider these examples, one from the middle phase and one from ending:

> *A patient in the middle phase of treatment says, "I have a funny feeling – as if I'm falling off a cliff." The therapist reflects that this is a new theme and says, "Can you tell me more about that?"*

> *A patient who is ending in two weeks says, "I have a funny feeling – as if I'm falling off a cliff." The therapist reflects that this is likely to be related to ending the therapy and says, "I wonder if this has to do with the fact that we won't be meeting after next week."*

The therapist will still do well to call for associations in order to make sure that the affect or fantasy is related to ending, but once this seems certain, it makes sense at this point in treatment to relate it to ending rather than just opening it up for further associations.

In psychodynamic psychotherapy we often adopt a neutral stance and steer clear of praise or judgments to facilitate the patient's ability to fantasize and associate freely. As this goal is somewhat less essential during this phase, ending is a time when the neutral stance can be somewhat relaxed. Remember that we aim for neutrality for a purpose, and when that purpose is less essential the therapist can be somewhat freed up to be less neutral. For example, we generally do not guide patients' associations *because* we want them to follow their thoughts freely. This is essential for uncovering in psychodynamic psychotherapy, since it helps us move toward unconscious material. However, a goal of the ending phase is consolidation of gains, and thus guiding the patient toward review of the treatment is an important technical tool. During this phase therapists actively help patients understand themselves, the treatment, and their gains:

Patient	*It was so funny at the party last night – I could see from 10 yards away that guy just wanted a one-night stand. So I just looked away and kept talking to my girlfriend.*
Therapist	*That's very different than the way you looked at things a year ago.*
Patient	*You're right – I didn't think of it that way – I guess that there has been a change.*
Therapist	*It's a big change – it's hard to see when you're in it, but we might take some time during these weeks to think about the ways in which you're seeing things differently.*

This technical maneuver is distinctly different from the technique we use during the middle phase of treatment, and it can be very helpful and consolidating for patients who are ending.

Relaxing some aspects of neutrality also means that the technique of the ending phase can be filled with a bit more humor and mutuality. By this stage of treatment, you and your patient have been working together a long time – there is a lot of trust and the therapeutic alliance is strong. Therapist and patient often have developed "short cuts" – ways of talking about things they've gone over many times. A comment like "there's that fear of commitment again" might be premature during the early phase of treatment, but once you've commented on it a few hundred times, you and your patient know exactly what you're talking about. Similarly, you may be able to interpret dreams and fantasies more quickly without as many associations once you and your patient both recognize certain patterns.

At the very end of the treatment, patients often ask us personal questions that we may be a bit more likely to answer than early in the treatment. Again, our decision during most of the treatment *not* to answer personal questions is not arbitrary – it has a rationale based in our theory of technique. Early in treatment, the goal is to allow patients to fantasize as broadly as possible about us in order to foster the development of transference. However, as therapy comes to a close, there is no reason not to answer the patient who asks, "So where are you going after your training?" As you reflect on how to answer, think about why you're saying what you're saying. No need to be a "blank slate" at this point – but also protect your boundaries. This is good for the patient, who doesn't need to be burdened by knowing too much about you, and it's good for you, since you deserve to have your own private life. So when the patient asks what you're doing next, you might say, "I'm going to be working on an inpatient unit" or "I'm going to work as a therapist in a community clinic." This amount of information tells them that you are a person whose life is continuing and that you value the relationship enough to share this piece of information. Remember, however, that patients who end therapy may return for treatment months or even years later. Continuing generally to maintain anonymity helps to keep the door open for future work with you [4].

Ending and supporting

It is important to recognize that for various reasons some patients cannot – and should not – be pressed to talk about their feelings of loss around ending the treatment. For patients who have trouble forming attachments, any admission that the therapist has become important to them may be intolerable; other patients need to think that they improved by themselves. With patients who continue to struggle with managing painful affects, the therapist might choose to **supportively bypass** the patient's difficult feelings about ending, emphasizing instead the gains made and the therapist's ongoing concern and availability. It may be useful in certain situations to taper visits gradually and plan to continue meeting at least intermittently until patients indicate they are ready to stop. As with people with persistent medical illnesses, ending may not be recommended for those patients who require ongoing support from the therapist to maintain stability [5].

Choreographing the last sessions

It is often useful to ask patients if they have any thoughts or fantasies about the last sessions. Some patients hope that you will hug them, while others fear that you will try to do so. Here, as before, good boundaries are key – the therapist should not initiate any physical contact beyond a handshake at the door. Don't underestimate how meaningful that handshake can be. Allowing patients to talk about the wish for a hug will usually allow the two of you to talk about it and what it means rather than actually having to engage in it. Patients may also give you a gift. (See Chapter 8 for more on gifts.) If they give it to you at the beginning of the last session, open it with them and have them tell you about it. No interpretations now – "thank you" will do. Again, the time for uncovering has come to a close. The gratitude may be tinged with a still not completely explored fantasy or expectation – but it is also real and should thus be acknowledged.

Communicating your thoughts about the treatment

Many therapists use the last session or the last few sessions to tell patients something about their impressions of the treatment. This often includes thoughts about changes that have occurred in the patient's emotional life and functioning in the world. It can also include ideas about what things might prove challenging to the patient in the future, as well as some thoughts about the therapist's experience of the therapy. Here is an example:

> In the last few weeks, you've been talking so much about what has changed over the course of therapy and what it's meant to you. But before we stop, I wanted to say something about that, too. When you first came, you were on the verge of losing your job and your relationship – and you've learned so much about why that was happening. It's been remarkable and rewarding to see the way in which learning more about yourself has helped you improve your relationships and so many other aspects of your life. As we've discussed, things may come up in the future that may put stress on you and make some of those "old ways" come back – but I have confidence that our work together will help you to recognize when that's happening. Those might be times that you want to drop in here for a few sessions to get back on track – that will always be fine. I also want you to know that it has been a pleasure to know you and to be your therapist, and that I've learned a great deal from our work together.

Of course, never say something you don't believe, but try to emphasize the positive in what you are able to say. All through the therapy, you presumably have been trying to help patients see that their relationship with you is real – now is the time to put your money where your mouth is. Real people in real relationships take leave of *each other* – so it's natural for the therapist to comment on leave-taking as well. Again, though, say just enough to convey this within the context of good boundaries.

In sum, the ending phase is marked by:

- listening for new things – like regression and mourning
- reflecting on how the patient's words can be linked to the work of ending
- intervening in ways that facilitate consolidation of gains, closure, and leave-taking
- strong transference and countertransference, so supervision can be very helpful during this time to help you metabolize your feelings and take leave of your patient in a meaningful way that also maintains boundaries

Suggested activity

Read the following and think about how you would respond if the patient were:

- in the middle phase of the therapy
- in the ending phase of the therapy

Patient # 1

Last night I was on the train going home from work and I had this memory of the last night of camp. You know, the bonfire – you look forward to that bonfire all summer – plan songs, and so on. But it's also sad – you won't see all of those close friends for another year. I haven't thought about that in a long time.

Patient # 2

You are really annoying me today. You're totally off base. You haven't annoyed me like this since we started treatment. Sometimes I wonder if you ever understood me at all.

Comment

Patient #1 is having a memory about the ambivalence of leave-taking. In the middle of the therapy, you might ask for more associations in order to understand why this is coming up at this time, or you might confront the temporal relationship between this memory and something happening in the patient's life and/or therapy. In the ending phase, you might first consider whether this memory is coming up in relation to ending. You might say:

This camp memory is about the ambivalence of leave-taking – it's exciting but also involves leaving people you care about. I wonder if that reflects something about the way you feel about leaving me?

Patient #2 is feeling angry about what she perceives as your inability to understand her. In the middle of therapy, you might validate her feelings and ask her to say more about them. You might also think about why these feelings are coming up at this time. In the ending phase, this is likely to be related to ending the treatment. It could relate to disappointment about things that were not fully worked through, or the patient's anger could be defensively covering feelings of mourning and loss. How you respond would depend, of course, on the therapeutic alliance you had with the patient throughout the treatment. Presuming that the patient generally felt that you did understand her, you might consider this to be a regression, particularly since the patient references her feelings about you from the earliest phase. You might say:

You're certainly very frustrated with me today, and it could be that I've been off base. But you're right – you haven't been this frustrated with me for a very long time. I wonder if it could be related to feelings you're having about the fact that we're only going to be meeting for a few more weeks?

Chapter 30: References

1. Gabbard, G.O. (2004) *Long-Term Psychodynamic Psychotherapy*, American Psychiatric Publishing, Washington, DC, p. 164–165.
2. Dewald, P.A. (1969) *Psychotherapy: A Dynamic Approach*, 2nd ed., Basic Books, New York, p. 282.
3. Dewald, P.A. (1982) The clinical importance of the termination phase. *Psychoanalytic Inquiry*, **2**, 441–461.
4. Gabbard, G.O. (2004) *Long-Term Psychodynamic Psychotherapy*, American Psychiatric Publishing, Washington, DC, p. 168.
5. Winston, A., Rosenthal, R., and Pinsker, H. (2004) *Introduction to Supportive Psychotherapy*, American Psychiatric Publishing, Washington, DC, p. 78–79.

Review Activity for Parts Six and Seven: "The Macroprocess Summary" – Understanding How Things Change in Treatment

Now it's time to put everything you have learned together to create a summary of a treatment. Your review activity after Part V focused on the **microprocess**; this review activity will focus on the **macroprocess**. While the microprocess is the moment-to-moment activity of the treatment, the macroprocess is the overarching story of change. Many things change in the course of a treatment, and tracking them helps you understand what happened with an individual patient and how psychodynamic psychotherapy leads to change in general. The Macroprocess Summary should track:

- **Changes in functioning:** How did the elements from Part Five (resistance, transference, countertransference, unconscious fantasy, and conflict), as well as the elements in Part Six (self-experience, relationships, characteristic ways of adapting to stress, cognition), change in the course of the treatment? What is your hypothesis about why this change happened?

- **Working through and (when applicable) ending:** What were the phases of the treatment? How did you know when you were in a new phase?

- **Transference and countertransference through the treatment:** What did you do in the course of treatment that made a difference? How did your patient respond? What is important here is that your story includes both you and your patient. This is a journey that the two of you have taken together, and your summary should reflect that.

As you read the following example of a Macroprocess Summary, notice that it:

- summarizes themes of each phase of treatment

- includes short segments of verbatim microprocess to give a sense of what happened in sessions

- includes hypotheses about why change happened. This is more than a report – it has to include your ideas about how and why change occurred

[Note to educators: see "A Guide for Educators" (Appendix 1) for more on using this exercise to assess advanced learners.]

*Dr Y is a 30-year-old psychology graduate student. This is her **Macroprocess Summary** of a two-year treatment with Ms B:*

Ms B, a 58-year-old gay high-school English teacher with two children, first presented for treatment two years ago saying she was unhappy in her relationship with her longtime partner, C. Ms B complained that C, a successful surgeon, with whom she had had a more than 30-year relationship during which they had each had a child, was not interested in her. Ms B said that she felt alone and neglected. The first session was in November, two months after their youngest child (of whom Ms B was the biological mother) went to college in a distant city. Although she was sad, Ms B did not have symptoms of a DSM mood or anxiety disorder, and had continued to teach. During the assessment phase, it was clear that Ms B had lifelong issues with self-esteem and tended to expect that others would not understand her. However, she generally handled stress with more adaptive defense mechanisms and was self-reflective. She reported that, despite having grown up in a stable household, she had always felt alone and "not close" to her parents and brother. In addition, she had had a difficult time in high school, teased for being a tomboy and inhibited about coming out as gay until matriculating at a women's college. Her first long-term relationship was with C, and she now wondered if she should have had more romantic experiences. I suggested to Ms B that, before making decisions about her relationship, we explore her feelings about herself and others to understand the way her early life and unconscious feelings might be related to her current unhappiness. She agreed and we began a twice-weekly psychodynamic psychotherapy.

Although Ms B was talkative and excited during the assessment, things changed once we began meeting regularly. Sessions in the first six months were characterized by silence, superficiality, and Ms B's sense that she "had nothing to say." She sometimes brought notes, listing things that C had done that upset her, saying "otherwise I'd forget." She sat rigidly in the chair, often asking me toward the end of the session, "What do you think I should do?" During these months, I wondered whether I had made a mistake during the assessment, since the self-reflection I saw initially had seemed to evaporate. I felt that she wanted me to pull words out of her. Her first dream, reported two months into the treatment, reflected these themes:

> *I was sitting in my office when Jane, one of my best students, came in. I thought she wanted to talk about her paper, but when she sat down and opened her mouth no sound came out. I couldn't tell whether she wasn't talking or I wasn't hearing. I felt like I was just supposed to know what she was saying. It was very disturbing.*

When I asked Ms B whether feeling that she couldn't communicate felt familiar, she could not connect it to her experience. At the time, I didn't ask whether she felt that way with me, although later in supervision I realized that the dream could have represented something about her experience of sitting with me in therapy. It certainly reflected something about my experience with her, and I wondered whether it also might reflect something about her early experience of her mother.

With my supervisor's guidance, I also realized that Ms B, who had never been in psychotherapy before, might need more support during this early part of treatment. Rather than waiting for her to associate at the beginning of sessions, I began to ask more questions, particularly about her relationship with C, and I empathized more with the difficulty she was having at home. This enlivened Ms B, and she looked more comfortable in her chair. Week after week, she told stories about the way C left early for the hospital, came home late, buried herself in journals and papers, and never asked Ms B about her work. "When the children were home, we tried to eat dinner together in the evenings, but even that has broken down," explained Ms B. " I just need something – some affection, some interest. I'm afraid this will never change." At Thanksgiving, she was buoyed by visits from her children – an older daughter who was a college senior and a younger son who was a freshman – although the four ate their holiday meal at a restaurant alone. "Neither C nor I can cook," she explained. "My mother kept me out of the kitchen. She thought that 'kids made a mess,' and so I never learned." This offered me an opportunity to learn more about Ms B's early relationships with her parents. She described her mother as "tough and beautiful" – a "country club lady" who "loved golf more than she loved us." I wondered to Ms B whether she felt that her mother couldn't understand her tomboyish, athletic daughter. "That's the understatement of the year – she had no idea who I was. I was acing school and captain of the field hockey team, but my brother, who was sort of a screw-up, was the apple of her eye." She described her father as warm but absent. "When he was around, I felt like he was interested, but he was constantly in the office – very successful." "Sounds a little bit like C," I offered. Ms B agreed and felt that she had been somewhat aware of that even when the two had met.

In the spring, my hours in the clinic changed and I had to change session times with Ms B. Instead of being able to see her in the late afternoon (after school), we now had one session in the early morning. She missed this session several times in the first weeks of that schedule. When I finally confronted this, it opened up transference feelings that Ms B had not previously discussed:

Therapist	It seems to me that since we've changed our session times you've missed many more sessions.
Ms B	It's just so hard to get here in the morning. And the whole parking thing is a nightmare.
Therapist	Of course there are difficulties related to getting here early, but do you think you might also have feelings about my needing to change the times?
Ms B	I know you said that your hours had changed in the clinic, but I'm embarrassed to admit that I wondered if you just had another patient who needed those times. Those are great times, and maybe you wanted someone else to have them.
Therapist	You're embarrassed to tell me that?
Ms B	Why should I care? But I do – it's been hard for me to believe that you're interested in me, and this made it harder.

This was the first time that Ms B was able to openly discuss her feelings about me – particularly her difficulty believing that I was interested in her and her fear that I would displace her with a favorite patient. With further discussion about this, Ms B stopped missing sessions and began talking more about her early relationship with C. When they met, she thought C was "this brilliant medical student," and she'd been "surprised" that C was interested in her. I was surprised that my comment, "that must have been very important to you, particularly since you hadn't felt that your mother was interested in you," resulted in some of the first tears of the treatment. "Yes, it was thrilling. I would have done anything for her." She began to realize, however, that some of C's interest in her might have stemmed from Ms B's "idol worship" of her:

Ms B	I'd have ironed her scrubs if she asked me to.
Therapist	You were excited by her interest. But you want more than that. You want to be taken care of, too.
Ms B	Babies are taken care of. I can take care of myself.
Therapist	Of course you can – but even grown-ups want to know that there's someone who takes care of them – at least a little.
Ms B	That makes me incredibly sad because I don't know if I've ever had that.

As Ms B became more comfortable with the idea that she longed for care, she became even sadder. For a few sessions, I was concerned that Ms B might be having a major depression, and I asked about symptoms like sleep and appetite. When she asked me why I was asking about sleeping and eating, I told her. Although I was concerned that this might make her even more upset, it actually had the reverse effect. In supervision, I realized that my concern demonstrated to her that I cared. She herself brought this up soon after, saying, "I'm so glad that I finally convinced myself to come to therapy. I'm starting to believe that you really have my back." Her mood improved.

During her summer vacation, Ms B busied herself with her children and attending to their needs. She discussed her pride in them – particularly her son – and the way they advocated for themselves. I suggested that this was due to their healthy self-esteem, something that she and C had helped them to develop. "I feel bad, but that makes me jealous," she said, "We accept them for who they are – that wasn't the case with my parents and me." She spent many sessions discussing her wish to be like other girls who were interested in boys, and her perennial feelings of being different. She began to tentatively ask C for more and was surprised when C was more forthcoming than she expected. For example, in August, as the family planned a vacation, Ms B advocated one plan more forcefully than usual and C agreed. This allowed me to wonder to Ms B whether some of her feeling of alienation might be the result of withdrawing from C, an idea that was newly interesting to her.

As we began our second year of treatment, I noticed how different things were in sessions. Ms B began sessions herself, full of associations and more assertive. I commented on this change to Ms B, who acknowledged it, saying, "Yes, it's true – I feel better – I can sense it at work, too. But with the kids gone again I'm back to feeling angry at C." I confronted the fact that although she said she was "back" to being angry at C, she'd never actually said that before. This surprised her, and she realized that while before she had been sad, now she was angry. "I deserve better," she said. "I'm a bright woman, a good teacher, and a great mom – she should realize that."

In January, Ms B developed a crush on one of the women in her book group. She realized that she was "fussing" about what to wear to the group, "something I never do." She asked the woman to coffee and, although she never revealed her feelings, had several months of fantasizing about whether the woman had feelings for her, too. Around this time, I noticed that she was dressing differently for sessions as well, and that she had grown her hair into a longer style. When watching the video in supervision, my supervisor commented that her hair now looked a lot like mine. My supervisor and I wondered together about the shift in the transference – was she identifying with me, or was it an erotic transference? Although I did not comment on this at the time, a few sessions later, after I made a comment that Ms B found helpful, she said, "I hope your husband appreciates you." We then had the following exchange:

Therapist	*Can you tell me more about that thought?*
Ms B	*You are a great person – so warm, so smart – I bet you are a great partner.*
Therapist	*Have you had thoughts about what it would be like to be my partner?*
Ms B	*Sometimes – of course, you are much younger than I am, and you're probably not gay, but I do think to myself – what if I had met someone like you instead of C? What would my life have been like?*

Interestingly, Ms B began to report that C had also noticed the change in her appearance. We wondered together whether she had kept herself from attending to herself for a reason. Ms B suggested that maybe she had needed to keep up her tomboyish look in order to hold on to her identity, but realized that she hadn't allowed herself to feel sexy. She associated to her mother's glamour and to her feeling that she could never compete with her. She and C gradually became more sexually intimate, and Ms B decided that they should have a "date night" like they did when the children were little. I realized that the transference was both an identification with me as a woman – her feeling that she could, in fact, compete with me in a way that she hadn't been able to with her mother – and an erotic transference. Staying with the transference, as uncomfortable as it was for both of us, had helped Ms B to work through her sexual inhibitions, grow into herself as a sexual woman, and improve her relationship.

The last phase of therapy was characterized by a return of Ms B's sadness. In March, I told Ms B that I would be leaving the clinic in June, as my training there was coming to an end. She missed a few of our early sessions, but quickly realized that it probably had something to do with her feelings about ending. I agreed, and commented on how well she was interpreting her own behavior. Although this made her feel good about our work, she soon provoked a major fight with C that brought her back to her feelings about the relationship:

Ms B   *Things are better with C, but they'll never be great. How come I'm losing you but get to keep her? I wish it were the other way around.*

Therapist   *Our work together has been so important to you, and so many things have changed. But faced with ending therapy, I think you created a crisis with C in order to demonstrate to me how much you feel you still need me. The fact is, though, that you're doing really well.*

Ms B   *Ugh! This is not easy. I do love C, but she'll never be perfect. (laugh) I guess I'm not either.*

As we neared the last weeks, we reviewed things that had happened during the treatment. Ms B was sad she hadn't spent more time thinking about her parents, whom she was now having somewhat different feelings about. She invited them to her daughter's college graduation, and found her mother to be quite warm with the children – this surprised and confused her and made her wonder about her perceptions of her. I suggested she had allowed herself to have many different feelings about me, and that this was allowing her to have a fuller picture of many people in her life. In the last sessions, she asked me about my future plans, and I told her that I had taken an academic job in a neighboring state. She expressed her gratitude and wished me well. I told her how much I had learned from her, and realized that I, too, was sad to end the treatment, as well as the supervision, which had been so helpful. We parted with a handshake and warm wishes.

31 Continuing to Learn

By this point, you've learned a tremendous amount about psychodynamic psychotherapy. You've learned to assess patients and begin the treatment; to listen to what patients say, reflect on what you've heard, and intervene to uncover unconscious thoughts, feelings, and fantasies or to support weakened function; and to use these tools to achieve important therapeutic goals such as improving self-esteem, relationships with others, and characteristic ways of adapting. Now you can take these skills into your clinics, offices, inpatient units, or wherever you work to continue the process of becoming a psychodynamic psychotherapist. Doing this work means learning something new every day. Each patient presents new challenges; each treatment teaches us new things. Ultimately we learn from our supervisors, our patients, and ourselves.

Learning from your supervisors

The best way to complement what you've learned by reading this manual is to conduct psychodynamic psychotherapy with patients of your own. In doing this, you will be greatly helped by supervision. There are many types of supervisors. Trainees generally have one or more assigned supervisors. Some of them may be experienced psychotherapists, although they may or may not have expertise in psychodynamic psychotherapy. Graduates sometimes seek out private supervision or they may present cases to peers.

There are several ways in which supervision will enhance your learning in psychodynamic psychotherapy. First, experience helps. Until you accumulate experience of your own, you can lean on your supervisor's expertise. Second, discussing the case with another person will foster reflection about it. This can be done with a more experienced person or with one or more peers. When you're very close to a case, you can't always accurately assess your countertransference, and thus talking to trusted teachers or colleagues is invaluable. Even after your training is completed, seeking out supervision for help with particularly challenging cases should be something that you always feel comfortable doing.

There are many ways to share your work with your supervisors. If you can make video recordings of sessions (with your patients' consent) and watch them with your supervisor, you will get the most out of supervision. Video captures not only what you and the patient really say, but also all of the non-verbal communication. Watch small sections at a time, stopping to analyze what you heard, how you reflected, how you chose your therapeutic strategy, and what interventions you made. Audio recordings, again made with your patients' consent, can also be useful. If you are unable to make recordings, general discussion of the case is helpful, as is examination of verbatim process notes. You and your supervisor can discuss what will work best in your

Psychodynamic Psychotherapy: A Clinical Manual, Second Edition. Deborah L. Cabaniss, Sabrina Cherry, Carolyn J. Douglas and Anna Schwartz.
© 2017 John Wiley & Sons, Ltd. Published 2017 by John Wiley & Sons, Ltd.

particular situation. If you take process notes, make sure to review them after sessions to include what you said but might not have been able to record.

However you share your work, being a proactive learner will help you get the most out of supervision. Too often, learners think their supervisors are there to "tell them what to do." Analogous to our "supplying and assisting" model of supporting interventions, sometimes a supervisor will make suggestions, but a collaborative model is generally most helpful. If you are a supervisor, you can foster collaboration by having clear goals for the learning experience. The various models presented in this manual can help structure supervision:

- **For assessment and formulation**: the Describe/Review/Link model (see also "Psychodynamic Formulation")
- **For technique**: the Listen/Reflect/Intervene model, the choosing and readiness principles, and the concept of uncovering and supporting interventions.

If you are a supervisee, try sharing some of what you've learned in this manual with your supervisors by asking them questions like:

- What did you hear when the patient said that?
- How would you reflect on that?
- How would you choose what to say?
- What did you think about what I said?
- I was confused about what to say there – can we hone in on that moment?
- How would you label that intervention?

Here is a segment from a session between a therapist and her supervisor:

> The therapist is a 40-year-old woman who has been treating a 28-year-old man in twice-weekly psychodynamic psychotherapy for two years. In the last few weeks, she has not been looking forward to this patient's sessions.

Therapist	It's interesting – I usually really enjoy working with this patient, but for the last few weeks I haven't felt that way. Once last week, I even thought, "Oh no, it's Monday – Mr A is coming today." But I'm not sure what's going on.
Supervisor	This is a great thing to talk about. Do you have any sense of something that's happening in his life or in the treatment?
Therapist	No – that's the funny thing – he's actually working more deeply in the treatment and feeling more connected. That's just what we've been working toward.
Supervisor	Let's hear some process to see if we can see what's happening. Can you read some material from one of the sessions in which you felt that way?
Therapist	Sure – here's a segment from yesterday's session:
Patient	I'm really getting into this now – I look forward to every session – I almost wish I could come every day. I had a dream that I was sleeping in your waiting area – like there was a little bed in that little alcove out there.

> *Therapist*   Can you say more about the dream?
>
> *Patient*   It was really cozy – like you were going to tuck me in.
>
> *Supervisor*   Let's stop there for a moment – what do you hear in this material and how did you reflect on it?
>
> *Therapist*   Well, there's the dream – being "tucked in" sounds like it's from childhood, so it probably has to do with an unconscious fantasy of having me take care of him the way his mother did. But we know his mother was quite neglectful. In the session, his surface affect was excitement – like he's excited to become so close to me.
>
> *Supervisor*   I hear that, too – your patient is almost breathlessly saying that he wants a tremendous amount from you – he's ready to figuratively "move in" – and you might be pulling back from that.
>
> *Therapist*   Well, as you know, I have two children of my own – I don't need another one! I mean, I know he wouldn't really be another child, but maybe I feel that way.
>
> *Supervisor*   Exactly – I think we're getting to some of your recent difficulties with him and learning a great deal about the patient as well.

Here the supervisor was able to help the therapist learn more about her counter-transference. The therapist's ability to discuss her feelings openly was key to the process. Notice that the listen/reflect/intervene method can work in supervision as well.

Communicating what you're learning in your classes or from this manual with your supervisor will help you be on the "same page" and will enhance the supervisory experience.

Learning from your patients

There's an old adage that "your patients are your best supervisors." In many ways, this is true. Each patient will teach you new things about people, their adaptations, their strengths, and their difficulties. Each therapeutic relationship will teach you about how to interact with patients in order to help them most. If you focus on something too deep, your patients will react by defending themselves in some way – if you attend to this, you can easily right yourself on a moment-to-moment basis. Here's an example:

> *Patient*   I was upset at the end of the last session because you started late and then you didn't give me extra time.
>
> *Therapist*   I reminded you of the way your mother focused more on your brother and left you feeling cheated.
>
> *Patient*   Whatever – I'm talking about you – my mother wasn't here last time – you were.
>
> *Therapist*   You're right – and I'm glad you were able to bring this up. Can you tell me more about the feeling you had?

This patient is an excellent supervisor: the affect was in the transference and the therapist focused on a genetic interpretation. Not the time to get defensive – if you listen to patients you can refocus on what feels most important to them.

Learning from yourself

Ultimately, understanding yourself is your best tool for your work as a psychodynamic psychotherapist. The degree to which you are aware of your feelings and reactions during sessions will directly correlate with your ability to help your patients. No need to think that you have to complete some process of self-awareness before you begin treating patients in psychodynamic psychotherapy – just as you will keep learning from your patients, you will continue to learn from and about yourself throughout your career. That said, it may be helpful, either at the beginning of your training or at any point along the way, to engage in your own personal psychotherapy in order to facilitate your ability to learn from yourself. Some therapists undertake this as a matter of course, while others seek out their own treatment in response to particular challenges they face as they mature as therapists. Some training programs, such as many of those that train psychoanalysts, require personal therapy or psychoanalysis as part of the educational experience. Clues that personal therapy might be helpful include strong negative or positive feelings to most or all of your patients, undue anxiety or depression related to your work, or the tendency to cross boundaries. Just as you will do for your patients, therapists will offer *you* confidential treatment that is likely to enhance your work and your life.

With or without personal therapy, ongoing self-reflection is key. We are all busy, but taking the time to reflect on our work is well worth it. This is as true in the middle of a session as it is between sessions – we are often so eager to "say something" that we don't always take the time when we are with patients to think about what's happening in the moment. These moments of reflection are time well spent and will turn you from a proficient to an outstanding psychodynamic psychotherapist.

Ending

People have searched for meaning since the beginning of time. Psychodynamic psychotherapy helps people find meaning within themselves – meaning that is present but out of awareness. This quest will always be relevant to people and to how they make sense of their lives. Learn from others, learn from your patients, and learn from yourself as you continue your journey as a psychodynamic psychotherapist.

Appendix 1

How to Use *Psychodynamic Psychotherapy: A Clinical Manual*

A Guide for Educators

Psychodynamic Psychotherapy: A Clinical Manual is a treatment manual that can be used as a primary text for teaching psychodynamic psychotherapy to learners in any mental health field, including counseling, nursing, psychology, psychiatry, social work, and postgraduate psychodynamic psychotherapy programs. Educators should also be aware that it has been translated into Mandarin, Korean, and Farsi. In this educators' guide, we first present some basic principles for the use of this manual as a teaching tool, as well as for teaching psychodynamic psychotherapy, and then offer suggested learning objectives, seminars, readings, and evaluation methods.

Basic principles for teaching psychodynamic psychotherapy

The Y model

We believe that learning to become a psychodynamic psychotherapist is a developmental process. Students need to learn fundamentals first, on which they can build more sophisticated skills. We have modeled our psychodynamic curriculum, and the structure of this book, on the Y model [1], which conceptualizes psychotherapeutic technique as based on common skills which then branch off into skills specific to different treatments:

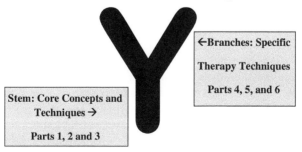

Psychodynamic Psychotherapy: A Clinical Manual, Second Edition. Deborah L. Cabaniss, Sabrina Cherry, Carolyn J. Douglas and Anna Schwartz.
© 2017 John Wiley & Sons, Ltd. Published 2017 by John Wiley & Sons, Ltd.

Core concepts and techniques roughly approximate the **common factors** that are part of all psychotherapeutic technique and are correlated with good clinical outcome [2]. We strongly believe that psychotherapy students should learn to use these core techniques, such as building a therapeutic alliance, listening empathically, and setting the frame and boundaries, *before* learning more specific psychotherapeutic techniques – including psychodynamic technique. This developmental sequence is echoed by the Accreditation Council for Graduate Medical Education's (ACGME) Psychotherapy Milestones for psychiatry residents [3]. Thus we use Parts 1, 2, and 3 of this book with early learners to teach core concepts, and Parts 4, 5, and 6 with more advanced learners to teach the specific techniques of psychodynamic psychotherapy.

The Y model also offers a clear way to coordinate instruction of psychodynamic psychotherapy with the student's general psychotherapy curriculum. Isolating one psychotherapy from others makes no sense in this day and age, and teaching different psychotherapeutic techniques in a coordinated way helps students to understand the way in which the various techniques and formulations are both similar and distinct. This enhances training and helps students to understand how and when to recommend different types of therapy in order to best treat their patients. Having a faculty member, such as a Director of Psychotherapy Training, who is able to oversee all of psychotherapy education in a training program is one way to ensure that this happens.

Teach technique and formulation together

Technique without formulation is shooting in the dark. Only by grounding one's technique in formulation can one really set goals and systematically achieve therapeutic aims. Thus, we teach technique and formulation side by side. While we briefly discuss formulation in this book, our companion book, *Psychodynamic Formulation*, is essential for truly learning this fundamental skill. In this educators' guide, we suggest how and when to use these books together in an integrated developmental sequence.

The flipped classroom

Informed by adult learning theory, we advocate active teaching methods for all of our psychotherapy didactic and supervisory instruction. We are heartbroken when we hear that people are "lecturing" from our books. Our manuals are specifically designed to promote a "flipped classroom" model of learning. The chapters are short, easy to digest, and headed by key concepts. Assign one or two chapters (at most), briefly review them for a few minutes at the outset of a class, and then launch into active learning techniques based on the material. Our "suggested activities" at the end of each chapter can be used for this purpose, and once you get the hang of them you can create more of your own. Divide classes into groups of two or three to work on vignettes, create short scripts to present to the class, or suggest formulations. If your students videotape their work, show clips from these videos (with appropriate consent) to illustrate concepts that you are teaching in class. Showing good student work is often better than showing expert videos, as it reminds students that they can do this work too. We have found that ongoing continuous case presentations are not particularly valuable, as they promote passive learning in everyone who is not presenting and they are not specifically geared to teaching skills.

Operationalizing and evaluation methods

The operationalization of skills in this manual naturally suggests evaluation techniques. Don't be afraid to assign some writing at the end of each seminar; it will help you to assess your learners and ensure that your teaching activities have achieved your learning objectives. We suggest learning objectives and evaluation techniques for all levels of learner in this educators' guide.

Course and lab

Finally, we strongly believe that didactic instructors and supervisors need to work together in a coordinated way to teach psychotherapy [4]. Too often, supervisors work in a diaspora that is disconnected from seminars, leading students to learn very different things in these venues. At best, this leads to disjointed learning; at worst, it leads to confusion and student disengagement. Having supervisors read this manual, as well as *Psychodynamic Formulation*, puts all of your instructors on the same page, enhancing learning and creating an integrated psychodynamic faculty. Our materials are designed to be accessible to all supervisors, from trained psychoanalysts to faculty who do not have specialty training in this area. Periodic communications (e.g., by email) to supervisors letting them know what students are learning in class help supervisors to know where their supervisees are in their learning process and to find teachable moments in clinical material [5]. We also recommend training supervisors for specific learner levels – for example, supervisors of junior learners should emphasize common factors, while supervisors of intermediate and senior learners should emphasize specific techniques (though not forgetting common factors). Faculty development workshops designed for specific supervisor levels can help to accomplish this. Just as some teachers are better at teaching 3rd grade while others should teach high school, some supervisors are excellent for junior levels while others excel at senior levels. Learning about your supervisors through observation, learner evaluations, and supervisory preference can help you to make more informed supervisory assignments.

Suggested curriculum materials

As already mentioned, we advocate a developmental approach to teaching and learning psychodynamic psychotherapy. It cannot be taught all at once, and thus we do not recommend reading straight through this manual in a single course. To help you plan your curriculum and use of the manual, we delineate Beginning, Intermediate, and Advanced level learners. Although educators can extrapolate to their different learning programs, Table 1 offers some suggestions as to how this might translate for different mental health programs:

Table 1 Guide to learner levels

Learner level	Mental health specialty	Year
Beginning	Social work	1st-year student
	Psychology	Beginning extern
	Nurse practitioner	1st year
	Psychiatry	PGY-I and II
	Postgrad psychotherapy	
Intermediate	Social work	2nd-year student
	Psychology	Advanced extern; master's level
	Nurse practitioner	1st year
	Psychiatry	PGY-III
	Postgrad psychotherapy	
Advanced	Social work	Postgraduate field work
	Psychology	Intern and post-doc
	Nurse practitioner	2nd year
	Psychiatry	PGY-III or IV
	Postgrad psychotherapy	

Beginning learners

Beginning learners are solidly in the stem of the Y model. They generally see patients who are in crisis, and they tend to work in clinics, emergency rooms, inpatient units, and consultation-liaison services. These are great places to begin to teach psychotherapy in general and psychodynamic psychotherapy in particular if the emphasis is on common factors. Thus, we emphasize core concepts and skills for beginning learners. Although this is a psychodynamic psychotherapy manual, we use many of our chapters to teach an introduction to psychotherapy in general.

Suggested learning objectives

Beginning learners will be able to:

- state what psychotherapy is and how it can be used in all clinical settings
- evaluate patients for psychotherapy, including making a DSM diagnosis, assessing function, and constructing an initial formulation
- set goals, give informed consent, establish a therapeutic frame and boundaries, and forge a therapeutic alliance
- discuss the basic skills of psychodynamic psychotherapy, including listening, reflecting, and intervening
- use supporting interventions with patients

Suggested seminars

Introduction to psychotherapy

This can be taught at the very beginning of training and should cover most of the core psychotherapy techniques, such as assessment, goal setting, establishing a frame and boundaries, technical neutrality, empathic listening, and initial formulation and treatment planning. We teach our students that they are using psychotherapy all the time, even when they are taking histories and working on discharge planning. We encourage them to discuss all the patients they are treating, not just patients who are designated "psychotherapy patients." All of the chapters in Parts Two and Three are appropriate for this teaching. Note that Chapter 12, "Our Patients' Feelings about Us and Our Feelings about Our Patients," does not use the terms transference and countertransference. This is intentional, since we believe that these concepts transcend psychodynamic psychotherapy. Specific psychodynamic use of transference and countertransference is discussed in Part Five.

Introduction to psychodynamic psychotherapy

Once core concepts are taught, beginning learners can start to learn the basics of psychodynamic psychotherapy. Assume nothing – reading some Freud in college has rarely taught your mental health trainees much about treating patients. We find that students are happy to really understand basic concepts, so start from the beginning. This is generally even true of learners in postgraduate psychodynamic psychotherapy programs. We introduce Listening, Reflecting, and Intervening at this stage, with an emphasis on the supporting techniques that students can use with the patients they are currently treating. Parts One and Four are most appropriate for this material. Although we encourage students to try to create an initial formulation in order to make a treatment recommendation (Chapter 5), our emphasis in terms of formulation at this phase is on **describing** the problem and the person's patterns. Chapters 4–8 from *Psychodynamic Formulation* are appropriate for this work.

Suggested evaluation methods

Try evaluating your students' ability to assess function by having them write a brief assessment of a short story character, describing the character's function in the five domains and characteristic defenses. You can have them write this about their patients as well, as long as you are familiar with the patients. Ask students to write a one-page initial formulation and discuss it with a supervisor. If your students videotape their clinical work, you can evaluate their ability to use common factors with the AADPRT Milestone Assessment for Psychotherapy (A-MAP), which can be accessed at www.aadprt.org.

Intermediate learners

Once students are grounded in the core psychotherapy techniques and the basics of psychodynamic psychotherapy, they are ready for their seminars in the various psychotherapies, including psychodynamic psychotherapy. At this stage of their train-ing, they are also likely to be treating outpatients with psychodynamic psychotherapy.

Suggested learning objectives

Intermediate learners will be able to:

- listen, reflect, and intervene when working with affect, resistance, transference, countertransference, unconscious conflict and defense, and dreams in psychodynamic psychotherapy
- use uncovering and supporting interventions, and explain their therapeutic strategy
- write a psychodynamic formulation for a patient in psychodynamic psychotherapy using the Describe/Review/Link method

Suggested seminars

Psychodynamic technique

This is when we teach psychodynamic technique, basing our seminars on the chapters in Part Five. We advocate teaching uncovering and supporting techniques side by side, rather than having separate courses in supportive and psychodynamic psychotherapies. This has made an enormous difference to our students' ability and willingness to use these techniques in a continually oscillating way. Teaching a psychodynamic psychotherapy course that truly integrates uncovering and supporting requires instructors to take time to teach both techniques; for example, seminars on transference should include management of the transference as well as interpretation of the transference [6].

Psychodynamic formulation

This continues the work started at the beginning level, adding Reviewing and Linking. Chapters 9–12 from *Psychodynamic Formulation* are appropriate for this teaching. Psychodynamic models of the mind can be taught at this point as well (*Psychodynamic Formulation*, Chapters 13–18).

Suggested evaluation methods

This is the time to review the **microprocess**, or the "she said, he said" of the treatment. The Review activity for Part Five – the "Microprocess Moment" – is a great way to see if your students can listen, reflect, and intervene in psychodynamic psychotherapy. Using the example in that activity as a guide, they can write up a moment in the treatment, specifying what they heard, explaining how they chose their therapeutic strategy based on the choosing and readiness principles, and labeling their interventions. Sharing this in class is a fun and productive way to encourage peer-to-peer learning. If your students videotape their clinical work, do a "Video Review." Watch 15 minutes of videotape with them and again ask them to tell you how they listened, reflected, and intervened. The summary table in Appendix 2 can be used for both the written "Microprocess Moment" and the Video Review.

Advanced learners

By this point in their training, your learners have a strong command of common factors and a solid ability to listen, reflect, and intervene in psychodynamic psychotherapy. They can now begin to consolidate their learning, can approach advanced topics, and can consider advanced training in psychodynamic treatments such as psychoanalysis, mentalization-based psychotherapy, and transference-focused psychotherapy. They can also begin to teach junior learners in this area.

Suggested learning objectives

Advanced learners will be able to:

- consolidate their learning in psychodynamic psychotherapy with ongoing individual or group supervision
- describe the way in which their patients change in psychodynamic psychotherapy to meet therapeutic goals
- describe the phases of working through and describe the phase a given patient is in
- apply their knowledge and skills to complex clinical situations such as stalemates, the erotic transference, and termination
- consider connections between psychodynamic psychotherapy and findings in neuroscience
- teach junior learners psychotherapeutic and psychodynamic knowledge and skills
- further explore psychodynamic models of the mind and apply them to clinical situations

Suggested seminars

Advanced psychodynamic technique

Learners should now have been treating patients in this modality for some time, and thus are ready to focus on how things change over time. Working through and termination are good topics, as is discussion of how we meet therapeutic goals (Parts Six and Seven). Learners may also be introduced to more advanced topics, such as stalemates and the erotic transference, and are often interested in further readings in psychodynamic theory and technique (see suggested readings at the end of this appendix).

Psychodynamic psychotherapy and neuroscience

Ideally, advanced learners should be introduced to the latest ideas about how psychodynamic psychotherapy can be understood through the lens of modern basic and cognitive neuroscience (see suggested readings at the end of this appendix).

Subspecialty psychodynamic techniques

When instructors are available, learners at this level will benefit from seminars in subspecialty psychodynamic techniques, such as brief dynamic therapy, mentalization-based therapy, panic-focused psychotherapy, and transference-focused psychotherapy (TFP). Learning these techniques not only augments the learner's therapy toolbox, it consolidates learning in core techniques. Suggested readings are at the end of this appendix, many of which are accessible and could be used by interested learners in the absence of a formal seminar.

Suggested evaluation methods

This is the time to focus on the **macroprocess**, or the overarching trajectory of the treatment, in order to assess your learners' understanding of meeting therapeutic goals and working through. The Review Activity for Part Seven – "The Macroprocess Treatment Summary" – is a good way to do this. As with the "Microprocess Moment," your students can use the example in the manual as a template for writing about their own patients. Encourage supervisors to help with this exercise. Consult Cabaniss and Graver's "Mapping the Macroprocess" for useful ways to help students conceptualize the trajectory of the treatment [7]. Once again, sharing de-identified material with peers encourages peer-to-peer learning and exposes learners to more patient experiences.

Suggested additional readings

Advanced technique and theory

Auchincloss, E.L. (2015) *The Psychoanalytic Model of the Mind*, American Psychiatric Press, Washington, DC.
Mitchell, S.A., and Black, M.J. (1995) *Freud and Beyond: A History of Modern Psychoanalytic Thought*, Basic Books, New York.
Schlesinger, H.J. (2003) *The Texture of Treatment: On the Matter of Psychoanalytic Technique*, Analytic Press, Hillsdale, NJ.

Psychodynamic psychotherapy and neuroscience

Demasio, A. (2010) *Self Comes to Mind: Constructing the Conscious Brain*, Vintage Books, New York.
Kandel, E.R. (2005) *Psychiatry, Psychoanalysis, and the New Biology of the Mind*, American Psychiatric Press, Washington, DC.
LeDoux, J. (2002) *Synaptic Self: How Our Brains Become Who We Are*, Penguin Books, New York.

Subspecialty psychodynamic techniques

Marmor, J. (1979) Short term dynamic psychotherapy. *American Journal of Psychiatry*, **136**, 149–155.
Milrod, B., Busch, F., Cooper, A., *et al.* (1997) *Manual of Panic-Focused Psychodynamic Psychotherapy*. American Psychiatric Press, Washington, DC.
Yeomans, F.E., Clarkin, J.F., and Kernberg, O.F. (2002) *A Primer of Transference-Focused Psychotherapy for the Borderline Patient*, Jason Aronson, Lanham, MD.

Appendix 1: References

1. Plakun, E., Sudak, D., and Goldberg, D. (2009) The Y model: An integrated, evidence-based approach to teaching psychotherapy competencies. *Journal of Psychiatric Practice*, **1**, 5–11.
2. DeFife, J.A., and Hilsenroth, M.J. (2011) Starting off on the right foot: Common factor elements in early psychotherapy process. *Journal of Psychotherapy Integration*, **21** (2), 172–191.
3. The Psychiatry Milestones Project, A Joint Initiative of the Accreditation Council for Graduate Medical Education and the American Board of Psychiatry and Neurology. July 2015. http:// acgme.org/acgmeweb/Portals/0/PDFs/Milestones/PsychiatryMilestones.pdf, accessed January 2016.
4. Cabaniss, D.L., and Arbuckle, M.A. (2011) Course and lab: A new model for supervision, *Academic Psychiatry*, **35**, 220–225.
5. Havinghurst, R.J. (1953) *Human Development and Education*, Longmans, Green, Oxford.
6. Cabaniss, D.L., Arbuckle, M.A., and Douglas, C.J. (2010) Beyond the supportive-expressive continuum: An integrated approach to psychodynamic psychotherapy in clinical practice, *Focus*, **8** (1), 25–31.
7. Cabaniss, D.L., and Graver, R. (2008) Mapping the Macroprocess, *Journal of the American Psychoanalytic Association*, **56**, 1249–1260.

Appendix 2
Template for Assessment of the Microprocess Moment and Video Review

Name of resident:

Psychodynamic skill:	Present in the exercise	Comment
LISTENING: **Affect**		
Resistance		
Transference		
Countertransference		
Unconscious themes		
REFLECTING: **Discussion of use of choosing principles (surface to depth, following affect, attention to countertransference)**		
Discussion of use of readiness principles (phase of treatment, state of the alliance, current function)		
INTERVENING: **Use of uncovering and/or supportive interventions**		
Labeling of interventions		

Reproduced with the permission of Springer from Cabaniss D.L., Havel L.K., Berger S., Deo A., and Arbuckle M.A. (2015) The Microprocess Moment: A tool for evaluating skills in psychodynamic psychotherapy, *Academic Psychiatry*, Dec 8, Epub ahead of press.

Psychodynamic Psychotherapy: A Clinical Manual, Second Edition. Deborah L. Cabaniss, Sabrina Cherry, Carolyn J. Douglas and Anna Schwartz.
© 2017 John Wiley & Sons, Ltd. Published 2017 by John Wiley & Sons, Ltd.

Appendix **3**

The Post-Evaluation Psychodynamic Psychotherapy Educational Resource – The "PEPPER"

What follows is a short psychoeducational resource about psychodynamic psychotherapy that we call the PEPPER (as above). You can use this with your patients during the informed consent process (see Chapter 7). This instrument was originally designed for patients in twice-weekly psychotherapy; you can amend it to reflect the frequency with which your patients are coming.

Based on what you have discussed with your therapist, including your problems and goals, you and your therapist have decided on a treatment called psychodynamic psychotherapy. This sheet will give you some information about what psychodynamic psychotherapy is and how we think it works. You should review this information and discuss it with your therapist to know what to expect and how to get the most out of this treatment.

Psychodynamic psychotherapy is a talking treatment based on the idea that thoughts and feelings that you may not be aware of can cause problems such as anxiety, depression, poor selfesteem, and difficulty with relationships. One way that we deal with painful or difficult thoughts and feelings is to put them out of our minds – that is, to make them unconscious. But even though we do not think about them, those unconscious thoughts and feelings affect how we think, feel, and behave. For example, it might be hard for you to have angry feelings towards someone you love because you think you shouldn't have them. Nevertheless, they might continue to affect your relationship.

Over the next few weeks, you and your therapist will develop goals that are specific for you, but in general the goals of psychodynamic psychotherapy include improving how you feel about yourself, how you relate to other people, and how you cope with stress. To accomplish these goals, you and your therapist will work together to help you become more aware of unconscious thoughts and feelings that are causing you to have difficulty and that may make it hard for you to feel happy, good about yourself, and satisfied with your job and relationships. You may also work on developing new,

Psychodynamic Psychotherapy: A Clinical Manual, Second Edition. Deborah L. Cabaniss, Sabrina Cherry, Carolyn J. Douglas and Anna Schwartz.
© 2017 John Wiley & Sons, Ltd. Published 2017 by John Wiley & Sons, Ltd.

healthier ways of dealing with painful thoughts and feelings, as well as with stress you may be experiencing in your daily life.

In psychodynamic psychotherapy, you will do several things to become more aware of unconscious thoughts and feelings:

- **Saying whatever comes to mind** helps you to move from thoughts you are aware of to related thoughts you're not aware of. It's not so easy to do, but your therapist will help you to notice when you're not allowing yourself to speak freely.
- **Talking about your feelings, not just your thoughts**, helps you to become more aware of what your feelings are. Just talking about feelings that were hidden can be helpful.
- **Talking about dreams and fantasies** helps unconscious thoughts and feelings come into your mind. Fantasies are not only your wishes and daydreams, they are also the underlying and often unconscious thoughts that you have about yourself and others. Learning about them can help you to think about yourself and others in new ways.
- **Talking about thoughts and feelings you have about your therapist** – yes, that's not a typo – we want you to talk to your therapist about the way you feel about him or her. These feelings are called your transference. Although it may not seem natural to talk directly to your therapist about these feelings, learning about them will help you to better understand the way you think and feel about others and can help to improve your relationships.
- **Talking about your whole life, particularly about people and events from your childhood**, helps you to remember early thoughts and feelings. This is important because feelings you have about people and situations in your current life may relate to feelings that you had when you were younger. Also, developing new ways of thinking about your life and how you came to be the way you are can lead to change in the way your think about yourself and others.

As you become aware of your unconscious thoughts and feelings, you will learn about patterns you have that are giving you difficulty, and, over time, you will learn new ways of thinking about yourself, coping with stress, and having relationships.

FAQs about Psychodynamic Psychotherapy

Why is it called psychodynamic psychotherapy? Psych means mind, and dynamic refers to moving forces. Your thoughts and feelings can be thought of as mental forces. They are constantly in motion and often conflict with one another. Learning about these forces and conflicts can help you to understand how you think, feel, and behave.

How long will this therapy take? Psychodynamic psychotherapy can be short term for specific problems like panic attacks, or long term for problems with self-esteem, relationships, and coping with stress. It's taken you a long time to develop these patterns, so they may take a while to change. Long term psychotherapy can last a year or longer. It is an "open ended" treatment, meaning that it lasts as long as needed to accomplish the goals that you and your therapist set. At the same time as you are working towards long term goals, you and your therapist may work on shorter term goals such as dealing with stress in your daily life.

Why do I need to come twice a week? Coming more frequently will help you become aware of thoughts and feelings underlying many types of problems. When you come less frequently, you are likely to spend most of your time just reporting on what happened since your last session.

Will my therapist talk? Of course. You do not do all of the work and your therapist does not do all of the work. You and your therapist will work together in a partnership. Your therapist may listen, take notes, ask questions, and help you to notice unconscious thoughts, feelings, and problematic patterns.

Should I really say whatever comes to mind? What if it's not relevant? Yes, you should really say whatever comes to mind, and you should not try to judge whether it is "relevant" or not. That "irrelevant" thought could lead you to an important thought or feeling you did not even know you had.

It feels strange to talk directly about my therapist – should I even say negative things? You are right – this is a strange thing to do – but it's an important way to learn about your relationships. For example, exploring why you get upset with your therapist might help you to understand why you get upset with other people. It may also help you to develop new and healthier ways to deal with other people in your life.

Can I be in psychodynamic psychotherapy and take medication at the same time? Absolutely – if you and your therapist think that you would benefit from taking medication, you can do both at the same time. In fact, it is very common for people to do both. If you are depressed or anxious, taking medication may help your symptoms and help the psychotherapy. If you are taking medication while you're in psychotherapy, talking about this with your therapist can help you to learn about your feelings about being anxious or depressed.

How come my therapist learns all about me and I don't learn much about him or her? Although you'd think that knowing a lot about your therapist would be helpful, the opposite is actually true. Not knowing much about your therapist allows you to really be yourself with him or her. For example, if you're very angry at your parents for getting divorced and you find out that your therapist is divorced, it might make it hard for you to speak freely about your parents. If you get frustrated about this, be sure to discuss it in a session.

By beginning this treatment, you have made an important decision to learn about yourself in order to improve things in your life. Thank you for reading this information sheet. If you have further questions about the treatment and how we think it works, be sure to ask your therapist.

Recommended Reading

Recommended Reading: Part One

Introduction

Gabbard, G.O. (ed.) (2005) *Psychodynamic Psychiatry in Clinical Practice*, 4th ed., American Psychiatric Publishing, Washington, DC.

Kandel, E.R. (2005) *Psychiatry, Psychoanalysis, and the New Biology of Mind*, American Psychiatric Publishing, Washington, DC.

Chapter 1

Mitchell, S.A., and Black, M.J. (1995) *Freud and Beyond: A History of Modern Psychoanalytic Thought*, Basic Books, New York.

Vaughan, S.C. (1998) *The Talking Cure: The Science Behind Psychotherapy*, Henry Holt, New York.

Chapter 2

Auchincloss, E.L. (2015) *The Psychoanalytic Model of the Mind*. American Psychiatric Publishing, Washington, DC.

Bender, S., and Messner, E. (2003) *Becoming a Therapist: What Do I Say, and Why?* Guilford Press, New York.

Bibring, G.L. (ed.) (1968) *The Teaching of Dynamic Psychiatry: A Reappraisal of the Goals and Techniques in the Teaching of Psychoanalytic Psychiatry*, International University Press, New York.

Bruch, H. (1974) *Learning Psychotherapy: Rationale and Ground Rules*, Harvard University Press, Cambridge, MA.

Caligor, E., Kernberg, O.F., and Clarkin, J.F. (2007) *Handbook of Dynamic Psychotherapy for Higher Level Personality Pathology*, American Psychiatric Publishing, Washington, DC.

Cozolino, L. (2010) *The Neuroscience of Psychotherapy*, Norton, New York.

Doidge, N. (2007) *The Brain That Changes Itself*, Penguin, New York.

Gabbard, G.O. (ed.) (2004) *Long-Term Psychodynamic Psychotherapy: A Basic Text*, American Psychiatric Publishing, Washington, DC.

Gabbard, G.O. (ed.) (2005) *Psychodynamic Psychiatry in Clinical Practice*, 4th ed., American Psychiatric Publishing, Washington, DC.

McWilliams, N. (2004) *Basic Therapy Processes in Psychoanalytic Psychotherapy: A Practitioner's Guide*, Guilford Press, New York.

Mitchell, S.A., and Black, M.J. (1996) *Freud and Beyond*, Basic Books, New York.

Storr, A. (1990) *The Art of Psychotherapy*, 2nd ed., Routledge, New York.

Ursano, R.J., Sonnenberg, S.M., and Lazar, S.G. (2004) *Concise Guide to Psychodynamic Psychotherapy: Principles and Techniques of Brief, Intermittent, and Long-Term Psychodynamic Psychotherapy*, 3rd ed., American Psychiatric Publishing, Washington, DC.

Recommended Reading: Part Two

Chapter 3

Bender, S., and Messer, E. (2003) *Becoming a Therapist: What Do I Say, And Why?* Guilford Press, New York.

Greenson, R.R. (1967) *The Technique and Practice of Psychoanalysis*, International Universities Press, New York.

MacKinnon, R.A., and Yudofsky, S.C. (1991) *Principles of the Psychiatric Evaluation*, Lippincott, Williams & Wilkins, Philadelphia.

MacKinnon, R.A., Michels, R., and Buckley, P. (2006) General principles of the interview, in *The Psychiatric Interview in Clinical Practice*, 2nd ed., American Psychiatric Publishing, Washington, DC, p. 3–77.

Winston, A., Rosenthal, A., and Pinsker, H. (2004) *Introduction to Supportive Psychotherapy*, American Psychiatric Publishing, Washington, DC.

Chapter 4

American Psychiatric Association (2000) Defensive functioning scale, in *Diagnostic and Statistical Manual of Mental Disorders: DSM-IV-R*, American Psychiatric Association, Washington DC, p. 807–813.

Bellak, L., (1988) *Ego Function Assessment (EFA): A Manual*, CPS, Larchmont, NY.

Bellak, L., and Goldsmith, L.A., (eds.) (1984) *The Broad Scope of Ego Function Assessment*, John Wiley & Sons, New York.

Caligor, E., Kernberg, O.F., and Clarkin, J.F., (2007) *Handbook of Dynamic Psychotherapy for Higher Level Personality Pathology*, American Psychiatric Publishing, Washington, DC.

Gabbard, G.O., (2005) *Psychodynamic Psychiatry in Clinical Practice*, 4th ed., American Psychiatric Publishing, Washington, DC.

MacKinnon, R.A., and Yudofsky, S.C. (1986) *The Psychiatric Evaluation in Clinical Practice*, Lippincott, Williams & Wilkins, Philadelphia.

Perry, J.C., and Bond, M. (2005) Defensive functioning, in *The American Psychiatric Publishing Textbook of Personality Disorders* (eds. J.M. Oldham, A.E. Skodol, and D.S. Bender), American Psychiatric Publishing, Washington, DC, p. 523–540.

Perry, C.J., Beck, S.M., Constantinides, P., *et al.* (2009) Studying change in defensive functioning in psychotherapy using the defense mechanism rating scales: Four hypotheses, four cases, in *The Handbook of Evidence-Based Psychodynamic Psychotherapy* (eds. R.A. Levy and J.S. Ablon), Humana Press, New York, p. 121–153.

Vaillant, G.E. (1977) *Adaptation to Life*, Little, Brown, Boston, MA.

Vaillant, G.E. (1992) *Ego Mechanisms of Defense: A Guide for Clinicians and Researchers*, American Psychiatric Press, Washington, DC.

Chapter 5

Cabaniss, D.L., Cherry, S., Douglas, C.J., Graver, R.L., and Schwartz, A.R. (2013) Psychodynamic Formulation, Wiley-Blackwell, Oxford.
Erikson, E. (1993) *Childhood and Society*, 2nd ed., Norton, New York.

Chapter 6

Buckley, P. (2009) Applications of individual supportive psychotherapy to psychiatric disorders, in *Textbook of Psychotherapeutic Treatments* (ed. G.O. Gabbard), American Psychiatric Publishing, Washington, DC, p. 447–463.
Leichsenring, F. (2009) Applications of psychodynamic psychotherapy to specific disorders, in *Textbook of Psychotherapeutic Treatments* (ed. G.O. Gabbard), American Psychiatric Publishing, Washington, DC, p. 97–132.
Pinsker, H. (2002) *A Primer of Supportive Psychotherapy*, 2nd ed., Routledge, New York.
Shedler, J. (2006) *That Was Then, This Is Now: An Introduction to Contemporary Psychodynamic Therapy.* http://www.jonathanshedler.com/PDFs/Shedler%20(2006)%20That%20was%20then,%20this%20is%20now%20R9.pdf, accessed April 2016.
Ursano, R.J., and Silberman, E.K. (2004) Psychoanalysis, psychoanalytic psychotherapy, and supportive psychotherapy, in *Essentials of Clinical Psychiatry*, 2nd ed. (eds. R.E. Hales and S.C. Yudofsky), American Psychiatric Publishing, Washington, DC, p. 899–914.
Winston, A., Rosenthal, A., and Pinsker, H. (2004) *Introduction to Supportive Psychotherapy*, American Psychiatric Publishing, Washington, DC.

Recommended Reading: Part Three

Chapter 7

Appelbaum, P.S. (1997) Informed consent to psychotherapy: Recent developments. *Psychiatric Services*, **48**, 445–446.
Beahrs, J.O., and Gutheil, T.G. (2001) Informed consent in psychotherapy. *American Journal of Psychiatry*, **158**, 4–10.
Croarkin, P., Berg, J., and Spira, J. (2003) Informed consent for psychotherapy: A look at therapists' understanding opinions, and practices. *American Journal of Psychotherapy*, **57**, 384–400.
Roberts, L.W., Geppert, C.M., and Bailey, R. (2002) Ethics in psychiatric practice: Essential ethics skills, informed consent, the therapeutic relationship, and confidentiality. *Journal of Psychiatric Practice*, **8**, 290–205.
Rutherford, B.R., Aizaga, K., Sneed, J., *et al.* (2007) A survey of psychiatry residents' informed consent practices. *Journal of Clinical Psychiatry*, **68**, 558–565.

Chapter 8

Bender, S., and Messner, E. (2003) *Becoming a Therapist: What Do I Say and Why?* Guilford Press, New York.
Bruch, H. (1974) *Learning Psychotherapy: Rationale and Ground Rules*, Harvard University Press, Cambridge, MA.

Gabbard, G.O. (2009) Professional boundaries in psychotherapy, in *Textbook of Psychotherapeutic Techniques*, American Psychiatric Publishing, Washington, DC, p. 818.

Gutheil, T.G., and Gabbard, G.O. (1993) The concept of boundaries in clinical practice: Theoretical and risk-management dimensions. *American Journal of Psychiatry*, **150** (2), 188–196.

MacKinnon, R.A., Michels, R., and Buckley, P.J. (2006) General principles of the interview, in: *The Psychiatric Interview in Clinical Practice*, (ed. R.A. MacKinnon), 2nd ed. American Psychiatric Publishing, Washington, DC, p. 3–77.

McWilliams, N. (2004) *Basic Therapy Processes in Psychoanalytic Psychotherapy: A Practitioner's Guide*, Guilford Press, New York.

McWilliams, N. (2004) Educating the patient about the therapy process, in *Psychoanalytic Psychotherapy: A Practitioner's Guide*, Guilford Press, New York, p. 86–96.

Schlesinger, H.J. (2003) *The Texture of Treatment: On the Matter of Psychoanalytic Technique*, Analytic Press, Hillsdale, NJ.

Chapter 9

Bender, D.S. (2005) Therapeutic alliance, in *The American Psychiatric Publishing Textbook of Personality Disorders* (eds. J. Oldham, D.S. Bender, and A.E. Skodol), American Psychiatric Publishing, Washington, DC, p. 405–420.

Gabbard, G.O. (2009) *Textbook of Psychotherapeutic Treatments*, American Psychiatric Publishing, Washington, DC.

Greenson, R.R. (1967) *The Technique and Practice of Psychoanalysis*, International Universities Press, New York.

Gutheil, T.G., and Havens, L.L. (1979) The therapeutic alliance: Contemporary meanings and confusions. *International Review of Psychoanalysis*, **6**, 447–481.

Hilsenroth, M.J., and Cromer, T.D. (2007) Clinician interventions related to alliance during the initial interview and psychological assessment. *Psychotherapy*, **44** (2), 205–218.

Horvath, A.O., and Bedi, R.P. (2002) The alliance, in *Psychotherapy Relationships That Work* (ed. J.C. Norcross), Oxford University Press, New York, p. 37–70.

Horvath, A.O., and Luborsky, L. (1993) The role of the therapeutic alliance in psychotherapy. *Journal of Consulting and Clinical Psychology*, **61** (4), 561–573.

Luborsky, L. (1976) Helping alliances in psychotherapy, in *Successful Psychotherapy* (ed. J.L. Clanghorn), Brunner/Mazel, New York.

Safran, J.D., and Muran, J.C. (2000) *Negotiating the Therapeutic Alliance: A Relational Treatment Guide*, Guilford Press, New York.

Safran, J.D., Muran, J.C., and Proskurov, B. (2009) Alliance, negotiation, and rupture resolution, in *Handbook of Evidence Based Psychodynamic Psychotherapy* (eds. R.A. Levy and J.S. Ablon), Humana Press, New York.

Sandler, J., Dare, C., and Holder, A. (1973) The treatment alliance, in *The Patient and the Analyst*, International Universities Press, New York, p. 27–36.

Chapter 10

Apfelbaum, B. (2005) Interpretive neutrality. *Journal of the American Psychoanalytic Association*, **53**, 917–943.

Caligor, E., Kernberg, O.F., and Clarkin, J.F. (2007) *Handbook of Dynamic Psychotherapy for Higher-Level Personality Disorders*, American Psychiatric Publishing, Washington, DC.

Gabbard, G.O. (2004) *Long-Term Psychodynamic Psychotherapy: A Basic Text*, American Psychiatric Publishing, Washington, DC.

Greenacre, P. (1954) The role of transference: Practical considerations in relation to psycho-analytic therapy. *Journal of the American Psychoanalytic Association*, **2**, 671–684.

Greenson, R.R. (1967) *The Technique and Practice of Psychoanalysis*, International Universities Press, New York.

Levy, S.T., and Inderbitzin, L.B. (1992) Neutrality, interpretation and therapeutic intent. *Journal of the American Psychoanalytic Association*, **40**, 989–1011.

Schlesinger, H.J. (2003) *The Texture of Treatment: On the Matter of Psychoanalytic Technique*, Analytic Press, Hillsdale, NJ.

Chapter 11

Barasch, A. (1999) Psychotherapy as a short story: Selection and focus in brief dynamic psychotherapy. *Journal of the American Academy of Psychoanalysis*, **24** (1), 47–59.

Bender, S., and Messner, E. (2003) *Becoming a Therapist: What Do I Say and Why?* Guilford Press, New York.

Binder, J. (2004) *Key Competencies in Brief Dynamic Psychotherapy*, Guilford Press, New York.

Bruch, H. (1974) *Learning Psychotherapy: Rationale and Ground Rules*, Harvard University Press, Cambridge, MA.

Crits-Christoph, P. and Barber, J. (1991) *Handbook of Short-Term Dynamic Psychotherapy*, Basic Books, New York.

Goldstein, W.N. (1997) *A Primer for Beginning Psychotherapy*, Brunner/Mazel, New York.

MacKinnon, R.A., Michels, R., and Buckley, P.J. (2006) General principles of the interview, in *The Psychiatric Interview in Clinical Practice*, 2nd ed. (ed. R.A. MacKinnon), American Psychiatric Publishing, Washington, DC, p. 62–63.

McWilliams, N. (2004) *Basic Therapy Processes in Psychoanalytic Psychotherapy: A Practitioner's Guide*, Guilford Press, New York, p. 132–162.

Chapter 12

Caligor, E., Kernberg, O.F., and Clarkin, J.F. (2007) The basic elements of DPHP, in *Handbook of Dynamic Psychotherapy for Higher Level Personality Pathology*, American Psychiatric Publishing, Washington, DC, p. 61–84.

Clarkin, J.F., Yeomans, F., and Kernberg, O.F. (1999) Strategies of treatment: The broad strokes, in *Psychotherapy for Borderline Personality*, John Wiley & Sons, New York, p. 29–46.

Freud, S. (1912) The dynamics of transference, in *The Standard Edition of the Complete Psychological Works of Sigmund Freud (1911–1913), The Case of Schreber, Papers on Technique and Other Works, Vol. XII*, Hogarth Press, London, p. 97–108.

Freud, S. (1914) Remembering, repeating and working-through (further recommendations on the technique of psycho-analysis II), in *The Standard Edition of the Complete Psychological Works of Sigmund Freud (1911–1913), The Case of Schreber, Papers on Technique and Other Works, Vol. XII*, Hogarth Press, London, p. 145–156.

Gabbard, G.O. (2004) Assessment, indications, and formulation, in *Long-Term Psychodynamic Psychotherapy: A Basic Text*, American Psychiatric Publishing, Washington, DC, p. 21–40.

Joseph, B. (1985) Transference: The total situation. *International Journal of Psycho-Analysis*, **66**, 447–454.

Kernberg, O.F. (1965) Notes on countertransference. *Journal of the American Psychoanalytic Association*, **13**, 38–56.

McWilliams, N. (2004) Educating the patient about the therapy process, in *Psychoanalytic Psychotherapy: A Practitioner's Guide*, Guilford Press, New York, p. 86–96.

Racker, H. (1957) The meanings and uses of countertransference. *Psychoanalytic Quarterly*, **26**, 303–357.

Chapter 13

Kohut, H. (1959) Introspection, empathy, and psychoanalysis: An examination of the relationship between mode of observation and theory. *Journal of the American Psychoanalytic Association*, **7**, 459–483.

McWilliams, N. (2004) *Basic Therapy Processes in Psychoanalytic Psychotherapy: A Practitioner's Guide*, Guilford Press, New York, p. 132–162.

Ornstein, P.H., and Ornstein, A. (1985) Clinical understanding and explaining: The empathic vantage point. *Progress in Self Psychology*, **1**, 43–61.

Schafer, R. (1983) The psychoanalyst's empathic activity, in *The Analytic Attitude*, Basic Books, New York, p. 34–57.

Schwaber, E.A. (1981) Empathy: A mode of analytic listening. *Psychoanalytic Inquiry*, **1**, 357–392.

Chapter 14

Gaylin, W. (2000) *Talk Is Not Enough: Why Psychotherapy Really Works*, Little, Brown, Boston, MA.

Nemiah, J. (1961) *Foundations of Psychopathology*, Oxford University Press, New York.

Chapter 15

Busch, F.N., and Sandberg, L.S. (2007) *Psychotherapy and Medication: The Challenge of Integration*, Analytic Press, New York.

Caligor, E., Kernberg, O.F., and Clarkin, J.F. (2007) Combining DPHP with medication management and other forms of treatment, in *Handbook of Dynamic Psychotherapy for Higher-Level Personality Pathology*, American Psychiatric Publishing, Washington, DC, p. 231–246.

Fosshage, J.L. (1997) Listening/experiencing perspectives and the quest for a facilitating responsiveness. *Progress in Self Psychology*, **13**, 33–55.

Gabbard, G.O. (2004) *Psychodynamic Psychiatry in Clinical Practice*, 4th ed., American Psychiatric Publishing, Washington, DC.

Kahn, D.A. (1991) Medication consultation and split treatment during psychotherapy. *Journal of the American Academy of Psychoanalysis*, **19** (1), 84–98.

Luborsky, L. (1984) *Principles of Psychoanalytic Psychotherapy: A Manual for Supportive-Expressive Treatment*, Basic Books, New York.

Riba, M.B., and Balon, R. (2005) *Competency in Combining Pharmacotherapy and Psychotherapy: Integrated and Split Treatment (Core Competencies in Psychotherapy)*, American Psychiatric Publishing, Washington, DC.

Roose, S.P., and Cabaniss, D.L. (2005) Psychoanalysis and psychopharmacology, in *The American Psychiatric Publishing Textbook of Psychoanalysis* (eds. E.S. Person, A.M. Cooper, and G.O. Gabbard), American Psychiatric Publishing, Washington, DC, pp. 255–266.

Sandberg, L. (1998) Analytic listening and the act of prescribing medication. *Psychoanalytic Inquiry*, **18**, 621–639.

Recommended Reading: Part Four

Chapter 16

Bruch, H. (1974) *Learning Psychotherapy, Rationale and Ground Rules*, Harvard University Press, Cambridge, MA.

Charon, R. (2006) *Narrative Medicine*, Oxford Univeristy Press, New York.

Copland, A. (1985) *What to Listen for in Music*, McGraw-Hill, New York.

Freud, S. (1912) Recommendations to physicians practising psycho-analysis, in *The Standard Edition of the Complete Psychological Works of Sigmund Freud (1911–1913), The Case of Schreber, Papers on Technique and Other Works, Vol.* **XII**, Hogarth Press, London, p. 109–120.

Freud, S. (1913) On beginning the treatment (further recommendations on the technique of psychoanalysis 1), in *The Standard Edition of the Complete Psychological Works of Sigmund Freud (1911–1913), The Case of Schreber, Papers on Technique and Other Works, Vol.* **XII**, Hogarth Press, London, pp. 121–144.

Greenson, R. (1967) *The Technique and Practice of Psychoanalysis*, International Universities Press, Madison, WI.

Schlesinger, H.J. (1994) How the analyst listens: The pre-stages of interpretation. *International Journal of Psychoanalysis*, **75**, 31–37.

Sullivan, H.S. (1954) *The Psychiatric Interview*, W.W. Norton, New York.

Chapter 17

Dewald, P.A. (1964) *Psychotherapy: A Dynamic Approach*, Basic Books, New York.

Fenichel, O. (1941) *Problems of Psychoanalytic Technique*, Psychoanalytic Quarterly Press, New York.

Gabbard, G. (2004) *Long-Term Psychodynamic Psychotherapy: A Basic Text*, American Psychiatric Publishing, Washington, DC.

Schlesinger, H.J. (2003) *The Texture of Treatment: On the Matter of Psychoanalytic Technique*, Analytic Press, Hillsdale, NJ.

Chapter 18

Appelbaum, A.H. (2005) Supportive psychotherapy, in *The American Psychiatric Publishing Textbook of Personality Disorders* (eds. R.E. Hales, S.C. Yudofsky, and L.W. Roberts, American Psychiatric Publishing, Washington, DC, p. 335–346.

Douglas, C.J. (2008) Teaching supportive psychotherapy to psychiatric residents. *American Journal of Psychiatry*, **165** (4), 445–452.

Gabbard, G. (2005) *Psychodynamic Psychiatry in Clinical Practice*, 4th ed., American Psychiatric Publishing, Washington, DC.

Greenson, R. (1967) *The Technique and Practice of Psychoanalysis*, International University Press, New York.

Misch, D.A. (2000) Basic strategies of dynamic supportive therapy. *Journal of Psychotherapy Practice and Research*, **9**, 173–189.

Pinsker, H. (1997) *A Primer of Supportive Psychotherapy*, Analytic Press, Hillsdale, NJ.

Rockland, L.H. (1989) *Supportive Psychotherapy: A Psychodynamic Approach*, Basic Books, New York.

Rockland, L.H. (1989) Psychoanalytically oriented supportive therapy: Literature review and techniques. *Journal of the American Academy of Psychoanalysis*, **17** (3), 451–462.

Rosenthal, R.N. (2009) Techniques of supportive psychotherapy, in *Textbook of Psychotherapeutic Treatments* (ed. G.O. Gabbard), American Psychiatric Publishing, Washington, DC, p. 417–445.

Sandler, H., Dare, C., and Holder, H. (1973) *The Patient and the Analyst*, International Universities Press, Madison, WI.

Winston, A., Rosenthal, R.N., and Pinsker, H. (2004) *Introduction to Supportive Psychotherapy (Core Competencies in Psychotherapy)*, American Psychiatric Publishing, Washington, DC.

Recommended Reading: Part Five

Chapter 19

Bion, W.R. (1962) *Learning from Experience*, Heinemann, London.

Caligor, E., Kernberg, O.F., and Clarkin, J.F. (2007) *Handbook of Dynamic Psychotherapy for Higher Level Personality Pathology*, American Psychiatric Publishing, Washington, DC.

Diener, M.J., and Hilsenroth, M.J. (2009) Affect focused techniques in psychodynamic psychotherapy, in *Handbook of Evidence-based Psychodynamic Psychotherapy* (eds. R.A. Levy and J.S. Ablon), Humana Press, New York, p. 227–248.

Fenichel, O. (1941) *Problems of Psychoanalytic Technique*, Psychoanalytic Quarterly, Albany, NY.

Fonagy, P., Steele, M., Steele, H., *et al.* (1995) Attachment, the reflective self, and borderline states: The predictive capacity of the adult attachment interview and pathological emotional development, in *Attachment Theory: Social, Developmental and Clinical Perspectives* (eds. S. Goldberg, R. Muir, and J. Kerr), Analytic Press, Hillsdale, NJ, p. 233–278.

Freud, S. (1893) The psychotherapy of hysteria, in *The Standard Edition of the Complete Psychological Works of Sigmund Freud (1893–1895), Studies on Hysteria*, Vol. **II**, Hogarth Press, London, p. 1–305.

Kernberg, O.F. (1988) Object relations theory in clinical practice. *Psychoanalytic Quarterly*, **57**, 481–504.

Klerman, G., Markowitz, J., Weissman M., *et al.* (2000) *Comprehensive Guide to Interpersonal Psychotherapy*, Basic Books, New York, p. 125–129.

Chapter 20

Freud, S. (1913) On beginning the treatment (further recommendations on the technique of psycho-analysis I), in *The Standard Edition of the Complete Psychological Works of Sigmund Freud (1911–1913), The Case of Schreber, Papers on Technique and Other Works*, Vol. **XII**, Hogarth Press, London, p. 121–144.

Gabbard, G.O. (2004) Working with resistance, in *Long Term Psychodynamic Psychotherapy*, American Psychiatric Publishing, Washington, DC, p. 99–16.

Gabbard, G.O., and Horowitz, M. (2009) Insight, transference, interpretation and therapeutic change in the dynamic psychotherapy of borderline personality disorder. *American Journal of Psychiatry*, **166** (5), 517–521.

Greenson, R. (1967) *The Technique and Practice of Psychoanalysis*, Vol. **1**, International Universities Press, New York.

Hellerstein, D.J., Rosenthal, R.N., Pinsker, H., *et al.* (1998) A randomized prospective study comparing supportive and dynamic therapies; outcome and alliance. *Journal of Psychotherapy Practice and Research*, **7**, 261–271.

Lowenstein, R.M. (1963) Some considerations on free association. *Journal of the American Psychoanalytic Association*, **11**, 451–473.

MacKinnon, R.A., Michels, R., and Buckley, P.J. (2006) *The Psychiatric Interview in Clinical Practice*, 2nd ed., American Psychiatric Publishing, Washington, DC.

Sandler, J., Dare, C., and Holder, A. (1973) Resistance, in *The Patient and the Analyst*, International Universities Press, Madison, WI, p. 71–83.

Schlesinger, H.J. (1982) Resistance as process, in *Resistance: Psychodynamic and Behavioral Approaches* (ed. P.L. Wachtel), Plenum Press, New York, p. 25–44.

Wallerstein, R. (1989) *Forty Two Lives in Treatment: A Study of Psychoanalysis and Psychotherapy*, Guilford Press, New York.

Chapter 21

Bender, S., and Messer, E. (2003) Transference and countertransference, in *Becoming a Therapist: What Do I Say, and Why?* Guilford Press, New York.

Caligor, E., Kernberg, O.F., and Clarkin, J. (2007) The techniques of DPHP, Part 2: Intervening, in *Handbook of Dynamic Psychotherapy*, American Psychiatric Publishing, Washington DC, p. 125–149.

Freud, S. (1914) Remembering, repeating and working-through (further recommendations on the technique of psycho-analysis II), in *The Standard Edition of the Complete Psychological Works of Sigmund Freud (1911–1913), The Case of Schreber, Papers on Technique and Other Works, Vol. XII*, Hogarth Press, London, p. 145–156.

Joseph, B. (1985) Transference: The total situation. *International Journal of Psycho-Analysis*, **66**, 447–454.

MacKinnon, R.A., Michels, R., and Buckley, P.J. (2006) *The Psychiatric Interview in Clinical Practice*, 2nd ed., American Psychiatric Publishing, Washington, DC.

Sandler, J., Dare, C., Holder, A. (1973) Special forms of transference, in *The Patient and the Analyst*, International Universities Press, Madison, WI, p. 49–60.

Schwaber, E. (ed.) (1985) *The Transference in Psychotherapy: Clinical Management*, International Universities Press, New York.

Chapter 22

Gabbard, G.O. (2004) Identifying and working with countertransference, in *Long Term Psychodynamic Psychotherapy*, American Psychiatric Publishing, Washington, DC, p. 131–151.

Kernberg, O. (1965) Notes on countertransference. *Journal of the American Psychoanalytic Association*, **13**, 38–56.

Michels, R., Abensour, L., Eizirik, C., *et al.* (eds.) (2002) *Key Papers on Countertransference*, Karnac, London.

Racker, H. (1957) The meaning and uses of countertransference. *Psychoanalytic Quarterly*, **26**, 303–357.

Sandler, J. (1978) Countertransference and role responsiveness. *International Review of Psychoanalysis*, **3**, 43–47.

Sandler, J., Dare, C., and Holder, A. (1973) Countertransference, in *The Patient and the Analyst*, International Universities Press, Madison, WI, p. 61–70.

Chapter 23

Brenner, C. (1973) *An Elementary Textbook of Psychoanalysis*, rev. and exp. ed., International Universities Press, New York.

Brenner, C. (1982) *The Mind in Conflict*, International Universities Press, New York.

Tucker, S.S. (2008) Current views of the oedipal complex: Panel report. *Journal of the American Psychoanalytic Association*, **56**, 263–271.

Chapter 24

Freud, S. (1900) The interpretation of dreams, in *The Standard Edition of the Complete Psychological Works of Sigmund Freud (1900), The Interpretation of Dreams (1st Part), Vol. IV*, Hogarth Press, London, p. ix–627.

Schlesinger, H.J. (2003) *The Texture of Treatment: On the Matter of Psychoanalytic Technique*, Analytic Press, Hillsdale, NJ.

Werman, D. (1978) The use of dreams in psychotherapy. *Journal of the Canadian Psychiatric Association*, **23**, 153–158.

Werman, D.S. (1984) The place of the dream in supportive psychotherapy, in *The Practice of Supportive Psychotherapy*, Brunner/Mazel, New York, p. 151–155.

Recommended Reading: Part Six

Chapter 25

Kohut, H. (1976) *The Analysis of the Self: A Systematic Approach to the Psychoanalytic Treatment of Narcissistic Personality Disorders*, 4th ed., International Universities Press, New York.

Kohut, H., and Wolf, E.S. (1978) The disorders of the self and their treatment: An outline. *International Journal of Psychoanalyis*, **59**, 413–425.

Pinsker, H. (1997) Self-esteem, in *A Primer of Supportive Psychotherapy*, Analytic Press, Hillsdale, NJ, p. 39–76.

Rosenthal, R.N. (2009) Techniques of individual supportive therapy, in *Textbook of Psychotherapeutic Treatments* (ed. G.O. Gabbard), American Psychiatric Publishing, Washington, DC, p. 427–431.

Siegel, A.M. (1996) *Heinz Kohut and the Psychology of the Self*, Routledge, London.

Stern, D.N. (1985) *The Interpersonal World of the Infant: A View from Psychoanalysis and Developmental Psychology*, Basic Books, New York.

Chapter 26

Caligor, E., Kernberg, O.F., and Clarkin, J.F. (2007) Internal object relations, mental organization, and subjective experience in personality pathology, in *Handbook of Dynamic Psychotherapy for Higher Level Personality Pathology*, American Psychiatric Publishing, Washington, DC, p. 37–58.

Kernberg, O.F. (1976) *Object Relations Theory and Clinical Psychoanalysis*, Jason Aronson, New York.

Luborsky, L., and Crits-Christoph, P. (1990) *Understanding Transference: The Core Conflictual Relationship Theme Method*, Basic Books, New York.

Mitchell, S.A. (1988) *Relational Concepts in Psychoanalysis: An Integration*, Harvard University Press, Cambridge, MA.

Pinsker, H., Rosenthal, R., and McCullough, L. (1991) Dynamic supportive psychotherapy, in *Handbook of Short-Term Dynamic Psychotherapy* (eds P. Crits-Christoph and P. Barber), Basic Books, New York, p. 220–247.

Rosenthal, R.N., Muran, J.C., Pinsker, H., *et al.* (1999) Interpersonal change in brief supportive psychotherapy. *Journal of Psychotherapy Practice and Research*, **8**, 55–63.

Chapter 27

Appelbaum, A. (2005) Supportive psychotherapy, in *The American Psychiatric Textbook of Personality Disorders* (eds. J.M. Oldham, A.E. Skodol, and D.S. Bender), American Psychiatric Publishing, Washington, DC, p. 335–346.

Caligor, E., Kernberg, O.F., Clarkin, J.F. (2007) A psychodynamic approach to personality pathology, in *Handbook of Dynamic Psychotherapy for Higher Level Personality Pathology*, American Psychiatric Publishing, Washington, DC, p. 24–31.

Hartmann, H. (1958) *Ego Psychology and the Problem of Adaptation*, International Universities Press, New York.

Pinsker, H. (1997) Adaptive skills, in *A Primer of Supportive Psychotherapy*, Analytic Press, Hillsdale, NJ, p. 115–131.

Vaillant, G.E. (1971) Theoretical hierarchy of adaptive ego mechanisms. *Psychiatry*, **24**, 107–118.

Vaillant, G.E. (1977) *Adaptation to Life: How the Best and Brightest Came of Age*, Little, Brown, Boston, MA.

Chapter 28

Pinsker, H. (1997) Ego functions, in *A Primer of Supportive Psychotherapy*, Analytic Press, Hillsdale, NJ, p. 99–114.

Werman, D. (1984) Typical situations and techniques, in *The Practice of Supportive Psychotherapy*, Brunner/Mazel, New York, p. 98–135.

Recommended Reading: Part Seven

Chapter 29

Caligor, E., Kernberg, O.F., Clarkin, J.F. (2007) Strategies of DPHP and the treatment setting, in *Handbook for Dynamic Psychotherapy for Higher-level Personality Pathology*, American Psychiatric Publishing, Washington, DC, p. 97–98.

Freud, S. (1914) Remembering, repeating and working-through (further recommendations on the technique of psycho-analysis II), in *The Standard Edition of the Complete Psychological Works of Sigmund Freud (1911–1913), The Case of Schreber, Papers on Technique and Other Works, Vol.* **XII**, Hogarth Press, London, p. 147–156.

Greenson, R.R. (1965) The problem of working through, in *Drives, Affects, Behavior* (ed. R. Loewenstein), International Universities Press, Madison, WI, p. 277–314.

Greenson, R.R. (1992) *The Technique and Practice of Psychoanalysis*, A Memorial Volume to Ralph R. Greenson, Monograph 1, Vol. **2**, International Universities Press, Madison, WI.

Karasu, T.B. (1977) Psychotherapies: An overview. *American Journal of Psychiatry*, **134**, 851–863.

Leichsenring, F. (2009) Applications of psychodynamic psychotherapy to specific disorders, in *Textbook of Psychotherapeutic Treatments* (ed. G.O. Gabbard), American Psychiatric Publishing, Washington, DC, p. 115–117.

Sandler, J., Dare, C., Holder, A., *et al.* (1992) Working through, in *The Patient and the Analyst*, 2nd ed., International Universities Press, Madison, WI, p. 121–132.

Werman, D.S. (1988) On the mode of therapeutic action of psychoanalytic supportive psycho-therapy, in *How Does Treatment Help?*, International Universities Press, Madison, WI, p. 157–167.

Chapter 30

Bender, S., and Messner, E. (2003) Termination, in *Becoming a Therapist: What Do I Say, and Why?* Guilford Press, New York, p. 291–307.

Caligor, E., Kernberg, O.F., Clarkin, J.F. (2007) The phases of treatment, in *Handbook for Dynamic Psychotherapy for Higher-level Personality Pathology*, American Psychiatric Publishing, Washington, DC, p. 222–227.

Firestein, S. (1978) *Termination in Psychoanalysis*, International Universities Press, New York.

Freud, S. (1937) Analysis terminable and interminable, in *The Standard Edition of the Complete Psychological Works of Sigmund Freud (1937–1939), Moses and Monotheism, An Outline of Psycho-Analysis and Other Works, Vol.* **XXIII**, Hogarth Press, London, p. 216–243.

Gabbard, G.O. (2004) *Long-Term Psychodynamic Psychotherapy: A Basic Text*, American Psychiatric Publishing, Washington, DC.

Gabbard, G.O. (2009) Techniques of psychodynamic psychotherapy, in *Textbook of Psychotherapeutic Treatments*, American Psychiatric Publishing, Washington, DC, p. 62–64.

Schlesinger, H.J. (2005) Endings for beginners, in *Endings and Beginnings: On Terminating Psychotherapy and Psychoanalysis*, Analytic Press, Hillsdale, NJ, p. 89–121.

Werman, D.S. (1984) Termination and interruption, in *The Practice of Supportive Psychotherapy*, Brunner/Mazel, New York, p. 176–181.

Chapter 31

Frawley-O'Dea, M.G., and Sarnat, J.E. (2001) *The Supervisory Relationship: A Contemporary Psychodynamic Approach*, Guilford Press, New York.

Hunter, J., and Pinsky, D.A. (1994) The supervisee's experience of supervision, in *Clinical Perspectives on Psychotherapy Supervision* (ed. S.E. Greben), American Psychiatric Publishing, Washington, DC, p. 85–98.

Jacobs, D., David, P., and Meyer, D.J. (1995) *The Supervisory Encounter: A Guide for Teachers of Psychodynamic Psychotherapy and Psychoanalysis*, Yale University Press, New Haven.

Pine, F. (2006) If I knew then what I know now: Theme and variations. *Psychoanalytic Psychology*, **23** (1), 1–7.

Index

Note: For brevity, subentries referring to "psychotherapy" imply psychodynamic psychotherapy unless otherwise mentioned.

Psychodynamic Psychotherapy: A Clinical Manual, Second Edition. Deborah L. Cabaniss, Sabrina Cherry,
Carolyn J. Douglas and Anna Schwartz.
© 2017 John Wiley & Sons, Ltd. Published 2017 by John Wiley & Sons, Ltd.